MANAGING

COMPUTERS

IN HEALTH CARE

A GUIDE
FOR PROFESSIONALS

Third Edition

MANAGING

COMPUTERS

IN HEALTH CARE

A GUIDE
FOR PROFESSIONALS

Third Edition

**John Abbott Worthley
& Philip S. DiSalvio**

Health Administration Press
Ann Arbor, Michigan 1995

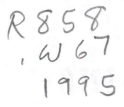

R 858
. W 67
1995

99 98 97 96 95   5 4 3 2 1

Library of Congress Cataloging-in-Publication Data

Worthley, John Abbott.
  Managing computers in health care : a guide for professionals / John Abbott Worthley, Philip S. DiSalvio. — 3rd ed.
      p.   cm.
  Includes bibliographical references and index.
  ISBN 1-56793-031-X (softbound : alk. paper)
  1. Medical informatics. I. DiSalvio, Philip S. II. Title.
  [DNLM: 1. Management Information Systems. 2. Health Services—organization & administration. W26.5 W934m 1995]
  R858.W67   1995   362.1'0285—dc20   95-8735 CIP

The paper used in this publication meets the minimum requirements of American National Standard for Information Sciences—Permanence of Paper for Printed Library Materials, ANSI Z39.48-1984. ♾ ™

Health Administration Press
A division of the Foundation of the
    American College of Healthcare Executives
1021 East Huron Street
Ann Arbor, Michigan 48104
(313) 764-1380

CONTENTS

PREFACE TO THE THIRD EDITION

A S AN OLD saw would say, some things change, while others remain the same. In the case of computer technology in health care organizations, some things have, indeed, changed drastically since we published the second edition six years ago; but other realities remain relentlessly similar. In particular, while the nature and use of computers in health care have developed enormously, the managerial challenges continue to be remarkably consistent. This third edition reflects both these changes and the continuity. It is offered as an assist to health care professionals seeking to manage the union of computers and health care into the next century.

My colleague and fellow health care professional, Phil DiSalvio, joins in this effort at updating, as he did for the second edition. Without his perseverance, this new edition might not have appeared before the second millenium. Together we have revised the text of each chapter and added an entirely new one, completed a major overhaul of the glossary, included new and revised cases, and appended more current and engaging readings following each chapter. Drawn from the likes of the *New York Times*, *Esquire*, the *New Yorker*, and the *Harvard Business Review*, these new readings are probably the most professionally focused within the three editions thus far.

While the changes we have incorporated are quite significant, we rigorously maintain the conceptual framework originally developed for the first edition. We do this for two related reasons: One, it has worked well. Feedback from students and professionals over the past 12 years has been uniformly positive regarding the unique approach of the book. Two, our continuing work as professors and consultants to health care managers convinces us more than ever of the practical wisdom of the original premise, namely—to quote the preface to the first edition—that "computer technology is a basically simple though tremendously powerful tool that desperately needs to be managed." We, therefore, begin with the three chapters designed to expose computers and information systems in their simplicity. The continual deluge of new technical developments and the sophistication of management information system books and designs more than ever tend to tempt professionals to overlook the basics that are key to sound understanding and management of the technology. So, rather than hesitate or apologize for our continued inclusion of these seemingly simplistic chapters, we stress their importance even more and refer readers to the companion volume for this book,* or similar texts, for more in-depth technical treatment.

Chapter 4 continues as a framework for the ensuing chapters. It emphasizes the basic simplicity of systematic analysis in an effort to highlight its profundity. Readers have, over the years, pointed to this chapter as the linchpin of the whole book. Chapters 5 through 10 proceed to probe the fundamental challenges that need to be managed if the potential of computer technology in health care management is to be furthered. Finally, we have added a chapter that explores further technological developments.

Once again, the text of each chapter provides concise and comprehensive treatment of the relevant subject, while the appended readings offer more in-depth views. Each chapter also includes an updated bibliography of some of the more useful writings on the concepts presented. A practical case study then challenges readers to apply knowledge obtained from the chapter to a commonly encountered scenario.

In completing this new edition we have drawn from the experience and insights of our students at Seton Hall University, Russell Sage College, and the Beijing (China) University of International Business and Economics, as well as our clients in numerous health-related organizations. We are grateful to them all for sharing their wisdom with us. We specifically would like to thank Sandra Crump and Marcia LaBrenz of Health Administration Press for their masterful oversight of this effort, and the two anonymous critics whose careful review of our draft revisions contributed significantly to what you are about to read. Godspeed!

John Abbott Worthley

---

*Austin, C. J. *Information Systems for Health Care Administration.* Ann Arbor: Health Administration Press, 1992.

TAMING COMPUTER TECHNOLOGY

THREE REALITIES underlie the focus of this book. The first is the general pervasiveness of computers. Computer technology is now a standard aspect of organizations in general, of health care organizations in particular, and, indeed, of our society at large. Computers are a reality from which twentieth-century health care managers, providers, and consumers can seldom escape. The second reality is that computers offer wonderful opportunities for significant improvements in organizational and social life, and in health care in particular. The potential benefits to be derived are enormous. The third reality is that experience with computers in organizations and in society often has been disappointing and problem-laden, a reality from which health care organizations have not been exempt. The road from potential benefits to actual improvements continues to be inordinately rocky. The world of health care professionals today, thus, continues to be a computerized environment characterized by great promise and hope, but sobered by struggles, frustration, and disappointment with the technology. As Kennedy suggests, there may be more questions than answers regarding information technology for health care in the next decade.[1]

Why are these realities so prevalent? Clearly, computer technology has become ubiquitous because its potential benefits are so significant. Computers can and have produced considerable advantages for health care organizations. The causes of our problematic experiences with computers, however, are not so clear. Typically, the technology itself is blamed when problems occur, as though computers were people responsible for their own actions. In truth, the technological challenge of building a sound and powerful electronic wonder has been well met. Thanks to scientists, computer technology today is highly sophisticated, reliable, and affordable. It is a powerful force, but one that has not yet been tamed by those who confront it in organizations and society. In brief, the technological challenge of computers has been met so well that we now are faced with a powerful tool that poses a major managerial challenge—how to reap the possible benefits and minimize associated problems by using and managing technology responsibly and wisely. This book is designed to help health care professionals tame computer technology. The importance of the subject is suggested by an astute commentator who, in reflecting on technology management in the 1990s, suggests that "while health care executives perceive great benefits from new technology, they often have problems managing it."[2] The emerging trends of a highly competitive, cost-conscious, environment additionally intensify the importance of effective information management.[3]

Given the frustrations, disappointments, and fears that are frequently generated by computers, health care professionals might prefer to delegate the challenge to someone else or, better yet, to stay away from computers altogether. However, the ubiquity of computer usage makes that approach unrealistic.

The Ubiquity of Computer Technology

In today's society computers are used for everything from analyzing football plays in Dallas to sorting political campaign messages in Washington. Microcomputer technology is now bringing the "black box" into the home where, according to many experts, the computer will be as common as a television set within a few years. Modern society is thoroughly inundated with the technology. A recent survey by the Times-Mirror Center for the People and the Press found that an increasing number of Americans are using technology, and that nearly one in three Americans has a personal computer.[4] "Not only have computers entered tens of millions of American homes, but they have become indispensable tools for people who use them," the survey finds. "Two out of three computer users (65 percent) said they would miss their personal computer 'a lot' if they no longer had it."[5] Clearly, these are signs that traffic is starting to thicken on the information highway.

Business usage of computers began in 1954 when a UNIVAC-I was installed in a General Electric plant in Kentucky. Since then, the technology has expanded so that today, even small, private business organizations employ computers for record-keeping, payroll, accounting, inventory control, and so forth.

Similarly, public agency use of computers has proliferated since the United States Census Bureau used a UNIVAC-I in 1951. Today, nearly all federal, state, and local government agencies are affected by computerization, and microcomputers have brought this technology to even the smallest agency. It is apparent that health care executives have embraced computers as well, and view technology as a solution to health care challenges. A recent study found that 93 percent of a representative sample of hospitals expects to increase their spending on information systems by an average of 10 percent a year on operations and almost 12 percent on capital projects. One in five respondents said they expect an average annual jump in capital spending of more than 20 percent.[6]

The situation is clear. Computers are everywhere, and health care professionals must deal with this reality in their organizations. To the long-recognized legal, fiscal, political, and organizational aspects of health care administration, there must be added a major new aspect—the technological.

The Potential of Computers

A second reality prompting this managerial challenge is the promised and proven benefits that computers can offer. A basic management challenge is to harness these benefits for health care. With the impetus to improve clinical care, connect with outside facilities, and install a financial link to claims processors, combined with the drive for patient information on demand, health service executives are awakening to the need to improve their information systems.[7]

A study from Lewin-VHI, commissioned by the Healthcare Financial Management Association, underscores the potential of computer technology. This study projects a total net saving of $2.6 billion to $5.2 billion per year from automating and standardizing just the total number of administrative transactions in health care.[8]

There is no shortage of information on the potential benefits of computer technology. Computer salespeople have reams of flashy brochures that tout the glory of their wares. To hear some vendors tell it, installation of their computer system in your organization will be like a "second coming"—a magic potion with almost limitless capability to improve your organizational systems. In fact, actual benefits often are considerably less than promised, but substantial nonetheless. Consider the following representative litany of success stories:

- The Western New York Health Sciences Consortium and New York Telephone Company have created a high-speed communication network or "superhighway" to improve data-sharing among consortium members, which include seven hospitals, a cancer center, and a medical school. The network will enhance medical education, research, and patient care. "Compared with our current data-sharing capabilities, its like expanding a highway from one to eight lanes," says the CEO of one member hospital.[9]

- The Harvard Community Health Plan has patients in about 150 households using home computers to receive medical advice and general health information. In use for about two years, the goal of the system is to improve patient education, raise the quality of health care, and lower costs by reducing the number of unnecessary visits to the doctor. Of households using the system, 90 percent gave it a high rating for usefulness, and participants' visits to the health center dropped by 5 percent.[10]

- Lutheran General Health System of Park Ridge, Illinois, is spending $7–8 million to install an "enterprise-wide network" as part of a $19 million project to automate all of its clinical data. This enterprise network links the computer systems within the entire system, a technology that will be essential in a post-reform era when shared information may mean the difference between life and death for both patients and the institutions that treat them.[11]

- Saint Joseph's Hospital and Medical Center of Paterson, New Jersey has implemented a new $25 million computerized patient-records network. This network of 500 personal computers within the hospital and affiliated out-patient centers will allow doctors to call up a patient's name to check on everything from the latest lab test results to a running tally of charges. Administrators will be able to calculate the exact cost of every variable of cardiac care or any other procedure. Nurses will be able to direct lab orders directly to the lab. Everyone from the cleaners in maintenance to the dieticians in food service will have on-line access for their departments.[12]

- Lakeland Regional Medical Center in Lakeland, Florida has automated a user-friendly, protocol-based charting system. By documenting only those times when a care decision departs from the protocol, Lakeland found that charting time dropped dramatically, from 25 to 30 percent of caregivers' time to 6 percent.[13]

- Physicians at Boston's Brigham and Women's Hospital can call up a patient's medical history—including a list of previously prescribed medications—by using a computer terminal in the internal medicine clinic. Before the electronic records, physicians would have to locate the patient's medical record from the central files and then search for the necessary information. According to the hospital, the system has made the ambulatory medical record the primary information resource for physicians in the clinics, and has saved money by substantially reducing the need to routinely pull files for the clinics from the medical records department.[14]

This is merely a sample of almost daily reports concerning benefits from automation. In health care, as well as in police work, education, transportation, research—indeed, nearly every functional aspect of government and non-profit organizations, as well as in business—computerization has provided significant benefits. One humorist pithily portrayed the apparent march of computer-related euphoria in a cartoon of an office meeting in which a project manager declared: "Computer Number 9 just discovered a cure for which there is no known disease!"[15]

All of these benefits, potential and actual, can be grouped into two categories: (1) administrative or processing benefits, and (2) decision-assisting benefits. That is, computers offer assistance in carrying out predetermined operations, and they can help decision makers clarify and plan. The benefits derive from computer characteristics, particularly speed, memory, and storage capacity, which are explained in Chapter 3. Computer speed facilitates extended calculations and the rapid retrieval of stored information; computer memory facilitates the storage and availability of enormous amounts of data.

Thus, the potential benefits of computers for organizations are tremendous. Health care professionals today face the task of harnessing the technology to realize these benefits; it is a prodigious challenge.

The Problems of Computers in Organizations

The most compelling reasons why health care professionals must tame computer technology are the serious problems that with remarkable, if alarming, consistency computer usage has engendered. Indicative of the overall situation is a classic *U.S. News and World Report* article that laments, "Those Computers Get Temperamental." It reports that computers are swallowing credit cards, delaying commuters and shoppers, raising havoc with bills, and generally disrupting life. "Americans are learning," the article concludes, "that electronic gadgets can be a curse as well as a blessing."[16] Anyone who has tried to correct an erroneous credit card bill (not to mention an automated hospital bill) or to get removed from a mailing list should well appreciate the story.

Some reports from health care would be laughable if they were not so alarming. At one eastern medical center, nurses noticed that automated patients' records were mysteriously disappearing. Nearly 40 percent of the records were destroyed.[17] Similarly, it is not uncommon to hear someone describe how their disk "crashed," or how they lost everything stored on their computer. One recent report tells of a common, disquieting occurrence: In a newly inaugurated system, the user, an occupational nurse, neglected to back up daily entries on a computer. When the disk on the new computer "crashed," the data could not be salvaged and four months of daily transactions were lost. Moreover, the individual responsible lost her job, because the company's operational quality assurance criteria required frequent software backups.[18] Another story reported a person "killed by computer." A New Jersey man was informed by Medicare that his medical bills would not be paid because it insisted he had died during a recent hospitalization.[19]

Furthermore, a recent newspaper article entitled "Workers Celebrate the Demise of a Balky Computer" provides an example of an attitude toward computers to which many health care managers undoubtedly can relate:

> Ames, Iowa (AP)—When it came time to retire a testy computer, office workers invited guests, dropped it from a cherrypicker and bashed it with sledgehammers.
>
> "It was a good feeling," said Cindy Jorgenson, office manager at Professional Property Management. The computer was dropped from 40 feet. Tenants of other buildings managed by the company were invited. Popcorn and soft drinks were served.
>
> "The computer," Jorgenson said, "caused us a lot of grief."

Employees first considered hiring a hearse to haul away the old computer, but decided that wasn't enough.[20] Some observers note that we, in fact, are being enslaved by technology, rather than harnessing these tools to serve our needs. In a recent survey that explored hospital executives' information expectations and impressions of how well their current information technology produces the kind of data they need and want, most reported they do not receive operational data in a form they can use to make decisions, and, as a result, many rely on personal instincts and experience in their decision making.[21] Over 85 percent of respondents report that they do not receive the factual information they are looking for to make decisions, and 82 percent declare that they want their computers to produce such information.[22]

Behind these tales of woe is a stark reality—computer usage in health care often has been difficult. In particular, fiscal, operational, organizational, psychological, legal, and socio-political problems have emerged as major challenges in this area.

Fiscal

The cost of computers always has been a difficulty. Until recently major investments in hardware have been required; now, with lower hardware prices, the issues are software and personnel costs. The salient problem has been the fiscal return on these investments and the fiscal efficiency with which the computer resource is handled. The New York City Board of Education, one of the largest users of this technology, has been criticized for uncontrolled spending on computers. One report summarized the Board's fiscal handling of the computer systems with the headline: "The Board of Education Has Spent $90 Million on Computer Systems and City's Schools Still: DO NOT COMPUTE."[23] Behind this story is a multitude of mistakes that essentially adds up to the Board of Education having dumped more than $90 million into two computer projects that are millions of dollars over budget and so far behind schedule that they are nearly obsolete.

Recent reports have crystallized the extent of this problem in health care organizations. Research shows that the paradigm shift in health care, characterized by changes in financing and delivery, is driving huge increases in spending on information technology.[24] At the same time, the primary concern appears no longer to be computerization's capital cost versus its benefits. As one information systems consultant notes, "It looks like people are spending money because they have no choice . . . people are thinking about spending more money to make themselves more efficient."[25] The *Wall Street Journal* estimates that over the next several years the total price tag for computer technology in health care will run into the billions of dollars.[26]

The Crozer-Keystone Health System in Pennsylvania exemplifies this kind of spending. Having recently installed an $80 million enterprise-wide data system, the CEO of the system revealed that, while it was somewhat difficult to justify to the Board of Directors such a large capital expenditure, future competitive and cost-containing pressures have forced the company to make such a choice in order to appear progressive.[27]

As health care institutions begin to invest heavily in technology, however, many run the risk of basing their investment on underestimated costs and overestimated payoffs. As a number of experts assert, there is no guarantee that the investment will pay off, but any institution not making it will not survive in the future U.S. health care system.[28] Clearly, the fiscal problems are imposing.

Operational

In an article titled "Air Traffic Computer System Still Grounded," a writer for the Los Angeles Times describes a $5 billion U.S. Government state-of-the art computer system that is supposed to let controllers better handle air traffic in the nation's increasingly crowded skies. He reports that the computer project is a disaster—a case of bureaucratic bumbling, corporate failings, repeated delays that have set back the project's completion at least two years, and one of the biggest potential cost-overruns in U.S. government history: $2 billion and counting.[29]

This notorious illustration of an operational problem, and others, have become so common that the terms "computer downtime" and "computer error" need little explanation in the modern lexicon. For example, patients are billed incorrectly, or not at all, because of "computer error"; clients become hypertensive while waiting to be issued a medical record number because a computer is "down."

Less recognized, but nonetheless common, are two other operational problems of computers: data pollution and security breakdowns. While new information technology has given health care managers unprecedented opportunity to tap into an organization's raw operational data, it is commonly reported that hospital executives are drowning in data. Take, for example, the case of the University of Chicago Hospitals, where executives who track trends in patient care must wade through more than one million computerized records of inpatient stays.[30] The sheer volume of information contained in these files is staggering. This is a classic example of an organization being overwhelmed by "information junk" and literally polluted with data. The information overload syndrome is pervasive. As health care operations have grown in volume and complexity, the extraneous has become common. Information systems that simplify rather than add to the complexity and confusion is the exception in health care administration, rather than the rule. As one experienced observer notes, "We still kill too many fleas with elephant hammers."[31]

Accompanying the inundation of data is the issue of security. While computer systems increase the amount and availability of information, wider access raises concerns about protecting an institution's information resources.[32] Security problems have become so widespread and serious that a separate chapter of this book is devoted to that challenge.

Finally, there is the ultimate operational problem—the computer that never becomes operational at all. Lurking in the basements of government buildings, hospitals, and clinics are more than a few computers, purchased months or years ago, that have never been uncrated.

Somehow when they arrived no one knew what to do with them. This occasional occurrence illustrates one fallout from a fairly pervasive operational problem that managers have had—dealing with smooth-talking computer vendors.

Organizational

Perhaps the greatest problems experienced thus far have been the organizational phenomena resulting from the introduction of computer technology. Such changes in structure as the establishment of a new unit for computing functions were anticipated and recognized, but much more unintended and subtle impacts have proven to be the nemesis of many computerization projects. Chief among these unanticipated consequences is the underappreciated phenomenon of user resistance to the technology. Inevitably, resistance to using computers has emerged as a powerful obstacle to their successful implementation and use in health care organizations. In certain instances caseworkers have refused to enter data onto computer-compatible forms, keypunch operators have intentionally jammed computer terminals, and doctors have clandestinely maintained their own written records rather than use computer printouts and terminals. Cards have been destructively folded, spindled and mutilated. The *New York Times* has reported that organizations are finding it harder to get management to accept the advanced technologies they must adopt to stay competitive. According to that paper, many managers simply do not like "the new order of accountability that technology has brought to their jobs."[33]

The effect of resistance is that technically sound computers do not work. The war of person versus machine has proven to be no contest—the machine may be smart, but a resisting person is clever. Related to the resistance problem are other informal organizational impacts that have tended to disrupt organizational life. Computerization has brought with it shifts in power and changes in informal groups. It has tended to relegate previously important file clerks to less significant roles, and to raise computer technicians to lofty heights. Antagonism between aloof technicians and intimidated users has been common, while the breakdown of informal organizational networks has disrupted other functions. The organizational impact of computers in health care has been considerable and, more often than not, dysfunctional.

Psychological

Closely connected with organizational difficulties are psychological reactions to computers. In a study commissioned by Dell Computers, a survey was taken to assess the attitudes of people toward computers. It revealed that one in four adults would not use a computer unless forced to, and that they miss the days when they only used typewriters.[34] Despite the preponderance of computers in society, there still appears to be widespread computerphobia. This dread, often termed "technophobia," may very well be the phobic disease of the 1990s. Larry Rosen, a psychology professor at California State University, who has been studying technophobia for over ten years, comments that, "We're talking about a phobia that in its worst form actually causes sweaty palms, heart palpitations and headaches."[35]

Such intimidation produces fear and paranoia that, in turn, can contribute to the operational problems of handling vendors and to the organizational difficulties of resistance. How many health program managers, doctors, hospital administrators, not to mention clients and patients, harbor a deep-seated uneasiness about the strange devices associated with computer technology? And how many, consequently, prefer to keep computers out of their lives?

Aggravating these psychological predispositions can be disillusionment and distrust generated by legions of bad experiences with vendors and computer systems. Computer users' fear and distrust of the technology can be fully exacerbated when the vendors' promises never materialize, when the terminal goes down in the middle of a transaction, and when printouts are incorrect. The psychological forces behind these negative attitudes toward computers have proven to be powerful obstacles to reaping the potential benefits of computers in organizations.

Legal

Two pieces of federal legislation, with counterparts in most state and local governments, further complicate the situation of computers in health care. Freedom of information, or "sunshine," laws have placed legal responsibilities on organizations to make available to the public information that they hold. On the other hand, privacy laws place legal restrictions on information processing. Health care professionals frequently are caught in the middle of these two categories of laws, and confront a dilemma. When computers are employed, more data tend to be collected and stored, which means under sunshine laws that more data must be made available, and under privacy laws that more data must be protected. In both cases "computer error" is considered to be an unacceptable excuse for breaking the law. Providers and payers that operate in more than one state must also comply with a multitude of "often inconsistent laws and regulations that are overly burdensome and costly."[36]

These legal requirements are becoming both more stringent and more applicable. Lawsuits and other legal proceedings under these laws are an increasing burden for health care organizations.

Socio-political

Over two decades ago, systems analyst Ida Hoos issued a caveat about computer use that is as relevant now as it was then: "Insensitivity to the special problems involved, preoccupation with the mechanistic formal model, and ignorance of the stuff and substance of the real-life situation can result . . . in designs for a neatly programmed future fraught with disaster."[37] Her warning points to the social and political implications of the use of computers; her incisive words have repeatedly proven to be prescient. Because of computer technology's seductive power to store and manipulate enormous quantities of data, and assuming that the economic future belongs to the information savvy, computer users are increasingly being looked at as a powerful elite.[38] While groups such as Computer Professionals for Social Responsibility (CPSR) continue to anticipate technology bringing much good, it's not a wild speculation to think that computerization could spawn bureaucracies (in health care and government, as well as in any public service enterprise) that are technically advanced, but indifferent and insensitive to people and society.

Implications for Health Care Professionals

It may seem remarkable that nearly all of the problems organizations have experienced with computers are not technical in nature, but that is the case. The basis of the problems encountered while seeking the benefits of computers is managerial—unenlightened use of the technology. Many chief executives of health organizations clearly are less than pleased with their investment in a computerized information system. The fundamental problem, however, may be that information technology often has been viewed as the answer, rather than as one part of an approach, to problem solving.[39] For practical purposes, the technology is nearly flawless. Management and use of that technology, however, are underdeveloped. Even "downtime" that appears to be a technical problem usually is caused by a user-managerial failure of control over the system. The challenge vis-à-vis computers, therefore, is a user-managerial one, and it is considerable. As Roger Spoelman, CEO of Muskegon (Michigan) General Hospital, observes, "Executives should manage their hospital's information as carefully as they oversee its financial results."[40]

Harvard professor Regina Herzlinger puts the same sentiment a bit more soberly: "The one factor accounting for most failures of information systems lies directly within the control of the organization: the characteristics and attitudes of top management."[41] This refrain is heard unfailingly among academics and practitioners alike—executive participation and involvement is vital in technology management in the 1990s.[42] A former graduate student, who now manages a health care agency, put it poetically:

> Dear Boss:
>
> The Computer is a wondrous thing
> A million benefits it can bring.
> It can store our files
> Eliminate our paper piles
> Save hours of calculation
> And enable data manipulation.
>
> But if we don't manage this thing
> A million headaches, it can bring.
> We'll need a well planned approach
> And ensure that our managers we coach.
> We'll need a user's point of view
> And, boss, the whole thing depends
> on you.
>
> —Julie Freestone

The key to managing "the whole thing" is prescribed in Carlyle's often quoted aphorism: "When a person kens, that person can." Understanding and appreciating computers and their ramifications, and developing managerial perspectives attuned to the realities of computer use, are needed to enable computer usage to facilitate health care and societal benefits.

Notes

1. O. G. Kennedy, "Info Systems Head Toward Central Decisionmaking," *Modern Healthcare*, 9 July 1990, 32.

2. S. B. Boxerman and R. E. Gribbins, "Technology Management in the 1990's," *Healthcare Executive*, January–February 1991, 21–23.

3. D. Johnson, "Hospitals Must Prepare for the Paradigm Shifts to Managed Care," *Healthcare Strategic Management*, December 1993, 10–13.

4. *USA Today*, 24 May 1994, 2D.

5. *Newark Star Ledger*, 24 May 1994, 10.

6. J. Morrisey, "Spending More on Computers to Help Keep Costs in Line," *Modern Healthcare*, 14 February 1994, 63–70.

7. Ibid, 63.

8. E. Gardner, "Automating and Standardizing Claims Processing," *Modern Healthcare*, 17 May 1993, 42.

9. *Hospitals & Health Networks*, 20 March 1994, 28.

10. Ibid, 52.

11. E. Gardner, "Hospitals on Road to Data 'Highways,'" *Modern Healthcare*, 7 June 1993, 32.

12. *New York Times*, 8 April 1994, B1.

13. *Hospitals*, "Pioneering Protocols: Hospitals Test the Computer Use in Patient Care Decisions," 5 May 1993, 18.

14. R. Bergman, "Electronic Medical Record Makes Life Simpler for Clinic Physicians," *Hospitals & Health Networks*, 20 July 1993, 60.

15. L. Lariar, cartoon in *Parade Magazine*, 21 January 1979, 24.

16. *U.S. News and World Report*, 20 August 1979, 54.

17. *Newsweek*, 1 February 1988.

18. K. Wolfe, "Getting a Grip on Computerphobia," *American Association of Occupational Health Nurses Journal*, July 1991, 352.

19. *Newark Star Ledger*, 10 July 1988, 26.

20. *Newark Sunday Star Ledger*, 27 March 1994, 31.

21. J. Johnson, "Information Overload: CEOs Seek New Tools for Effective Decisionmaking," *Hospitals*, 20 October 1991, 24.

22. Ibid, 27.

23. *New York Daily News*, 8 November 1992, 3.

24. Morrisey, 64.

25. Ibid.

26. *Wall Street Journal*, 8 October 1993, B-9.

27. *New York Times*, 2 May 1993, 8.

28. *Wall Street Journal*, 8 October 1993, B-10.

29. *Newark Star Ledger*, 1 May 1994, Sections 8–10.

30. Johnson, 24.

31. J. Kanter, "The Role of Senior Management in MIS," *Journal of Systems Management*, April 1986, 37–45.

32. R. Hard, "Keeping Patient Data Secure Within Hospitals," *Hospitals*, 20 October 1992, 50.

33. *New York Times*, 7 February, 1988, B-1.

34. *USA Today*, 3 August 1993, 2B.

35. Ibid.

36. *Hospitals & Health Networks*, 20 November 1993, 14.

37. I. Hoos, "Information Systems and Public Planning," *Management Science*, June 1971, B-671.

38. H. Brody, "Of Bytes and Rights," *Technology Review*, November–December 1992, 23–29.

39. D. Ryckman, "Information Technology Is Not Enough," *Healthcare Executive*, May–June 1991, 39.

40. Johnson, 24.

41. R. Herzlinger, "Why Data Systems in Nonprofit Organizations Fail," *Harvard Business Review*, January–February 1977, 83.

42. Boxerman and Gribbens, 23.

Selected Readings

Bergman, R. "Electronic Medical Record Makes Life Simpler for Clinic Physicians." *Hospitals & Health Networks*, 20 July 1993, 60.

Brody, H. "Of Bytes and Rights." *Technology Review*. (November–December 1992): 23–29.

Boxerman, S., and R. E. Gribbins. "Technology Management in the 1990's." *Healthcare Executive* (January–February 1991): 21–23.

Darnell, J. "LIS Technologies Must Grow Into the 21st Century." *Computers in Healthcare* (September 1993): 41–42.

Elliot, B. "Executive Information Management Strategies to Improve Care and Control Costs." *Healthcare Executive* (January–February 1992): 29.

Freund, L. M. "Information Technology Conference: Technology's Expanding Role." *Healthcare Executive* (July–August 1991): 30–31.

Gardner, E. "Automating and Standardizing Claims Processing." *Modern Healthcare* (17 May 1993): 42.

Gardner, E. "Hospitals on Road to Data 'Highways.'" *Modern Healthcare* (7 June 1993): 32.

Gross, M., and B. Cassidy. "Information Technology and Today's Health Care Management." *Topics in Health Information Management* (August 1992): 1–10.

Hard, R. "Keeping Patient Data Secure within Hospitals." *Hospitals* (20 October 1992): 50.

Herzlinger, R. "Management Non-Information Systems in Health Care Organizations." *Health Care Management Review* (Spring 1976): 71–76.

———. "Why Data Systems in Nonprofit Organizations Fail." *Harvard Business Review* (January–February 1977): 81–86.

Johnson, D. "Hospitals Must Prepare for the Paradigm Shifts to Managed Care." *Healthcare Strategic Management* (December 1993): 10–13.

Johnson, J. "Information Overload: CEOs Seek New Tools for Effective Decisionmaking." *Hospitals* (20 October 1991): 24.

Kennedy, G. "Info Systems Head Toward Central Decisionmaking." *Modern Healthcare* (9 July 1990): 32.

Kortbawi, P. "From Manual Charting to Computers: Easing the Transition." *Nursing Management* (November 1993): 89–90.

Lumsdon, K. "Computerized Patient Records Gain Converts." *Hospitals* (5 April 1993): 44.

Montrose, G., and K. Marcoux. "Management by Information: A New Imperative." *Computers in Healthcare* (November 1991): 49–54.

Morrisey, J. "Spending More on Computers to Help Keep Costs in Line." *Modern Healthcare* (14 February 1994): 63–70.

Ryckman, D. "Information Technology Is Not Enough." *Healthcare Executive* (May–June 1991): 39.

Sherer, J. L. "Clinical Information Systems: Up to Par?" *Hospitals & Health Networks* (20 August 1993): 28.

Takeda, Y. "Managing Technology in the 21st Century." *Research-Technology Management* (November–December 1993): 8.

READING

T HE FOLLOWING *New York Times* special report chronicles the actual experience of a large medical center in trying to tame computer technology. Kirk Johnson's insightful narrative reveals practical problems encountered while seeking to reap the benefits of computers in the health care environment of the 1990s. His empirical report highlights the managerial challenge addressed throughout the book.

Computers in a Community Hospital:
New York Times Special Series

Kirk Johnson

Anthony R. Macaluso's delicately timid techno-ballet of batch files and interface gates will reach its moment of truth at exactly 1 p.m. on Saturday at St. Joseph's Hospital and Medical Center. That's when technicians will throw the switch to take the hospital's new computerized patient-records network fully on line for the first time.

Nearly all of the hospital's 3,500 employees will have been trained. Debugging SWAT teams will be roving the labs and nurses' stations for trouble. Every foreseeable contingency has been planned for. But for Mr. Macaluso, a hospital vice president overseeing this hospital's unusual transformation, the nagging worry is what he hasn't thought of. And this is not a business where you can shut down and tinker for a while if things don't fly.

'It's like trying to change a flat tire on a car that's hurling down the road at 60 miles per hour,' he said. 'You don't have the luxury of stopping.'

Hospitals everywhere are on this high-tech road, propelled by the changes in the health-care industry that have transformed the once-mundane functions of the back office—filing, billing, supply, communications—into matters of institutional survival. Hospitals like St. Joseph's need to monitor their costs more closely and to trim expenses to compete for group-care contracts, patients and the loyalty of the doctors who refer those patients. And that requires new technology that may not change a hospital's mission, but does change how the place works and how its people do their jobs.

'Computerized records will change health care more than anything in the last 30 years,' said Everett Hines, a partner at Coopers & Lybrand, the accounting firm, which served as a consultant to St. Joseph's. 'And institutions are being forced—there's a tremendous squeeze.'

Most hospitals do this sort of surgery in a less radical fashion than St. Joseph's, putting in integrated systems one at a time. Here, they're calling it the Big Bang: Over the course of one Saturday shift, three years of planning, preparation and employee training, not to mention $25 million in computers, software and fiber-optic cable, will come glowing to life all at once.

It is an approach dictated both by costs and technologies. A more deliberate changeover from an existing obsolete network would require many costly temporary computer solutions. So the shock of the new is being crammed into a single day.

'My son did a cartoon drawing for me, what we're going to look like on April 10,' said Maureen Romoser, the hospital's administrative director for nursing services. 'It's a picture of Wile E. Coyote with a little firecracker—Bang!'

St. Joseph's new computer system—essentially a network of about 500 personal computers in the hospital and affiliated out-patient centers—will ultimately change just about everyone's job here. The immediate jolt will be a tidal surge of information. Through a group-computing package created and managed by Shared Medical Systems Corporation, a Pennsylvania medical software company, doctors will be able to call up a patient's name to check on everything from the latest lab test results to a running tally of the charges.

In coming months, expansions will include an artificial intelligence 'protocol' program that compares past patients and procedures with the facts in the current case. Full electronic patients charts, offering the latest blood pressure and medication information from the patient's bedside, will come next year.

As of Saturday, administrators will be able to calculate the exact cost of every variable of cardiac care or any other procedure. Nurses will zap lab orders directly to the lab. Everyone from the cleaners in maintenance, to the dietitians in food service will have on-line access for their departments. In the materials supply department, the goal is a 'just in time' inventory system—possible now because hospital-wide use of any item, from rubber gloves to Robitussin, will be trackable.

Some Anxiety

As in any institution, the prospect of all this change worries people, despite repeated practice runs.

'Everybody is anxious,' said Colleen Weber, a registered nurse in the intermediate respiratory therapy ward. 'A lot of the information that we may need is now on paper—hopefully we'll be able to get it on the screen.'

St. Joseph's crash course also provides something of a mirror for the New York metropolitan region. Health care experts say many hospitals in the region, especially in New York City, have lagged behind the rest of the nation in accepting how managed care will drive the market to greater awareness of costs and how to control them.

Some have been able to keep their beds full and so stay insulated from the competition that is gripping hospitals like St. Joseph's. Others lack the resources. Many are stepping in one toe at a time. New Britain Hospital in Connecticut, for example, has recently adopted imaging technologies that can absorb written records—even doctors' handwriting technologies—for an archive of patient information that administrators say will form the foundation of an on-line interactive system.

'I don't think there's a hospital in the country that doesn't want this—but there's some caution,' said Dr. Clement J. McDonald, a professor at Indiana University who studies hospital technologies. 'And it's just hard,' he added. 'It's like a brain transplant—that's what it's like putting in a medical-records system—hundreds of millions of nerves, all those sources of input.'

Lessons Learned

And the lessons learned by St. Joseph's in reaching this threshold day are sobering as well. The hospital put in a partial network in the late 1980s that didn't work as it was supposed to. Burned by that experience, administrators embarked on a quest for fiber-optic infrastructure that could embrace the full interactive medical frontier, from bedside terminals to on-line patient charts and multi-media electronic physician consultations. They also insisted on elaborate backup systems. St. Joseph's computers, while linked by fiber optics, will have roof-top laser connections between buildings that can take over if the cable breaks.

'We're going to be one of the hospitals that survives, and survives well,' said Sister Jane Frances Brady, the hospital's president. That all this is happening in downtown Paterson—'a city in struggle,' as Sister Jane put it—and in an old traditional-minded hospital with many poor and uninsured patients, is the story within the story.

St. Joseph's, which was founded just after the Civil War by the Roman Catholic Sisters of Charity of St. Elizabeth with the specific mission of caring for this city's immigrant population, has—like Paterson itself—teetered on the edge of insolvency repeatedly. In the 1960s it saved itself by specializing in health services like dialysis and pediatrics and by transforming itself into a teaching hospital. The new network, to make the hospital competitive in a new era, is being paid off over nine years, with some of the hardware leased, to make the monthly carrying charge manageable.

'We're not looking at some white middle-class, upper-middle-class community hospital,' said Dr. Patrick E. Ryan, a dentist who headed the steering committee charged with devising the new computer system. 'If you can do it here, you can do it anywhere.'

But technology does not change an institution's culture, and some things will continue to be done the old-fashioned way. Tests for HIV, the virus that causes AIDS, for example, will not be entered on the St. Joseph's network out of concern that the system will not be fully secure. Those records will remain paper-bound in files that doctors and nurses will have to paw through.

And Dr. Ryan said a decision was also made early on that doctors would not have to use the computers if they didn't want to. There will still be paper records and charts for the traditionalists. And there will still be demanding, very human bosses.

'As I told Tony, it better work or else,' said Sister Jane, referring to Mr. Macaluso. 'I didn't want to put him under any pressure.'

A Little Nursing Gets Hospital's Computers Up and Running

Monitors were not plugged in. Printers were not on line. The names of some discharged patients could not be found in the system. Some employees, who had somehow not been trained, phoned for help.

But after some debugging, an extra 18 hours of labor and many cups of coffee, St. Joseph's Hospital and Medical Center's computerized record-keeping network was finally on line just after 7 a.m. Sunday.

'We just have our normal chaos now,' said Anthony R. Macaluso, a hospital administrator who oversaw the change and had dark circles under his eyes to prove it.

Nursing the Bottom Line

The technology is the easy part. What begins now is a new engine of change that will affect the lives of the people who work here and their patients. The network, essentially a central nervous system for the hospital, is intended to shape every job and every decision around the new realities of health care: competition and cost control.

Because of health care competitors like HMOs, who can buy in bulk and drive down costs—administrators say changing the hospital in this way is the key to survival and to maintaining the 127-year-old mission of never turning away a patient, however poor and uninsured.

Finding Patients and Patience

But for the next few weeks, at least, it also means a great deal of hand-holding and patience. Most of the newly bewildered will end up on the phone with people like Mercy Cobo, a system coordinator who took calls on Saturday at the Help Desk, a windowless fifth floor room crammed with personal computers and crisscrossed telephone wires and adorned with a single, small wood-and-gold crucifix on one wall.

Most of the problems fielded by Ms. Cobo and other phone line workers were basic: I forgot my password. I forgot how to sign on. The printer doesn't work. Are we live yet?

But the last great hurdle was a mystery: finding out what had happened to people who, according to backup records, had been discharged from the hospital in the 48 hours before 1 p.m. on Saturday, which had been scheduled as the zero hour for going on line. Those patients' names were absent from the record.

The Shared Medical Systems Corporation of Malvern, Pa., which designed the system and which will also operate it for the hospital, found the problem late Saturday night: the space for the patient's name on the electronic form had been filled instead, apparently through a programmers error, with symbols that prevented the information from being entered.

Solving that problem meant doing a new census of the hospital through early Sunday morning, to make sure that any new, moved or discharged patients were where the computer said they were.

'The system is pretty stable—it's the people who are nervous,' said Natalie Contaldi, an associate at Coopers & Lybrand, a consultant to the hospital, who was working the Help Desk this weekend.

Some Doctors Face Computer Age Warily

The computer age may have arrived at St. Joseph's Hospital and Medical Center, but the bits and bytes have not changed a basic truth of hospital life: there are doctors, and there is everybody else.

Hospital administrators, in putting a new computerized hospital-records network on line here in April, decided early not to require physicians to type their orders into the computers. It would doom the effort, they said. That has put clerical workers like Alisa McClendon, a unit receptionist in the first-floor geriatric ward, in the vanguard of the hospital's march toward automation. An alternative point of view is that clerks and nurses have simply been saddled with the work.

'They, I think, will never change, no matter how much you give them,' Ms. McClendon said, referring to the doctors who troop by her post every day, trying to extract information from the computer. 'It seems like one little step they might not be familiar with, so instead of them just trying it on their own, they'll try to find the unit receptionist or the unit manager,' she said. 'Do you think it's possible to get this for me? Is there any chance you're not busy?'

Old and new coexist everywhere in the special geriatrics unit known as Regan One West. The new computers are plunked down on tables in the crowded nursing station next to an ancient-looking Executone patient intercom. Nurses, aides and doctors whirl in and out through the corridors, checking computer screens one minute, dog-eared paper charts the next.

It is a hospital of time-honored traditions. Founded after the Civil War by the Roman Catholic Sisters of Charity to treat the immigrant poor, St. Joseph's has grown into one of the largest teaching hospitals in the region, with 792 beds and advanced treatment in areas like neonatal care and dialysis. Nurses, doctors and administrators say the old guard of physicians is still strong. Many do not deign to type.

And because administrators made the conscious decision not to force the issue, the anxieties that some doctors might have in dealing with computers have simply been avoided as an issue: no one has asked or required them to learn even the elementary step of signing on, not to mention requiring them to type in their own orders for hospital procedures, called physician order entries.

'I don't think it will ever come to a point where using the computer will be mandatory, because there will always be some physicians who do not want to do it,' said Maureen Romoser, the administrative director for nursing services. 'Maybe I should clarify that,' she added. 'Maybe in 50 years.'

'It Takes Time to Learn'

Other people said that the hospital, having leaped into the information age with a $25 million network that went completely on line in a single weekend this spring, should not expect miracles.

'To have 'physician order entry,' you have to have the physician staff capable of using the computer, and I'm not sure everyone is capable,' said Dr. Gary Kosc, a gastroenterologist from West Paterson, who was checking on one of his geriatric patients on a recent afternoon. 'It takes time to learn,' he said, and time to embrace it as a useful tool.

Every hospital's culture is different. So too are the paths they take in adopting the tools of cost control, managed care and automated records systems, a transformation being forced on hospitals everywhere by insurance companies, big health care buyers like health maintenance organizations, and the prospect of a Federal health care overhaul from Washington.

At St. Luke's-Roosevelt Hospital Center in Manhattan, for example, the hospital is installing a new internal records network similar to St. Joseph's, but will leap directly to doctors' typing in their own orders in late 1995. At other hospitals, like New York University— perhaps the most automated hospital in the region—computer literacy for physicians has been a requirement for years.

Hospital experts say that places like St. Joseph's—in an area with many hospitals—have less leverage in compelling doctors, who can take their business elsewhere if they are unhappy. And the less a physician is tied to any one hospital, the less incentive to learn its computer system.

Challenging the Old Ways

But there is no question, they add, that hospital records systems are threats to old bases of power.

'It challenges the old ways of doing things,' said Dr. Patricia Flatley Brennan, an associate professor of nursing and systems engineering at Case Western Reserve University. 'Once you change the way information flows, you change the way people work together—you change who is in power and who has the right to make decisions.'

But even here, some doctors are urging that they be required to participate fully.

Dr. John J. Farkas, a wiry, bearded gastroenterology and hepatology specialist, said he sees himself as a catalyst of sorts, prodding the administration to move faster on the road it has set for itself. While he understands the hospital's reluctance to compound confusion by forcing old ways to change too fast, he maintains that delaying a cultural adaptation by physicians will not make it easier. 'Without physician order entry, the system is a big miss,' he said.

But there is also fear, in various varieties.

The new network, essentially a nerve system for the hospital, now only allows coordination of medical supplies, lab results, admissions, transfers and dozens of other basic functions. Add-on components scheduled for introduction in coming months, however, will create a whole new push into matters of medical judgment, a function called 'decision support.'

Before the network came on line, orders for things like blood tests or radiology were handwritten and dispatched by messengers who roamed the hospital corridors; individual departments and labs had computers, but they were never coordinated. Under the new regime, the connections—from the administrative offices to the warehouse—are like nerves extending through every limb.

The computer will be able to assist doctors in diagnoses. It will schedule operating rooms by calculating how fast or slow a surgeon has performed a particular procedure in the past. It will allow administrators to know much more than they do now about who exactly does what.

Doing that also requires the assigning of numerical values to things that have always been done on human need and intuition. One software program scheduled to come on line early next year, for example, will calculate how many hours a day of hands-on nursing time should be required for a particular patient with a particular health problem.

For some, the computer symbolizes bureaucracy and intrusion.

'It's getting worse and worse,' said Tammy Gundlah, a 28-year-old registered nurse, sitting in her office, a converted coat closet she shares with another nurse in geriatrics. 'Everything is so legal, you need all this documentation all the time. It's disappointing, you're always afraid somebody's going to sue for this, you've got to make sure you write everything down, everything's got to be charted. And this computer thing; it's like you're more out at the desk dealing with the computers than with the patients.'

In this unit, in particular, where the patients are older, sicker and likely to stay longer, health care providers worry that all the data will ultimately make it harder for the hospital to subsidize long-term and indigent patients.

As the computer system is able to collect very precise statistics on every cost, many doctors and nurses worry that administrators, armed with vast new amounts of information and under pressure to economize, could find it harder to justify providing treatment without regard to cost.

How, exactly, do you measure the treatment received by Stella Zober? Mrs. Zober, a wispy-haired 79-year-old Wallington resident, was admitted in late May, barely able to move after her arthritis suddenly worsened. Through therapy in the geriatrics unit, she has regained the ability to get about with a walker, but she is not ready to go back to her apartment, or to a nursing home. And no one is pushing to have her discharged.

'I think, always, that the quality of care, the quality of life, will prevail,' said Dr. Belinda Vicioso, the chief of geriatric medicine. Then she paused for moment. 'I'm hoping.'

Dr. Vicioso also believes that physicians at the keyboard will ultimately be common at St. Joseph's, though she concedes it will not be painless.

'The old guard is dying off,' she said. 'It will happen; it has to happen. If we can cut down on the number of steps, the delivery of care will be more efficient, and cheaper, hopefully.'

Hope is plentiful. Nurses who deplored the changes they see and fear, like Mrs. Gundlah, also said just as often that they couldn't envision working anywhere else. Some who seem to have inherited the burden of the work in the new electronic order have also observed that information is power, even if you have to work harder.

'Like they say, one hand washes the other. You be nice to me, I'll be nice to you; treat me with respect, I'll treat you with respect,' said Ms. McClendon, the unit receptionist. 'Even the doctors figure that out eventually,' she added, smiling, 'So it's not that bad.'

Kirk Johnson is a *New York Times* correspondent based in Connecticut.

CASE 1
Snug Harbor Pediatric Hospital

FRED HARTLEY reflected over the events of the last six months and wondered whether he had, in fact, really lost his "fast ball." He always thought his strongest asset as a manager was his ability to motivate and bring people together (i.e., his interpersonal skills). The recent low morale, tensions and overall poor productivity in the hospital was a total reversal of the esprit de corps he felt during the first few months of his tenure. Snug Harbor, a 160-bed pediatric facility located in suburban Connecticut, hired Fred ten months ago as Administrator. Armed with his graduate degree in Public Administration and three years experience as an assistant administrator in a large rehabilitation institution, he was convinced that the Board chose him over the other applicants because of his academic credentials, his experience in a larger institution, and his willingness to initiate and implement change. Norman Jones, Chairman of the Board, summarized it best during the initial interview when he said " . . . Snug Harbor has a long, proud tradition of providing care to the children of this area. The staff are devoted to these kids and committed to rendering the best care possible. But, with increasing financial pressures, competition from other health facilities, and dwindling resources, we need to upgrade our technological and administrative capabilities, beginning with our management information systems."

Fred's mission was clear. Introduce a centralized computer management information system into the facility, and do it as quickly as possible. His predecessor had succeeded in avoiding this task, although it had become increasingly evident to everyone that such an undertaking was necessary. The manual information systems used in such areas as medical records, accounts receivable, accounts payable, purchasing, payroll and cost-accounting were becoming burdensome and difficult to manage. The storage of data was primitive and transmission of data was plagued with errors and omissions. The pressure for change came both from within the organization and from outside. Most key employees talked frequently about how a computerized data base and information system could better handle the rapidly growing information load. Pressure from outside came from fiscal intermediaries, accrediting agencies, and financial institutions, demanding that procedures be streamlined.

Fred initiated the change by hiring a manager of data processing, Ginger Martin. Deciding on the hardware and software seemed a relatively straightforward task—choosing that which Ginger had worked before under a similar situation had seemed a logical first step. Fred compared the cost of the package chosen with other packages and was pleased to learn that not only was this package one of the best on the market, but the cost was 10 percent less than the list price. Despite all this, things did not appear to be going smoothly.

Fred recalled a number of conversations with his staff and attempted to make sense of what went wrong.

Ginger Martin, Manager of Data Processing

After choosing the hardware and software packages for the new computerized management information system, I called a meeting for all department heads. At that meeting I explained the benefits of the new system and distributed questionnaires for every department to fill out. These questionnaires were to help ascertain departmental needs. They were to complete the forms for the next meeting, which was to be held in one week. Not only did they fail to return the forms, but half of the department heads missed the meeting. The excuses were amazing. One department head told me the reason he didn't complete the questionnaire was because he didn't have the time! Because of the lack of interest I decided to circulate the conversion schedule by memo. Don't these people realize this new system will make their job easier?

Dennis Jones, Accounts Receivable Manager

I've worked with a computerized MIS before, at my previous job. I don't know why everyone is making such a big deal about this.

Although I was surprised that their information systems were not computerized, most people catch on quickly, and see the benefit. If the computer people (Ginger) will just do their job, we can do ours. I would think that they should do all the work up until D-Day and then let us learn the system after it's ready for use. I know I speak for most people here when I say we are cooperative. I know at the last place I worked they gave us manuals, conversion schedules, forms and flow charts. I'm not sure who prepared them, but they seemed to represent a great deal of work. The instruction manual for this system is probably similar to the one at the other place.

Sharon Johnson, Director of Inventory and Purchasing

I'm not convinced that the new system is better than my system. I've been here for fifteen years and no one has complained about my department. All these new forms and new procedures have created more work, not less. I've been here every night until 8 p.m. trying to figure this out. I know supplies are not getting up to the floors as quickly and I'm really not sure how much stock I have at this point. The new system gives me different information than the old system. And it's not because I'm scared of computers. My ten-year-old son has a computer and we work with it together at home.

Mary Michaels, Payroll Manager

They promised these wonderful reports when the conversion came. It took my staff three weeks to prepare the input documents, and I haven't seen anything yet. We had to do our ordinary work and on top of that, do these computer forms, too. We all were pretty tired of this new system even before it started. I'm also uncomfortable with the fact that all the pay roll records and pay statistics now "belong" to the new data processing department. I've talked to the director of human resources and the nursing director. They also feel that personnel records and nursing records belong in the respective departments, not somewhere else.

Janice Anderson, Director of Nursing

Look, I'm all for making the job easier for my staff, but I have some real problems with this, and I'm not sure a data processing manager can understand. My medical records are sensitive and contain life and death information. I feel they should be easily accessed by my staff and *only* my staff. This information is not just accounting ledgers or inventory amounts but vital information that should only be within reach of my staff. I hope that the administration is not putting efficiency ahead of patient care. I will not let another, less important, department tell my nurses what to do. One of the nurses actually couldn't access patient information the other day and demanded that data processing come up to the floor to get the information. They actually told her to look in the manual. My nurses don't have time to look in a manual, they are giving care to sick children. I'm short of staff as it is.

Tom Smith, Medical Records Supervisor

I'm not sure that converting the management information system in every department all at once was the best way to approach this. Ginger thought that converting the entire hospital simultaneously would be quicker. Perhaps if they converted one department at a time it would have stopped much of the bickering between departments. Of course medical records should be first because we have the most to gain.

Questions for Discussion

1. What factors have led to the problems that now exist in the full implementation of the system?
2. How could these problems have been avoided in the preimplementation phase?
3. Appraise the ramifications of the use of computers in an organization such as this.
4. What do you recommend that Fred do now? Why?
5. What constraints and opportunities are related to implementing your recommendations?

UNDERSTANDING INFORMATION CONCEPTS

RECENTLY, A 1,200-bed health care complex in San Antonio reported that, despite a large in-house computer department and a major outside computer service contract, its information system was unreliable. Information provided to managers within the complex was found to be inconsistent and incomplete. In the words of its president, the information system "could not respond to the current health care environment, resulting in high cost, duplication and lack of relevant information."[1]

In a related situation some years ago, New York City computerized a "match-up" system designed to detect and reduce welfare fraud. The computer was viewed as a godsend well worth the considerable investment. It would, after all, detect and eliminate millions of dollars in welfare cheating by matching welfare rolls against payrolls and other lists, and also greatly simplify record keeping. Instead, according to an internal report, the system caused "tremendous confusion" because clients identified as fraudulent turned out to be legitimate. It seems that errors in recording and transcribing data were, with automation, aggravated rather than diminished. Typically, computers, not computer users, were blamed for the problem.[2]

Similarly, a physician in the Midwest spent $50,000 on an automated patient accounting system that, he was told, would tremendously simplify his record keeping and billing. Instead, his accounts receivable are larger than ever, bills are frequently erroneous, and patient records more difficult to maintain. He, too, blames the computer.

Each of these cases, and thousands of others like them, illustrate the prevalence of the dangerous myth that the key to better information is a computer and, concomitantly, that the cause of information problems is "computer error." One commentator goes so far as to suggest that the myth of "computer error" has become so mired that many organizations buy a computer just to have a credible object to blame problems on.[3]

A second pervasive myth is that the more data that are available, the better off we are. Witness the reams of computer printouts that fill office bookshelves, even though they are seldom used. In noting the plethora of data generated within health care organizations today, many health care executives acknowledge that these data are often not worth the computer paper they are printed on.[4] One insightful health care executive suggests that *"How* people use the information is much more important than *what* the computers spit out—if management is given data and those data are not relevant for decision making, then the data are worthless for everybody."[5] Unfortunately, "data proliferation" is a major reality, and many agree that health care executives are drowning in it.[6]

A third myth is that everyone understands the meaning of "computerese," at least basic jargon such as "on-line," "batch," and "real-time," and certainly the frequently heard "management information system." In truth, the jargon of computerized information systems is often misused and misunderstood, and sometimes altogether unfathomed. Technology—in the guise of jargon, acronyms, incomplete sentences, and codes—often puts the nonexpert user in a position of maximum uncertainty and minimum productivity.[7]

These three myths, and others, stem from an underappreciation of information as a resource that needs to be managed by its users. This and the following concepts provide a foundation for undertaking the task of information management.

Data versus Information

The Los Angeles phone directory is a collection of names, addresses, and phone numbers that have been printed on paper. Does it contain data or information? Many health care professionals receive daily printouts with words and numbers printed on large, thin paper. Do these printouts contain data or information? The answer is: probably both.

Data are the raw material from which information can be generated. Information is the relevant, usable commodity needed by the phone caller, the manager, the health care provider—the user. If I need to call someone in the Los Angeles area, the phone book may very well be a source of information for me if from among those thousands of words and numbers (data) I am able to derive the one correct number (information) I need within the time period in which I need it.

Similarly, a printout may be intended to contain a needed piece of information. If it is there and I am able to derive it, then the printout has been a source of information for me. If it is not there, or if I am unable to decipher it, then the printout is a mere collection of data to me.

There are three important points to note from these examples. One is that information is something that a user can effectively use; words and numbers are merely data unless we can effectively use them. Second, users need information to do their jobs; data that cannot be effectively used are not needed. Third, most modern professionals seem to receive a lot of data and not nearly enough information. They are deluged with reams of printed sheets and rays of bright computer screens that at best waste time, and at worst may conceal needed information. Anyone can produce data, but only the user can produce information.

Modern health care professionals receive more data than their predecessors and are entirely too patient with the situation. If information is what is needed, then workers should demand more information and less data. What, then, distinguishes information from data?

Characteristics of Information

Every information user has particular substantive information needs. That is, a nurse manager needs words and numbers concerning patients on the floor, a government personnel manager needs words and numbers concerning worker performance, a food services manager needs words and numbers concerning prices and availability. However, in addition to such particular substantive information needs, all users also have "generic" needs.

Generic information needs are the characteristics that distinguish data from information. Substantive words and numbers that bear on a user's job remain mere data if they lack these distinguishing characteristics—accuracy, timeliness, completeness, conciseness, and relevancy.

Accuracy

Did you ever get a wrong number from a phone book? When that happens, what would otherwise be a good piece of information becomes mere data, a row of digits, because it lacks accuracy. More commonly, printouts of accounting numbers are inaccurate or patient files contain incorrect words.

Timeliness

Several years ago a stockbroker sent a client a report about a company that analysts argued was a prime takeover prospect. The client received the report on Thursday and immediately called the broker to place a buy order. He was informed that a takeover had been announced on Wednesday, and that the stock price had doubled. The client lost a chance to invest profitably because the report was not timely and, therefore, could not be effectively used; failing the timeliness need, it remained mere data. Similarly, accounting reports can be useful to help manage finances, but not if they are received two months late.

Completeness

We once discovered that the phone book we were using had a corner of a page missing, so that the number we needed was missing its last digit. We had an accurate, timely six-digit number, but were unable to effectively meet our needs because it was incomplete. Patient files that have a thorough medical history but lack the most recent laboratory test results make decision making difficult, if not impossible. Incomplete, the files are mere collections of data, instead of useful sources of information.

Conciseness

Too often professional reports are unnecessarily lengthy. Frequently they do contain important information, but require so much of the reader's time that the information is difficult to absorb.

Medical records often are similarly flawed. Records with years of notes that are unindexed, for example, are unwieldy. Lacking conciseness, they remain data, unread and unused.

Relevancy

A report, printout, or screen display must be relevant to a user's needs or interests to be information. Equally important, a report may be substantively relevant, but presented in such an irrelevant format—for example, it contains meaningless codes and symbols—that it is not understandable. The Los Angeles phone book would be irrelevant if it did not format the thousands of names and numbers by alphabetic code.

While there sometimes are other required characteristics of information, such as confidentiality in politically sensitive programs, the absence of generic characteristics that distinguish information from data often is a major reason why health care professionals are inundated with data and starved for information. A significant task of information management is to ensure that these distinguishing characteristics are provided.

Information Systems

Every administrator has heard of an information system. But just what, exactly, is an information system?

An information system is a network of steps taken to collect and transform data into information. That is, it is a series of actions to collect words and numbers and transform them into something needed and usable by an information user. Many so-called "information systems" actually are data systems—they collect and transform data into more data. Too many health care administrators tolerate data systems when information systems are what they need to do their jobs well.

At least nine basic steps are included in the network that forms an information system. Understanding what is involved in each step is necessary for effective information management.

Classifying

The essential first step in an information system is identifying information needs and the kinds or classes of data needed to generate that information. In running a public health clinic hypertension program we may need to collect blood pressure readings so that progress can be evaluated, to know how to contact people for follow-up visits, and to track medications prescribed in the program. To meet these information needs it would probably be necessary for us to have data on periodic blood pressures; on addresses and phone numbers on prescriptions written; and to have it all in a certain understandable format. Determining these kinds of data and format needs is the first step—the classifying step—in an information system. In this case we have identified several classifications of data: blood pressure readings, addresses, phone numbers, prescriptions, and the format in which we need them. This step is a thinking step, not a mechanistic one—it takes place in the mind of the person needing information.

Collecting

Armed with specifics on what is needed, we can then provide for collecting the data. We might design a form and use either clinicians, clerks, or both to collect the data, or we might retrieve it from the medical record and patient registration form. In most cases, however, data should be collected from as close to the source as possible.

Recording

A third step is the actual recording of the data. It might involve pencil and paper, a tape recording, the use of codes, or several recordings such as an original handwritten form that is then typed or keypunched. Anyone might do the data recording.

Sorting

The recorded data frequently are sorted or organized to facilitate processing. We could sort the hypertension clinic data by day collected, by alphabetical order of patients' last names, or by range of blood pressure readings.

Calculating

The recorded and sorted data can be further organized, summarized, or analyzed. For example, we might want to count the number of blood pressure readings in each range, the number of patients who live in each town, the number of patients taking a certain prescribed drug, or simply the number of patients.

Storing

Information systems usually involve some kind of storage capability. We might use folders and file drawers, a card file, or a computer to store information.

Retrieving

Retrieval might involve written notations on the tab of a folder or labels on file drawers—whatever is required to be able to find information when we need it.

Reproducing

Reproduction could involve carbon paper, duplicating machines, mimeographs, or printouts.

Communicating

The final essential step in an information system is delivering output to the information user. This could involve a routing slip, a distribution list, or a terminal placed at the proper desk.

Understanding these steps can facilitate the construction and diagnosis of an information system. For example, which step is the most important? It can convincingly be argued that communicating is critical because failure in this area means the system fails in its purpose of providing needed information. One could also argue that classifying is the key because even the most sophisticated system will fail if needs are not properly identified. Actually, an information system is only as good as its weakest link. An otherwise perfect system will fail if one element fails—if just the retrieval step is faulty or data collection is incomplete. Each step in the chain must be carefully managed.

We could also analyze each step in terms of its effect on the generic characteristics of information. Where is accuracy most likely to be lost or gained? If timeliness is missing in an information system, at which step would you look for the problem?

Certainly relevance is affected at the classifying stage. If the user is not involved in determining classifications, the selected classifications may not be relevant to his or her needs. If the collecting stage is done in an interview and the collector forgets to ask one of the items, the resulting data may be incomplete. Or, if a form is used and the data provider does not understand it or resists providing information, the resulting data may be incomplete or inaccurate.

If a form and a pencil are used for recording, any number of disruptive contingencies could occur. If the recording is done illegibly, accuracy could be completely lost. Conciseness can be promoted at the sorting and calculating stages. A faulty retrieval step could cause delay and reduce timeliness, and blurred reproduction can impede accuracy and completeness.

Of course, each of the generic characteristics of information can be affected to some degree at nearly every step in an information system, but in designing or diagnosing an information system it can help to focus on certain steps for certain information characteristics. For example, an accuracy problem might suggest that a verifying mechanism should be built into the recording stage, a relevancy problem might mean more user involvement is required, a timeliness loss might be remedied by improvements in the retrieval or collection steps.

Finally, we can ask at which steps in an information system a computer might be helpful. Without doubt, a computer can sort large amounts of data, conduct complex, error-free calculations, and store more data than a warehouse full of file cabinets. However, a computer cannot determine our information needs or collect needed data. That takes a human being, unless the data have already been collected and stored in machine-readable form. Can a computer communicate the output to the user? It certainly can hasten retrieval and greatly facilitate reproduction, but a person is needed to decide where, when, and how it will occur.

In other words, there is no such thing as a "computerized information system." There are only partially computerized information systems. A computer is useful at only some of the steps in an information system. Placing a million-dollar computer in an information system, therefore, can improve parts of the information system, but the overall system will still be only as strong as its weakest link.

Management Information System

Few terms are more bandied about in organizations today than "management information system," better known under the acronym MIS. There seems to be some sort of MIS for nearly everything. We have HISs (hospital information systems), WMISs (welfare management information systems), SSISs (social service information systems), LISs (library information systems), and so on.

But just what is an MIS? The term is so overused and misused that its lack of conceptual clarity contributes to the problems of dealing with MISs in organizations.

First, it is important to remember that an MIS is supposed to be an information system. That is, it is supposed to produce information (not merely data); therefore, it consists of a network of steps something like that described above.

Second, an MIS is supposed to be management oriented; that is, it is intended to meet managerial information needs, more particularly, decision making needs. Most information systems are designed to meet clerical information needs. A system to develop and maintain a roster, for example, is routine oriented. A payroll system and a billing system are usually intended for specific, routine purposes of concern to clerks and many others. Management information systems, on the other hand, are intended to assist the decision making functions of professionals.[8] Some writers distinguish between electronic data processing (EDP) and decision support systems (DSS), the former being geared to reporting and consistency needs (routine), the latter to ad hoc and flexibility needs (decision making).[9]

Third, because of its decisions-assisting purpose, the concept of MIS is information unity. It is intended to bring together in one system various data that are relevant to managerial level functions. The administrator of a family practice, for example, needs information on finances, staff patients, doctors, and so on when planning next year's activity. Without an MIS the administrator must pull vital information from various sources and places, and then try to interrelate the data. With an MIS the data are standardized and interrelated so that required information can be easily and quickly retrieved.

Fourth, to facilitate the kind of data integration described above, the concept of MIS nearly always entails computerization.

There are two major kinds of management information systems: special purpose or limited systems, and data base management or total systems.

Special Purpose Systems

These are information systems that integrate some files into one system to facilitate well-defined, repetitive decision-making tasks. A special purpose system in a health care agency might integrate patient history data with administrative data to facilitate admissions processing, much like airlines use special purpose systems to facilitate flight reservation decisions. Some commonly used, and misused, jargon stems from this kind of MIS. Since these systems usually are geared to quick feedback for quick decisions, they are almost always "on-line." To say that a system is on-line means that a user can directly and immediately access a file. In practice this means a user can type at a terminal and a screen will display the requested file. For example, airline clerks can call up a flight number on a screen and immediately determine whether there are seats available.

A "batch" system does not provide direct access to a file. Many modern libraries, for example, have computerized periodical research services. Typically, the most recent years are on-line—the researcher can go to the terminal in the library, type in the subject of research interest, and see on the screen a list of relevant articles. For older articles, however, the researcher might have to fill out a form requesting those files, and return the next day for a printout listing the relevant articles. The researcher must wait overnight because those files are in batch mode.

The term batch can have two meanings—it can refer to the method of sorting or to the method of recording data. In the example above, data on older articles are stored in batch mode—the data are on tapes or disks that are "batched" or stored on shelves, off-line, until a request arrives at the data center for information from those batched files; at that time the tape or disk is placed on a machine and the resulting printout is sent to the library. The term batch is also used to describe the method of recording data. Most credit card sales, for example, are not recorded immediately on our computerized bill file. Instead, after we sign a credit card slip, it is sent to the central billing office, where it is placed in a pile of other slips. When this batch of sales slips reaches a certain size, or at a certain time of day, the data is then recorded and the transactions appear on our monthly statement.

Note that an on-line system, then, must have on-line storage, but it might also reflect a batch recording mode. That is, in an on-line system the user has direct access to the file, but the file may not be up-to-date if the data in it are entered through a batch mode. A "real-time" system does not have this condition. It provides not only the on-line capability of immediately viewing a file, but also the capability of making immediate entries or recordings in the file. A typical example of this capability is the airline reservations system. The reservations clerk uses a real-time capability to book a seat so that every person who accesses that file now knows there is one less seat available.

Batch systems are still the most common types employed because they are less expensive and adequate for many purposes. Waiting over-night for a printout is perfectly fine for all sorts of functions. Most management information systems, however, are on-line because decision making frequently requires quick information. On-line systems are considerably more expensive than batch systems, though not nearly as costly as real-time systems, which require special software and hardware (this will be discussed in Chapter 3). On-line systems without real-time capability are, however, adequate in most cases for health care organizations. Airlines, clearly, need real-time systems to manage their reservations function because it requires instant updating, but relatively few other functions are sufficiently improved by a real-time capability to warrant the additional cost.

Other important concepts and terms associated with management information systems are "timesharing" and "distributed systems," both of which are usually on-line systems. In timesharing, many users are connected to (i.e., share time on) the same computer; in distributed systems several computers are linked with each other so that the resources and capabilities of one are available to all. Many hospitals have a large computer which is the data processing resource for all the separate users in the institution; the users are engaged in timesharing, and each has allotted space and time on the computer. Some hospitals have several separate computers—one used by the laboratories, one by the finance office—with no link between them. These computers would be linked in a distributed system.

Additionally, workstations and distributed computing systems continue to play an important role in the evolution of computer networking. With one computer for each user in a network, workstations bear little resemblance to dumb terminals (i.e., where on-line terminals are connected to one mainframe or central computer). Workstations can have as much processing power as the mainframe computers of a decade ago, and can give users unprecedented control over what information they see and how they see it. Unlike stand-alone personal computers, workstations can be linked to form networks that share information among many computers. In a distributed computing network, there are many computers for each user, forming a web of specialized services. Each user's computer functions as a window into a number of systems and the mainframe computer. The network schedules when programs are run, communicates between programs and various devices inside of the computer, manages the computer's memory space and decides how best to allocate its resources.

Total Systems

Until recently, total systems have proven to be very difficult to realize. However, with health care reform has become an increased awareness that information sharing between financial, clinical, and administrative components is essential to future viability of health care organizations. Concomitantly, there is an expanding interest in implementing total systems or, as they are sometimes called, integrated data base systems (DBS) or enterprise-wide systems.[10] A total system is a profound step beyond a distributed system. Whereas a distributed system provides for separate, independent systems to be linked or networked, a total system provides for complete integration and standardization so that, in effect, the entire organization works out of one file cabinet. In government it would mean that if the health department collected your name and address, that data would be available to the motor vehicle department when you applied for a license—you would not have to fill out another address form since it would already be entered in the government's "total system." And if you changed addresses, the change would only have to be reported and recorded once—every user would then have the change.

A hypothetical example can illustrate both the concept and problems with implementing a total system. It is technically possible today to automate all typewriters in the world, to link them with a computer, and to link all the computers in the world into a total system. Since most of the data in the world today passes through a typewriter at some stage in its generation, it is technically possible to have most of the world's data available in one common system. Of course, to make this workable, everyone would have to use compatible typewriters and the same computer language. There are a number of health service organizations that are on the road to having one total system in which any and all data collected anywhere in the organization are available to everyone.[11]

Some suggest that hospitals, health care systems, and health care service organizations are steering toward integrating disparate systems in their organization in order to speed the flow of data.[12] While few total systems exist now, many "partially total" systems do exist; they are commonly called "database systems." A database system builds one file by drawing pieces from other files. Managers may need financial data from the accounting department, staffing data from the personnel department, and client data from various operating departments. A database system draws the needed data into one file so that the managers can access and interrelate the various data for their decision-assisting purposes.

Of course, a database system might also be called a special purpose system, except that database systems are designed to be contingent and flexible, to respond to ad hoc managerial information needs. And although, as the *Wall Street Journal* notes, the health care industry is becoming increasingly "data driven,"[13] it must be appreciated that database systems, on-line systems, and the rest are merely resources at a manager's disposal to help in the task of information management. Alone, these tools can cause more confusion than clarity.[14] When used to implement the concepts discussed above, they can indeed be an ally of health care professionals.

Notes

1. T. H. Rockers and L. R. Vaughn, "Audit Helps Transform Inefficient Information Systems," *Health Care Financial Management*, June 1989, 127.

2. M. Sherry, "Making Computers the Goat for All Our Woes," *Newsday*, 2 December 1979, 41.

3. J. Johnson, "Information Overload: CEOs Seek New Tools for Effective Decisionmaking," *Hospitals*, 20 October 1991, 24–27.

4. Ibid.

5. Ibid, 24.

6. Ibid, 24.

7. J. Bell and W. Richter, "Needed: Better Communication from Data Processors," *Personnel*, May 1986, 20–26.

8. R. Simpson, "Benchmarking MIS Performance," *Nursing Management*, January 1994, 20–21.

9. S. L. Alter, "How Effective Managers Use Information Systems," *Harvard Business Review*, November–December 1976, 98.

10. T. Binius, "Conference Report: Executive Forum on Information Management," *Healthcare Executive*, September–October 1992, 38–39.

11. *New York Times*, 2 May 1993, F-8.

12. R. Bergman, "Integrated Information Paves the Way to Better Decisionmaking on Patient Care," *Hospitals & Health Networks*, 5 January 1994, 56.

13. *Wall Street Journal*, 8 October 1993, B-11.

14. "Databases Learn to Hop, Skip, and Jump," *The Economist*, 22 February 1986, 76–77.

Selected Readings

Barlow, J. F. "Structuring Informal Information." *Journal of Systems Management* (January 1988): 28–33.

Beaumont, J. R., and C. D. Beaumont. "Applied Management Information Systems." *Futures* (August 1987): 442–45.

Bex, M. "Management Information Systems—Definition and Status." *Computers in Healthcare* (February 1985): 26–30.

Bradbury, A. "Computerized Medical Records: The Need for A Standard." *Journal of the American Medical Records Association* 61 (March 1990): 25–35.

Ducker, J. "Electronic Information—Impact of the Database." *Futures* (April 1985): 164–69.

Holmberg, C. "Evaluation of Mainframe Database Management Systems." *Bulletin of the American Society For Information Science* (October–November 1986): 22–24.

Howell, J. "Merger of Clinical and Financial Databases to Support Strategic Planning and Marketing in an Academic Medical Center: A Case Study." *Topics in Health Record Management* (March 1986): 21–23.

Lemon, R., and J. Crudele. "Systems Integration: Tying It All Together." *Health Care Financial Management* (June 1987): 46–53.

Montrose, G., and K. Marcoux. "Management by Information: A New Imperative." *Computers in Healthcare* (November 1991): 49–54.

Nolan, R., et al. "Ten Principals Transforms I-S Operation into Information Utility." *Data Management* (January 1986): 18–26.

Packer, C. L. "Management Information Systems: Key Tools for CEOs." *Hospitals* (16 November 1984): 107–10.

Pickett, G. C. "DP to MIS: Making the Transition." *Data Management* (December 1986): 46–47.

Porter, M., and V. Millar. "How Information Gives You Competitive Advantage." *Harvard Business Review* (July–August 1985): 149–60.

Raco, R., C. Shapleigh, and D. Cook. "Decision Support in the 1990's: The Future Is Now." *Computers in Healthcare* (December 1989): 26–29.

Riggs, R. "Twelve DP Myths that Just Won't Die." *Computer World* (6 October 1986): 77–83.

Shangraw, R. "How Public Managers Use Information: Examining Choices of Computer and Printed Information." *Public Administration Review* (November 1986): 506–15.

Steinwachs, D. M. "Management Information Systems—New Challenges to Meet Changing Needs." *Medical Care* (May 1985): 607–22.

Vong, J. "Information Systems for Planning and Control." *Management Decision* (Winter 1986): 17–20.

Vitale, M. "The Growing Risks of Information Systems Success." *MIS Quarterly* (December 1986): 327–34.

Wysong, E. M. "MIS in Perspective." *Journal of Systems Management* (October 1985): 32–37.

READING

THE FOUNDATION concepts presented in this chapter are further probed by Sandra Hendren. She applies the database concept to an emerging health information structure that she calls a community health information network. In emphasizing the need to manage information systems toward results, her article provides understanding of how health care information systems might be designed to better meet the market and political demands of the current health care environment.

Community Health Information Management Systems

Sandra J. Hendren

Every time you buy a bag of Frito-Lays corn chips, information regarding your purchase becomes part of a customer database within hours. America's snack food "needs" are analyzed and decisions are made about filling the shelves of every corner convenience store in the nation with exactly the right product. This system has saved the company more than $20 million a year through increased efficiency.

But when you buy a diagnostic test to identify a potentially life-treatening condition, results can remain unavailable for days.

If we can bring computerized efficiencies to marketing corn chips, why aren't we doing it for healthcare?

Imagine—managers of community health systems who know their customers' needs so precisely that they "fill the shelves" of local "convenience health stops" with exactly the right services to maximize the health of the customers. As a by-product, they save a few million dollars per year in costs.

Managers of other industries use information technology to deliver the right product or service to customers at just the right time, to differentiate their services by adding value, to compete effectively on cost and/or quality. Many members of the healthcare industry, where only 2.6 percent of expenditures go to information systems (compared to 5 percent in manufacturing and 7 percent in banking) and where the basic unit of work—the patient record—is still a manual process, are years behind in their thinking about how information systems can make their business better.

The New Organization—The Community Health Network

Healthcare is in a period of consolidation. As market and political demands for integrated systems of healthcare increase, community health networks emerge as effective structures for integrating care. But we have no chance of integrating care delivery without simultaneously integrating information systems.

A quick retrospective of the U.S. healthcare industry in this century is shown in [Figures 2.1–2.3]. The bold line in each figure between consumers and providers shows the delivery of the basic service—healthcare; the lines with a dollar sign ("$") show the flow of money to pay for that service; double lines show the information flow to support the service.

When I display [Figure 2.3] to civic groups and other nonhealthcare professionals who want to understand healthcare costs, the audience

Figure 2.1 Healthcare Industry before the 1940s

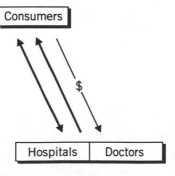

Providers

Figure 2.2 Healthcare Industry, 1940s to 1970s

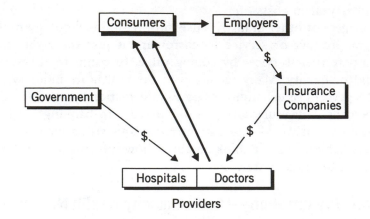

Figure 2.3 Healthcare Industry Developments in 1980s

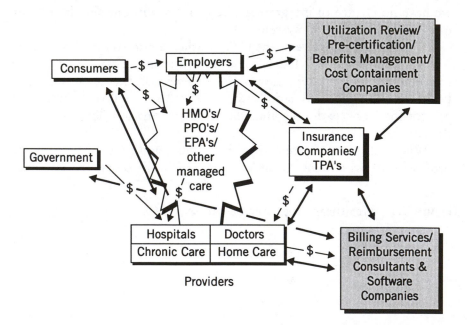

breaks into laughter. The complexity, circularity and untold number of hand-offs in the system show clearly why the market demands change in the way we deliver care.

Figure 2.3 shows a system in which we have lost our way. It no longer provides efficient, effective healthcare, the purpose for which it was intended. It became side-tracked as short-sighted patches and fixes were applied, often addressing the wrong problems. We in healthcare must reexamine the original intent of the system and collaborate to deliver the basic service more efficiently and effectively. This implies dramatically different roles and a blurring of old boundaries.

While such periods of change are painful, they also present rare opportunities for innovation within the industry. And no matter what the final form of our healthcare system, one thing already is clear— integration of the management and delivery of healthcare is critical. As Peter Drucker said: "Building the information-based organization is the management challenge of the future." For healthcare, the future is now, and you—the information systems professional—are in a leadership position, whether or not you want to be.

The Promise of Community Health Information Management Systems

The promise of community health information management systems is that they can drive a new business model for delivering healthcare. But for them to fulfill the promise, we must stop thinking of information systems as a support function and an overhead of doing business, and start thinking of them as a way to leverage our business.

The promise of community management information systems is to put us back in touch with our customers, to learn to micro-market healthcare services like Frito-Lay micro-markets snacks. As a by-product, we also can expect to increase the efficiency and effectiveness of our services, allowing us to compete ethically and appropriately on cost and quality measures.

Having been involved as an information systems management consultant in innumerable projects—to use information systems for strategic or competitive advantage, to reengineer work processes or to measure and monitor total quality management programs—I recognize that one overriding concept permeates all these initiatives: In all successful systems it is the relationships—both formal and informal— that define how well organizations run and how they create value for their customers. Information systems' real benefit, therefore, is to add value to those relationships. No matter if the original business intent of the system was to speed delivery, cut costs, improve quality or provide integration of services, information systems' value resides in their ability to get the right people (not the computers) to talk to each other more efficiently and effectively.

Take this simple premise, apply it to the emergence of community health networks and ask, "What relationships matter and how can technology most effectively enhance them? The answer, combined with the need to deliver high quality, lowest possible cost healthcare, is the promise of community health management information systems.

This approach may seem overly simplistic for information systems professionals who design complex systems for complex business needs. But I contend that we have been looking through the wrong end of the binoculars in such efforts and use our information systems to support activities that remove us farther and farther from the real purpose of our business—to add value to our service for our customers. The result is our contribution to [Figure 2.3] (shown by the double lines— information passing), where often we have automated bad practices. And we will continue to do so as long as each of the separate players continue to think and act independently. The promise of community health management information systems is that by nature of defining the information flows, we help define the effectiveness and the efficiency of the business.

This approach leads to [Figure 2.4], which shows a process analysis of the major business activities of a community health network. Unlike the previous diagrams, which showed a functional approach to our business, the process approach allows the design of an integrated, value-added model of the business.

Figure 2.4 Community Health Networks

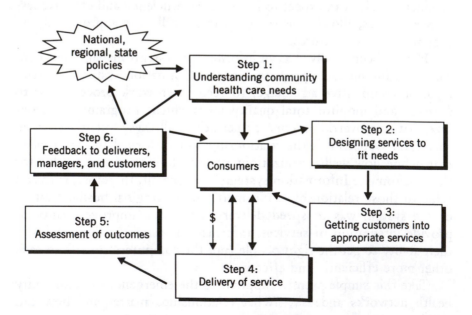

There are inherent advantages to this model. Foremost, information flow and the flow of actions to deliver the product of the organization match. In healthy organizations, in systems that are effective and efficient, these flows match. Second, this model implies a major restructuring/consolidation of the functions of providers, employers, insurers and government. Indeed, they can no longer be identified—they are no longer divided into camps of checks and balances in a system of unclear tasks, diffuse decision-making and high uncertainty. Where each of the players fit into this diagram remains to be determined. Some functions and roles may be dissolved or merged into others; all will likely change. In our current healthcare system, where there is a public and political consensus that we are delivering too little service at too high a cost, no room exists for functions that add no value to the basic service—the delivery of healthcare.

An examination of the core competencies of each of the existing players in the healthcare system points to strengths that, when joined in a collaborative fashion, could assist in the transition from [Figure 2.3 to Figure 2.4]. Historically, insurers have used the most sophisticated information systems; managed care groups and insurers have been the best marketers; providers have clinical data, the most important information in the system; the intermediaries have played the role of changing data into information and handling/reporting it for their clients. The following six steps could help combine the core competencies of all the players into an efficient community health information management network.

Step 1: Understanding Community Healthcare Needs

The healthcare industry has been terribly unsophisticated in systematically understanding community healthcare needs and designing services to meet them. For years, we paid no attention to community needs and continued to create general purpose, "me-too" healthcare delivery systems as if it were a field of dreams—"If we build it they will come." More recently, with the idea of healthcare being a competitive industry, we jumped directly to a model of corporate marketing with the glossy-ads-and-catchy-jingles approach to penetrating a market, instead of understanding it. I am talking about a completely different approach than either of these, using commonly accepted, low cost techniques of ascertaining customers' healthcare needs and feeding that data into a customer database.

A variety of techniques could be used to accomplish this, including pre-registrations to the system through health fairs and supermarket and shopping mall booths where health questionnaires can be administered. While Americans seem tired of the use of such marketing techniques for a new cereal or laundry detergent, I think there would be an overwhelmingly positive response to this approach when asked about their healthcare needs. These data would begin to feed a customer database.

Step 2: Designing Services to Fit Needs

Then the database would be analyzed to construct community and individual health profiles and design specific services for each community, just as Frito-Lay does with snack foods. The services could be more comprehensive than our old diagnose-and-treat model of healthcare. The need to "predict and manage" health expands one's thinking to a host of educational and special purpose programs given in a variety of formats—classes, interactive videos, ask-a-nurse phone lines, chronic pain clinics, self-directed physical therapy and physical fitness for the elderly.

Step 3: Getting Customers into Appropriate Service

The community health network's managers could use the customer database to select customers with specific needs and mail personal invitations to them for specific programs. Another approach is to take the service to where the individuals congregate, the equivalent to Frito-Lay putting the right snack food on the right shelf of every convenience store. For healthcare, such locations might be homes for the elderly, waiting areas for commuter trains or facilities adjacent to sports medicine clinics. As it becomes richer with data collected over time, the customer database provides greater capabilities to micro-market services.

Step 4: Delivery of Service

There is extensive literature and hundreds of software vendors who concentrate on this aspect of healthcare information systems. In addition, much effort now is being devoted to creating the computer-based patient record. As these system evolve, they must be easy to integrate with the community health network's customer database in order to provide the continuum of information that is the crux of the network. Point-of-service information systems, when integrated with information from the customer database, make it possible to consistently deliver personalized, customized service.

Step 5: Assessment of Outcome

Work has begun in earnest on this aspect of the healthcare system within the last couple years. Functional assessments of clinical and service outcomes, both immediately following each delivery of service and over time, will clearly identify the community health network's strengths and areas for improvement. New, clearer measures of efficiency and effectiveness based on comparisons to the initial individual and community health profiles, will become possible.

Step 6: Feedback to Deliverers, Managers and Customers

Information from the assessment of outcomes feeds back into the first step, adding data to the customer database to refine and update the understanding of community health needs as well as to provide to state, regional, and nation health policy decision makers information on the efficiency, and effectiveness of systems' delivery of care. One day potential customers may be able to access such information from public kiosks, for example, for their own evaluation of cost and outcomes information.

The Technology Platform

The technology platform for this model of community health networks calls for a three-tiered model—a transaction-oriented, high-performance database with a search-and-query front end, an analytic engine with a relational or multidimensional relational database for decision support and a suite of desktop office automation tools with interfaces to the decision support database—with a communications backbone connecting all sites involved in the service.

The transaction-oriented database with an easy-to-use, intuitive user interface is needed for Step 4, the delivery of the service. This is where information systems professionals typically have the most knowledge and experience and where most software vendor activity occurs. Steps 3 and 6, getting customers into services and feedback about the results, can be supported by basic office automation tools as long as there is a reliable way for them to access the data from the other systems. The first two and last two steps—understanding needs, designing services to fit needs, assessment of outcomes, and feedback of results—demand an analytic engine running off of a decision support database, either relational or multidimensional, depending upon various issues such as size of the database and number of users.

Too often I have seen information systems professionals try to get by on a single-tiered platform, using transition-oriented databases with a search-and-query front end (usually SQL-based) for their analysis needs. This cripples their analytic and reporting capability, which is needed on the front end and back end of the business, and leads to the "technology trap," where the platform defines and limits the business instead of the business defining the platform. The decision support tier is necessary for administrative and management reports and "what-if" analyses. It is tuned for number-crunching and provides flexible views of data. The proficiency of this tier defines the predict-and-manage capabilities of the entire organization.

The information, and therefore the technology platform, should be a distributed architecture with a communications network tying the deliverers, managers and customers together. The network minimally includes e-mail and/or automated fax capabilities, possibly with voice and image transmission. It can be a real-time or a store-and-forward model, or a combination of both, depending on specific needs.

The Charge for Information Systems Professionals

For years now I have heard healthcare information systems professionals talk about what they cannot do because there are still no standards and because no consensus has been reached on patient identification numbers. I believe that these are issues that need to be resolved, but they are not show-stoppers. I have developed many systems over the years, without resolution of such technical details. That meant that we had to create smart, data-driven designs to minimize the pain of future changes; it meant we sometimes had to do tedious crosswalks from old codes to new codes; occasionally, we had to delay adding functionality to a system. But other industries have rejected such technical issues as justification for failing to get on with business!

Neither have other industries been so dependent upon software vendors to fulfill their needs with standardized products; their programmers develop customized systems. In today's world with the wide selection of database management systems on the market, robust fourth-generation application development languages and proven rapid-development techniques that enable small programming teams to achieve 3-to-6-month development cycles, there's no reason for you not to do the same thing.

Comparing my experience both in healthcare and in other industries, I would proffer the following advice—if you don't stop asking, "How do you want this report to look?" and start saying, "This is how we could deliver the business better," soon you will have no job. Neither will anyone around you. Your entire organization will be gone. In the current economic and political climate, where the number one national topic is that healthcare costs too much and delivers too little, only organizations that address problems appropriately and rapidly will survive. In 1993, in an information-intensive business like healthcare, all solutions are information systems-dependent. Laggards will be road kill.

To avoid such a fate, get started with the steps outlined here:

1. Be an active participant in creating the business vision for community health networks and operate from the perspective of using information systems to add value to the business relationships.
2. Establish a three-tiered, open systems technology platform and get a communications infrastructure in place.
3. Put together a portfolio of applications that combines customized and purchased systems to best meet your needs.

If you follow these steps, interesting things will happen. You will find that your paradigm has shifted; you will exhibit system thinking; you will become a member of a learning organization; you will practice total quality management; and you will link the business plan to the information systems plan. By adopting a process view of your business and designing the system from the perspective of adding value to the customer, you will have reengineered the system for more efficiency and effectiveness. All the things the current literature tells you to do, you will have done.

So turn those binoculars around and look through them the right way! Get it straight what information systems are all about—adding value to the relationships that make up your business.

Sandra J. Hendren is Founder and President of Healthcare Management Systems Inc., Boston. An information systems professional with 20 years experience, she has developed customized decision support, executive support, sales and marketing, and customer service systems for the insurance, pharmaceutical, banking, shipping and healthcare industries.

CASE 2
HomeCare, Inc.

RUTH CONTINUED to stare at the computer printout on her desk, as she had for the last fifteen minutes, and then placed it with the rest of the printouts she had received since the implementation of the new data processing system. She euphemistically called the file cabinet where she placed these printouts "computer heaven," because she assumed God only knew what the numbers on the printout really meant.

Ruth Anthony, executive director of HomeCare, Inc., a nonprofit home health care organization, had no doubt that the recently installed data processing systems would be a boon to her organization, and well worth the investment. She observed how other home health agencies had begun the inexorable move towards computerization and welcomed the new technology. Her organization had grown dramatically in the past five years, a reflection of the current state of health care delivery. Many families were choosing home care as an alternative to institutionalizing their relatives, hospitals were utilizing the home care model more frequently, and third-party payers were increasingly recognizing the cost-effectiveness of noninstitutionalization.

Recognizing the obvious connection between automated data processing and simplicity and efficiency, Ruth was determined that HomeCare, Inc. would lead the way in the booming home health care business.

A memo to the board on her intentions to fully automate carefully outlined the major data processing systems and their applications. The

Table 2.1   HomeCare, Inc. Data Processing Systems and Applications within Each System

Financial Management	Payroll
	General Ledger
	Patient Billing
	Accounts Receivable
	Accounts Payable
	Materials Management
Patient Care	Clients
	Medical Records
	Nursing Care Plans
	Medication Orders
	Physician Orders
Strategic Planning	Marketing
	Word Processing
	Decision-Making
	Forecasting and Modeling
	Budgeting

chart that accompanied the memo helped to clarify how each of the systems would be used to support the specific applications or types of activities.

Not only were applications of this in-house computer system extensive, but they were integrated. Ruth recalled her visits to other home health care agencies and noted that those agencies that were computerized had only single-application systems that focused on specific areas of activity, such as accounts receivable or patient records. This new system not only had the capacity to retrieve and process increased flows of data, but had the advantage of giving concurrent information from the different data processing subsystems so as to increase decision-making capabilities (e.g., budgeting data could be used in conjunction with long-range planning). Originally envisioning a system that could support and respond to a view from the "mountain top," in order to understand the organization and make decisions, Ruth soon found that computer errors, computer jargon, and meaningless "information" generated by the system had forced her to rethink this vision.

Trouble in Paradise

"Computerese", the high-tech vocabulary associated with computer technology gave Ruth ambivalent feelings. On one hand, the jargon gave validity to the notion that it was the language of the future. In fact, the lingo had slipped into everyday usage. Words like "interfacing," "on-line," "real-time," and "software" were used pervasively. On the other hand, Ruth was not completely comfortable with all the words the computer technicians so deftly threw at her during the preimplementation phase. At times she would shake her head, half pretending to understand everything they were saying, knowing that she would eventually have a clear understanding as she acquired experience with the technology.

For their part the computer professionals saw their job as bridging the knowledge gap between what the technology could do and what the organization needed. The three half-day sessions that Ruth and her staff attended seemed adequate. Although they thought the interchange of information was sufficient, Ruth seemed to think that the language the data processing professionals used was awkward. Recalling a conversation with one fellow, she cringed when the answer to one of her questions was: "The syntax of the current set of permanent control commands is unaffected by the change, but new commands have been added. The new READ, SAVE, KILL, and LIST commands are the counterparts of READPF, SAVEPF, KILLPF, but they do not accept the PF set of IDs or password. . . ." Ruth wondered why these "techies" couldn't speak in everyday language. Why must they use these arcane words?

These questions became especially poignant one day when Ruth's assistant, Joan, came storming out of her office after the system was installed. Apparently, Joan had been having a heated discussion with one of the data processing professionals who had come to "get the bugs out of the system." Joan, director of finance, had been attempting for the past week to clear up billing errors that occurred after the installation of the system. Some clients were overbilled, others were given credit when they shouldn't have been, and still others were inadvertently sent "lawyer" letters for failure to pay. When Ruth cornered Joan at the coffee machine and asked her if she was having a "nice day," she was barraged with a not altogether unexpected rant:

> I'm sick and tired of listening to that guy. He makes me feel like an old, uneducated fuddy-duddy, flying by the seat of my pants and standing in the way of progress. I ask him a question and all I get from him is: "Work with the system . . . it will do what you want it to. . . ." I've tried time and time again. The result is that my receivables are all messed up, clients are calling me the wicked witch of the west, I can't identify the problem accounts, and I'm sure the account ledgers and trial balance for this month are way off. I'm also receiving word that there are mistakes in payroll this week, so I

examined the payroll printouts and I'm not sure whether they're completely accurate. There are so many numbers and abbreviations on that printout. . . .

Soon after that encounter, Scott Howell, the data processor, knocked on Ruth's door.

> Joan's people blame the computer system for their mistakes. Apparently the inputs to the system were in error or missing and naturally the output was wrong. Now she's behind schedule and she blames the system. She keeps going back to the manual system to check the input and I keep telling her that if she continues to do that, we'll never get this off the ground. I told her that during the shakedown period we would work together to get the kind of information she wants. She thinks she has to adapt to the computer, when in reality we can design output to fulfill her needs. I've continued to give her suggestions on what she might need. In fact, she has the opportunity to use a huge volume of output that can accelerate her decision making. She can control and use the form, content, and volume of the information.

Ruth listened intently and thought twice about asking Scott to again explain the data on the printouts in her file cabinet. Instead, she switched on the baseball game and heard the announcer screaming " . . . this has been the second home run this inning. Last time at bat the Yankees' designated hitter sacrificed by hitting a Texas leaguer to the right-fielder. His RBIs for this season has matched last year's output, but since his rotator cuff injury in spring training (when he was picked off in a double-play in an extra-inning game), he has been ice-cold at the plate. . . ."

Ruth wished she were at Yankee Stadium enjoying the game.

Questions for Discussion

1. What assumptions have Ruth, Joan, and Scott made concerning the nature of data and information?
2. What communication dynamics exist between users and the data processing professionals? How are they manifested in the case?
3. How important is it for Ruth and Joan to understand the capabilities and potential of the system? How important is it for them to communicate to the staff the capabilities and potential of the system?
4. Identify the factors that necessitate MIS replacement. Discuss issues of feasibility and justifiability.

UNDERSTANDING COMPUTER TECHNOLOGY

HOW WOULD you draw a computer? In workshops for managers we frequently ask participants this question and direct them to sketch what hardware and software look like. Inevitably, the hardware drawings turn out as either plain boxes, keyboards, squares with tape reels on them, or terminals with screens. The software sketches usually pose more of a challenge, but typically result in depictions of diskettes or printouts. The exercise often suggests that many of us have little understanding of what a computer really is and how it works. This chapter provides a basic understanding of computer technology. It explains how the "black box" works and dispels the "magic" that technicians have a tendency to hide behind.

Evolution of the Technology

Given the pervasiveness of computerization today, it is somewhat astonishing to remember that the first actual electronic computer came on the scene only in 1951. Since then, the organizational use of computers has become so prevalent that it is a significant component of management in all organizations, including health care enterprises. Today there are thousands of major computer systems in the United States and innumerable "micro-" computers in use. Some observers note that personal computers (PCs) are "spreading in hospitals like a virus." The features that have made PCs popular in other industries—user friendliness and more computer power for the dollar—are some of the contributing factors behind the explosive growth in health care.[1]

For health care today, the major impetus behind this growth in computerization appears to be the pressure from government and payers to control costs. As one expert points out regarding the current state of health care technology, "External pressures are causing internal concerns that only (computerized) information systems can begin to address."[2]

The enormous increase in computer usage is matched by an enormous decrease in the cost of computing. The figures change rapidly, but it is safe to say that computer processing costs today are more than a thousand times lower than they were in the 1950s. As one expert puts it: "If automobile costs and technological improvements had changes at a rate comparable with computer hardware over the last 15 years, you would now be able to buy a self-steering car for $20 that could attain speeds up to 500 mph and could travel the entire length of California on one gallon of gas."[3] Depending on to whom you talk—consultants, vendor sales representatives, or software company CEOs—prices for health care information systems will increase modestly, grow rapidly, stabilize, or even drop in years to come. Although most agree that prices will increase over the short term, estimates on the size of the increase—and causes behind it—vary. Health care executives, according to Management Science America (MSA), see a need for new applications and rank pricing as less important than functionality and flexibility.[4] In a recent survey looking at information systems trends conducted for *Modern Healthcare*, data from a sample of 688 hospitals indicated that the primary rationale in buying decisions is moving away from the traditional preoccupation with price to "open architecture" considerations, i.e., whether a computer system can mesh with that of other vendors and whether the system can integrate future technological innovation.[5] This attention toward protecting the computer investment against early obsolescence has rapidly surpassed the price issue in this time of steady technological advancement.

Several aspects of the evolution of computer technology are remarkable. Singling them out can help clarify the unusual nature of the evolution and help explain why our experience with computers has been so arduous.

Physical Aspects

The physical size, speed, and capacity of computers have evolved dramatically. The early large computers are now equated with small hand-held calculators. Today, small computers can contain billions of circuits. So thorough has been the process of miniaturization that over the last

25 years the size of a computer with the same capability has been halved, on the average, every year.

The physical speed of computers has evolved to the point that new words are needed to describe the phenomenon. Early computers were measured in milliseconds (thousandths of a second); by 1960, it was microseconds (millionths of a second); in the 1970s it was nanoseconds (billionths of a second); today it is picoseconds (trillionths of a second). This kind of speed defies comprehension. For example, it would take 30 years of seconds to equal the number of nanoseconds that there are in one second.

In terms of storage capacity, suffice it to say that a computer that could store 20,000 characters in the 1950s can today store millions of characters. This kind of spectacular progress has resulted from developments in electronic physics. The early computers, like early televisions, used vacuum tubes that required a good deal of space. In the late 1950s, transistors were developed, which significantly reduced space requirements. In the late 1960s, physicists and engineers developed "chips," sometimes called "microprocessors," which miniaturized transistor circuitry through a process called large-scale integration (LSI). Significant advances have been made in storage capacities for the internal chip memory of the computer and the amount of storage for data and files. Recent announcements of the availability of a one-million-byte memory on a dime-size computer chip is evidence of the increase in computer power. In many computer workstations today, we find an increased prevalence of the RISC chip (reduced instruction set computing). The RISC chip is a type of microprocessor that makes for faster, more powerful, cheaper computers. Many vendors and users estimate that for the same price, RISC-based systems offer four to ten times the processing power of traditional computers.[6] And as with computer chips generally, prices continue to fall even as the power and sophistication increase.[7] With this kind of technology, a health care professional can store up to hundreds of millions of bytes of information in a desk-sized microcomputer.[8]

Indeed, for practical purposes the old concepts of time and space are nearly inapplicable today. Computers are now so fast and so small that few physical limitations exist.

Time Aspects

The time aspects of the evolution, in turn, requires a new jargon. For example, the term "generation" was given new meaning by the computer. While a generation of people is usually 25 years, a new generation of computers has appeared every five years or less. Thus, the same group of computer users has experienced six generations of computers.

This is significant, especially when contrasted with the evolution of organizations and of pre-computer information technology. Modern organizational structures and techniques originated in the late nineteenth century, about the same time that the typewriter and other pre-computer information processing tools were introduced. While information processing tools remained basically the same, organizations matured through the insights of Taylorism and the "human relations" work of Follet, Mayo, and others. By the time computers were introduced, organizations were matured and "set in their ways," one of which was information processing based on pre-computer, manual technologies.

Industrial Aspects

Some unusual phenomena in the computer industry have further complicated the evolution of computer technology. Remarkably, the first computer company to produce a working machine for both business and government—Remington-Rand—did not become the leader in the field. IBM not only took hold, but became a giant, dominating the industry with, at one point, more than 80 percent of the market. This market domination severely limited purchasing options for consumers. Additionally, the industry has experienced considerable instability due to high technological and research costs. Three major computer producers—RCA, GE, and Xerox SDS—dropped out of the market. These occurrences further complicated the efforts of organizations trying to harness the computer because of the subsequent confusion caused by the re-alignment of the industry.

People Aspects

Personnel realities are another complicating factor in computer evolution. A *Dun's Review* comment on the private sector experience is equally applicable to health care organizations: "In many ways the rapidity of the computer revolution has left a 'computer gap' between those who manage most of our businesses today and the people who run data processing departments—a gap that is not the fault of anyone, but rather was caused solely by historical circumstance."[9]

Computer specialists, with their specialized jargon, focused on technical aspects and frequently were ignorant of organizational goals and needs. They have dominated the evolution of computers in organizations. Kitta MacPherson, a noted writer on science and technology, offers some sage advice to these computer experts, who speak in a strange language known as "mystical mumbo-jumbo":

> Just as a patient should not tolerate medical gibberish from a doctor who is attempting to explain an illness or course of treatment, consumers of computer equipment should also demand clear statements.... When communicating with the outside world, lose the techno-jargon ... it intimidates and confuses and, frankly, promotes resentment.[10]

Thus, managers are often distrustful and disillusioned. They have also been slow to gain a basic understanding of the nature of computers and the rudimentary jargon associated with them. On the other hand, with the proliferation of the PC we have now seen a move of computer resources from the technician's basement to the manager's desk.

The Nature of the Technology

Most of us commonly use two high technology items today—the telephone and the automobile. What do we need to know to control and use these machines well? To use a telephone we need to know what a dial tone is, which end of the phone to speak into, how to read a touch-tone pad, and so forth—things we take for granted, but that are actually technical aspects of telephone technology that a user must know. To manage the use of our phone we need to understand long-distance service options, how to use an area code, how to get a conference call, and other such phone technology concepts. Similarly, to use a car effectively we do not need to understand principles of internal combustion, hydraulics, and electricity, but we do need to be able to read a fuel gauge, know where the brake pedal is, and, on a manual transmission, understand the relationship between a clutch and shift lever.

The same kinds of requisites apply to the effective use of computers. Health care professionals do not need to know and understand the principles of electronics or computer programming in order to use and control a computer effectively. However, they must know and understand basic computer jargon and concepts—the equivalents of dial tone, brake pedal, area code, and miles per hour. As one observer puts it, computer literacy for health care managers is simply "understanding the capabilities and potential of computer systems."[11] This includes knowing how to make a system respond to organizational needs and opportunities, knowing what a computer can do, and being able to communicate what you want it to do. It requires a basic, not a technical, knowledge of computer technology.[12]

Computers can be understood, described, and conceptualized in several ways. First, a computer can be accurately viewed as a system. Like all systems, a computer consists of input, process, and output. Something is put in, something is done with what goes in, and, as a result, something comes out. In the system that is a computer, this process is controlled by established procedures, or instructions, and uses records or files.

Second, a computer can be correctly perceived as a package of components. That package consists of five basic components: (1) input, (2) processing, (3) storage, (4) instructional, and (5) output. Every computer has these components, even a small hand-held one, although in that type the components are all in one casing so that it seems like a single component. On hand-held computers the input component may consist of numbered buttons that are pushed or a handwriting pad and stylus (as in some Personal Digital Assistants). The processing component is a small chip inside the casing, the storage component is also a chip either inside the casing or inserted through a slot, the output component is the clear screen on which the numbers or letters appear, and the instructional component is material stored on the chips. On large computers, these components are physically separate devices that are described below.

Third, a computer can be understood as a set of operations or capacities. This is similar to a stereo music system, which has the capacity to convert electronic signals into sound signals and to modulate them. As a result of these capacities or operations the music system can "magically" provide all sorts of music in soft or loud tones and send it instantly to any number of speakers. Similarly, a computer has only two fundamental capacities—it can perform mathematical calculations and it can perform logical functions based upon comparisons. That is all a computer can do. However, because it can do these things so fast (at the speed of light) and in such volume, it can produce sophisticated reports as if by magic. Programming uses these basic capacities and, therefore, must reduce instructions to a series of comparisons and calculations.

Fourth, a computer can be understood in terms of physical definition. In essence, a computer is an electronic computational device that is controlled by a program, is utilized through electromechanical input devices, and displays results through electromechanical output devices. Its computations are "electronic" in that it employs no moving parts, and therefore can function at the speed of light. However, its input and output devices are "electromechanical," using moving parts along with electric signals and, therefore, are subject to the much slower speeds owing to friction. The keys on a keyboard, for example, are mechanical—they must be moved to produce the electronic impulses. A printer can receive output at the speed of light, but can print it only as fast as the printing device can move. While laser printers are not constrained with the kind of speed limitations common to mechanical printers, they still have speed limitations. Computers are slowed down considerably because of the mechanical aspects of their input and output devices.

What are these devices? Explanation of them clarifies the meaning of some common computer jargon with which all health care professionals should be familiar. There are two basic types of computer devices: hardware and software.

Hardware

Hardware is any and all of the visible, touchable, physical items or devices that are associated with a computer. There are several kinds of hardware:

Input Devices

Input devices are machines used for entering the computer system. Perhaps the most commonly recognized input device today is the keyboard part of a terminal, the component that resembles a typewriter. Other pieces of hardware that are input devices are tape drives and disk drives, onto which tapes and disks are loaded; optical scanners, which "read" penciled forms or, in supermarkets today, cans and boxes with a coded label attached, and mouses. Other examples are hand-held personal digital assistants (PDAs) that convert handwriting to typed messages, as well as audio or voice input devices that are now emerging.

Output Devices

Output devices are machines used to display results of a processed input. A line printer is an output device that produces an organization's computer printouts. Some line printers are relatively slow because they use an impression ball similar to that of a typewriter. Such devices can produce output ranging from several hundred to over a thousand lines per minute. Extremely high-speed line printers reduce reliance on moving parts by using a laser beam that can produce printed material at as many as 20,000 lines per minute. Even this technique, however, relies on a mechanically moving laser, and is thus much slower than the electronic computer's processor component, which will be described below.

A second major kind of output device is the cathode ray tube (CRT), which is similar to a television screen. Often encased with an input device (the keyboard), a CRT terminal is sometimes referred to as an I/O (input/output) device because it seems to be one machine. Actually, the keyboard and the screen are two separate items.

A third kind of output device, called a data plotter, is similar to the tracing mechanism of an electrocardiogram. Instead of producing output in letters and numbers, it draws the result on paper. These output devices normally are used for specialized purposes like map making. However, computer graphics using CRTs is a rapidly developing aspect of computer systems. The Washington state legislature, for example, has employed a system for several years that responds to "what-if" inquiries with drawings on a CRT. A legislator's request for information on what would happen to the state budget if a certain bill were passed is answered with a pie diagram.

Audio or voice output devices are also available, but are very limited in use. Phone companies are using them to have a recording tell us how much money to deposit for the call we just placed.

Processing Devices

Processing devices are machines that actually conduct the procedure requested. These are called central processing units or, simply, CPUs, and form "the computer" part of computers. There is one stored on a silicon chip inside the casing of your hand-held calculator, just as there is one or more in the computer center of large organizations. The brain of a computer system, a CPU performs the logic function that produces the output, whether that be retrieving a desired file or conducting a complex calculation.

CPUs come in different sizes. The term "mainframe" has traditionally been used to refer to a large computer system with a large CPU, i.e., one capable of dealing with very large amounts of data. Advances in technology, however, have led to the introduction of a new line of mainframe computers that utilize the same chips used in PCs. A minicomputer is a smaller, more limited CPU (and, of course, is less expensive), and a microcomputer is the smallest variety, associated with the desktop PCs so commonly available today. Describing computers using these classifications is fast becoming dated, however. Technological advances in speed and size are making the distinctions formerly attributed to mainframe, minicomputers, and microcomputers blurred.

Size can be measured in weight or in cost. For example, microcomputers usually weigh less than 50 pounds, while mainframes can weigh hundreds. Minicomputers are typically priced between $2,500 and $25,000, while many stand-alone microcomputers are priced under $1,000. More accurately, size is measured in capacity, and the capacity of a CPU is expressed in kilobytes (k) or megabytes (mb) of data it can handle. Miniaturization is enabling more and more capacity to be available in smaller and smaller packages. The larger the capacity (the greater the kilobytes or megabytes), the more procedures a computer can perform. A 200mb computer, for example, is more powerful than a 60mb computer. The power, or processing speed, is usually measured in megahertz or mips (millions of instructions per second). The more megahertz (or mips), the faster (or more powerful) the computer is.

To better understand how a computer works, you should visit a computer center and ask a technician to remove the cover or casing from the CPU. You will then be able to see that a CPU consists of microcircuitry. Removing the casing from your hand-held calculator will reveal the same scene on a smaller scale. Technically, the circuits are usually made of silicon "miracle chips" or "magnetic bubbles." Conceptually, the circuitry is like a mass of tiny light bulbs grouped together. As you know, a light bulb can be in only one of two possible states—it can be on or it can be off. In computer jargon this condition of having only two possible states is called "binary coding," which, following the binary numbering system, uses only the digits 0 and 1. Data are stored in the CPU as a series of "bits" (binary digits) that are either "on" or "off," which is represented by "1" for "on" or "0" for "off." The computer's electronics determines whether the bits are on or off; it is this ability that allows the CPU to store and process data.

These bits are grouped to represent alphanumeric characters and other special characters and symbols. A group of bits is called a byte. There are many ways of grouping bits; one of the most commonly used is the coding scheme called EBCDIC (extended binary coded decimal interchange code), which uses a group of eight bits to make a byte. For example, the grouping, or byte, 11000001 represents the letter "A", and the byte 11110001 represents the number "1". Thus, it usually requires several bytes to form a word. The number of bits a CPU can hold determines its capacity, which is measured in kilos (thousands) or megas (millions). If a desired calculation requires that hundreds of words and numbers be handled simultaneously, the CPU must have the capacity (kilos of bits) to do this.

Finally, the CPU is further organized into three sections: a control section, a logic section, and an internal storage section that is called memory. The control section is used to direct and coordinate the workings of the computer. It controls the input and output devices so that, for example, they are coordinated.

The logic section is used to actually conduct the calculations or procedures desired. The memory stores the instructions or program being run and the data needed for the run. What is not stored in the "main" memory or "core" of the CPU is stored on secondary storage devices for access when needed.

Secondary Storage Devices

Secondary storage devices are items used to hold data outside of the CPU. To carry out a process, a CPU needs in its memory the instructions and relevant data only at the exact instant at which the process is being executed. The instructions and data can then be stored until they are to be used again. Instead of storing them in the expensive "main" memory of the CPU, however, they are stored on inexpensive secondary storage devices that can be linked to the CPU when needed. The most common of these storage devices are diskettes (floppy disks), tapes, and optical disks. When a disk is put on a disk drive connected to the CPU, the material stored on that disk is available to the CPU's memory; that is to say, it is on-line. This increase gives the CPU a "virtual memory" capacity much greater than its internal memory alone. Another form of storage, known as "cache" storage, also provides secondary access. An amount of internal "main" memory is set aside to hold data that is expected to be accessed again. This second access, which finds the data in the main memory, is very fast.

Note, then, that while the data on the diskettes, tapes and optical disks are not hardware, the diskettes, tapes, and optical disks themselves are hardware. Note also the difference in retrieving data stored on a disk as opposed to a tape. The CPU can work at the speed of light, but a tape must physically move to the part containing the needed data, and the "needle," called a read/write head, of a disk must move to the appropriate groove of the disk.

Which storage device is faster? Tapes employ sequential storage, which means that the entire tape must be wound to the section in which the desired data is located. Diskettes, too, can use sequential storage, but they can also employ direct access storage that allows data to be retrieved "randomly," without reading through all the other data preceding it on that disk (just as you can move the stereo needle to the part of the record containing your favorite song). Optical disks, using laser-driven optical technology, employ direct access storage. For some purposes in hospitals and health agencies, speed is essential, and is worth the extra cost of direct access storage; for other functions, sequential storage, less expensive but slower, is adequate.

Peripherals

Peripherals are other hardware devices that can be used in a computer system. They include card sorters, keypunch machines, and communications equipment, and are called auxiliaries or peripherals, although the latter term is sometimes used to mean everything other than the CPU. Most important in this category of hardware is the modem, which connects individual terminals to a central processing unit through phone lines, and which is needed for on-line systems and networks that are not "hard-wired". In a hard-wired network, on-line terminals (sometimes called "dumb terminals") are connected by a direct line to a central processing unit or central computer. In many other networks, however, the terminals are connected to the CPU by telephone lines. In these cases, input from the terminal is converted by a modem from an electronic signal into an audio signal that is transmitted then "demodulated" back into the original electronic signal that the CPU can process. While most networked on-line systems are connected by a direct line or through a modem, wireless networks are attracting a great deal of interest. A system called Wavelan, developed by NCR, connects computers by wireless technology through spread spectrum radio transmission. This system allows users to share files, programs, electronic mail, laser printers, and other common computer resources.[13]

Software

If you ask a technician to show you software (or a "program"), or, if you buy a software package, you are likely to be given a disk and documentation for the software package. However, strictly speaking, software is invisible. Software (or programs) are the instructions to the hardware about what to do—a set of electronic impulses, organized in a precise way, that activate a computer process. Programming, or software development, is the process of generating the desired impulses, and it is in programming that the visible items, which many of us associate with software, are employed.

The development of software begins with mental identification of a need for information. This information is transformed through programming into the appropriate electronic impulses. The process usually includes a written outline and a flow chart, which graphically depicts what will happen. Typically, this is followed by manually written code forms in which the instruction is expressed in an appropriate computer language; these instructions are then keyed onto disks or tapes, which are placed on the appropriate input device. Finally, the instructions are converted into electronic impulses. This process is tedious and complex because the instruction desired must be reduced to bits and to functions of calculation and comparison for use by the computer. When an organization buys a software package it is buying the final step in the process, the physical devices on which the instructions are stored. Documentation of the previous steps is needed to understand the organization of those impulses when, for example, a change in the program is desired. There are several kinds of software.

Translation Programs

Translation programs are software that converts, or translates, the language of the programmer into machine language, that is, into binary codes. These special programs significantly ease the task of programming because they save the programmer from having to manually convert letter and number into binary codes, an incredibly long and tedious task.

There are two basic kinds of translation programs: assemblers and compilers. Assemblers translate symbols into machine language and are usually used today for technical purposes involving the operation of a computer. Compilers translate "high-level" languages (those that people can easily use) into machine language. Computer languages such as FORTRAN, COBOL, BASIC, and RPG are examples of such high-level languages. Each requires a compiler in order to be used on a computer. Compilers are also being developed that permit instructions to be given by spoken word, that is, that translate vocal sounds into machine language.

Application Programs

Application programs are software that harness the computer for applied tasks. Application programs are the key link between a user's needs and the power of computer technology. They are the instructions to the computer to provide specified output or to complete certain tasks, such as payroll and laboratory analyses. Programmers write application software, but packaged or canned programs are generally purchased. These packages are typically for common applications, such as administrative (e.g., collecting, storing, and manipulating financial data), clinical (e.g., medical record storage/retrieval and clinical decision making), and management support programs (e.g., inventory and strategic planning).[14]

There is also public domain software—programs developed primarily by government funds that are available to the public. One premier example of this is COSTAR (Computer Stored Ambulatory Record

System), a public domain system developed by the government for about $10 million over a ten-year period. This system handles ambulatory record maintenance, patient appointment scheduling, accounts receivable, and medical and management reporting.[15] In addition, there is increasing mutual sharing of application programs in the hospital industry. For example, Brockton Hospital solved a serious management problem by borrowing an inventory application program from Mother Frances Hospital in Texas.[16] The trend toward managing physician practice patterns is driving the adoption of "expert systems," as part of health care computing.[17] As the name implies, expert systems incorporate the experience of experts in certain areas and offers it as a guide to the system's user. If a physician orders a certain drug or therapy, an expert system might check to see whether the order is an accepted treatment for the patient's condition.

Despite these developments, there remains a "software support gap" of considerable dimensions. Developments in hardware have far surpassed application software developments. As a result, the full power of hardware is not being utilized, and many organizations have hardware capability that far exceeds their software resources.

Control System Programs

Control system programs are software, usually provided with hardware, that direct the operation of the computer system. Also known as operating system (OS) programs, these software packages use the control section of the CPU to regulate and coordinate the various devices in the computer system and to perform various "housekeeping" functions. If, for example, a CPU has ten terminals connected to it, the control system recognizes and coordinates each one. Most control systems provide for capabilities like multiprogramming, which permits the CPU to run several application programs at the same time.

Special kinds of control programs, called probes or monitors, are available; they monitor the efficiency of hardware utilization and of program construction. These software packages, which are becoming fairly sophisticated, can be useful in evaluating the management of the computer system per se.

Recent technological advances in computer communication have led to increasing application of LAN (local area network) technology. Using a LAN architecture allows communication between computers of different vendors with different communication protocols and operating systems. The LAN at Vancouver General Hospital, for example, allows micro-to-mainframe communication between 15 major computer systems which support over 400 terminals and 50 microcomputer systems. Rather than a "monolithic mainframe approach" where one mainframe is hard-wired to every device used (with all hardware normally supplied by one vendor), the system specialists at Vancouver General customized the network to accommodate a wide variety of hardware by developing software tools that simplify protocol conversions and intercomputer transmissions.[18] This next fundamental shift in computing, called component software, will allow users to mix and match pieces of software from different developers to create custom software configuration, much the way an audiophile might combine stereo components.[19]

The result of all this technology for health care organizations is that the configuration of information in most medical facilities today has six pillars: One, there is data processing, which provides information in the form of numbers on printouts and screens, largely through on-line terminals. Two, there is word processing, which provides information in the form of written words (letters, reports, and so on), largely through personal, desktop computers. Three, there is image processing, which provides information in the form of visual pictures, largely through graphics software. Four, there is audio processing, which provides information in the form of spoken words, mostly through telephones (teleconferencing, answering machines), but also through voice recognition computers. Five, there is network processing, which provides shared information, largely through distributed systems and communications technology such as modems and LANs. Six, there is video teleconferencing, which provides information in the form of interactive video through the transmission of digital images. Managing all of this toward the organizational mission is a formidable and exciting challenge.

Notes

1. F. Cerne, "PCs Proliferate," *Hospitals*, 5 June 1988, 74.
2. T. Zinn, "Spending More on Computers to Help Keep Costs in Line," *Modern Healthcare*, 14 February 1994, 64.
3. D. H. Sanders and S. J. Birkin, *Computers and Management* (New York: McGraw Hill, 1980), 62.
4. F. Cerne, "Prices Stabilize," *Hospitals*, 5 June 1988, 70–72.
5. *Modern Healthcare*, 14 February 1994, 63–70.
6. E. Gardner, "New RISC Systems Boast Processing Prowess," *Modern Healthcare*, 12 February 1990, 40.
7. *New York Times*, 2 January 1994, F-9.
8. P. Lefort, "Health Information Systems: Creating the Competitive Edge," *Healthcare Financial Management*, June 1988, 34.

9. *Dun's Review*, July 1977, 65.

10. *Newark Star Ledger*, 11 December 1990, 23.

11. T. G. Roovers, "Executive Managers, Take Note!" *Computers in Healthcare*, February 1985, 33–34.

12. "Ignore Computers at Your Own Risk—Managers Need to Be Computer Literate," *Business Week*, 14 October 1985, 170.

13. *New York Times*, 23 September 1990, F-8.

14. J. K. H. Tan, "Graduate Education in Health Information Systems," *The Journal of Health Administration Education*, Winter 1993, 35–36.

15. S. LaViolette, "Public Domain Computer Software," *Modern Healthcare*, August 1980, 26.

16. S. L. Priest, "Borrowed Package Eases Computerization Inventory," *Hospital Financial Management*, October 1979, 62–64.

17. *Modern Healthcare*, 12 February 1990, 43.

18. G. Minot, "Applications for LAN Technology," *Computers in Healthcare*, November 1986, 22.

19. *New York Times*, 22 May 1994, F-10.

Selected Readings

Austin, C. J. *Information Systems for Health Services Administration*, 4th Ed. Ann Arbor, MI: Health Administration Press, 1992.

Brightbill, T. "Disk Contentment?" *Healthweek* (24 September 1990): 21.

Coolidge, G. "The Operating System: Your PC's Middle Manager." *PC Novice* (January 1992): 16–22.

Gardner, E. "The Coming Evolution in Computer Systems." *Modern Healthcare* (12 February 1990): 29–44.

Harrison, S. L. "Technology at Work: What Works?" *Association Management* (February 1992): 20.

McEwan, C. E. "Computer Graphics: Getting More from a Management Information System." *Data Management* (July 1981): 30–32.

Morrisey, J. "Spending More on Computers to Help Keep Costs in Line." *Modern Healthcare* (14 February 1994): 64.

Omiya, E. H. "Technology Increases Microcomputer Performance." *Healthcare Financial Management* (July 1987): 112.

Schroeder, M. A. "Computers in Nursing: Applications for Ambulatory Care." *Nursing Economics* (January–February 1987): 27–31.

Staggers, N. "Human Factors: The Missing Element in Computer Technology." *Computers in Nursing* (March–April 1991): 47–49.

READING

THOMAS CRISTO'S article provides an awareness of the nature of acquiring computer technology. He describes various "scams" that computer salespeople have been known to employ, and suggests some ways of dealing with the task of shopping for computer hardware and software.

How to Fold and Spindle Crooked Computer Salesmen

Thomas K. Christo

When you buy a piece of medical equipment, you know how it's supposed to work and what to check on before you give a salesman your order. But when you shop for an office computer system, you're likely to be short on expertise and a pigeon for any salesman's pitch. If you happen to get mixed up with a slick operator, you could be conned into the wrong deal faster than you can say "on-line."

I know. As an attorney specializing in computer malpractice, I've represented plenty of doctors who didn't recognize a scam when they saw one. You'll find their unhappy experiences instructive if you're considering automating your own office.

Note at the start that you can con yourself, with no assistance from a salesman. It's amazing how many doctors with offices neither large enough nor complicated enough to warrant owning their own computer are lured into buying one out of vanity or lack of a sense of proportion. So before you go shopping in the computer market, ask yourself: Is this purchase really necessary? You may be better off modifying your manual processes or letting a computer service do your work.

If you still feel that a computer will serve you well, don't make it easy for the seller. A fast-buck operator will bring a parade of technicians into your office, for instance, and will snow you with impressive diagrams and statistics. Don't accept them on blind faith. Over and over, I've uncovered not only cases of sloppy analysis and incorrect computer design, but cases of outright fraud.

The Super-Saver Scan

You're ripe for a rip-off if you go by price alone, which is too often the prime determinant in a smaller office. An exceptionally low quote for a computer system should be an automatic danger signal. If you've passed up some reputable companies because their systems were too expensive, beware when a little outfit promises to give you "practically" the same thing for half the price.

The salesman may tell you that his computer system will do all the things you want it to do, but the odds are that you'll end up as did a six-physician internal-medicine group in the Midwest that I represented.

The doctors paid $25,000 for what was sold to them as a general accounting and patient-scheduling system—a system that would handle their total office operations. Nine months after it was installed, the doctors realized that it would never perform all the jobs it was guaranteed to do. I was able to establish in court that they'd been defrauded because the capabilities of the computer system they'd bought had been grossly misrepresented.

The Bait-and-Switch Scam

This age-old sales ruse is a corollary of the super-saver pitch. The salesman knows that if he submits a bid on equipment of the appropriate size he probably won't make the sale, so he purposely sells you on a smaller system that can't possibly do the job. He figures that once you've changed your entire billing procedures over to the new computer, you'll be so far down the implementation path that you'll have no choice but to upgrade.

That was the scam used on one of my clients, a computer service bureau in the South that did data processing exclusively for doctors. The bureau's four owners, three of whom were physicians, wanted to set up an on-line system. Via terminals in their offices, customers could then enter data directly and get back instant readings on the status of their accounts receivable, their scheduling, their patient histories, and so forth.

A representative of a large company came along and sold them hardware—that is, the computer itself—that he knew was too small to handle the load. He was banking on the fact that if the service bureau wanted to stay in business it would be forced to move up to a more expensive machine. We sued and won a hefty settlement: the larger system for free plus money to compensate the physicians' bureau for employee overtime and other expenses incurred while it was trying to manage with the inadequate equipment.

The Flagship-Account Scam

In a gimmick frequently used by smaller companies the vendor offers to custom-design a complete system for you from scratch. It won't cost you a lot, he tells you, because your system will serve as a demonstration model that they can sell later to other doctors' offices around the country. You get it cheap because you're their "flagship account." Read it as: their guinea pig.

You're likely to run into this if you deal with a company that buys the computer machinery from a manufacturer at a discount and then develops its own software—or programming—and sells the whole system for a package price.

Without a program, of course, the computer can do nothing. Developing good programs takes a tremendous amount of skilled man-hours—and correspondingly large outlay of cash. If the company isn't heavily capitalized, it can't afford to do that properly, and you're the loser.

A Virginia orthopedic group that bought a computer and prototype software from such a firm ended up as one of my clients. The doctors had contracted with the company for a system that would take care of all their accounting and billing. What they didn't perceive was that the outfit didn't have the resources to do the development job it guaranteed. It had put in a low bid expecting to fund the process from future sales; when these didn't materialize, it passed off a shoddy job on the doctors.

Signing up for a new system is always risky at best. If you're willing to take the risk, find out if the company is sufficiently capitalized to fund the development effort.

There's another risk to consider: The creation of any new software package entails a long shakedown period. All kinds of bugs can surface from six months to several years after your system is in place, despite successful initial testing. This is so even when you're dealing with a highly reputable and well-capitalized company.

The Fully Tested Scam

Unfortunately, you're not necessarily con-proof if you buy an existing software package. The salesman, of course, will assure you that his is a fully tested program, so you won't have to go through a long shakedown phase.

Doctors at one Colorado medical clinic bought a patient-billing package that was sold to them as fully tested, but when they attempted to operate it, an inordinate number of bugs cropped up. Patients were misbilled or not billed at all. Entire files of some patients just disappeared. If there were, say, 12 patient accounts on-line at one time and a thirteenth was added, account No. 8 might be dropped. It was chaos.

When I got into the case, I found out that, contrary to what the sales brochure stated and what the salesman had told the doctors, the system had never been adequately tested. When the company couldn't document the tests it claimed to have done, it agreed to give the clinic all its money back. That didn't make up for the months of inconvenience the doctors had to put up with, to say nothing of the loss of patient goodwill. They'd have avoided the whole hassle if they'd asked to see the test results before committing themselves to the purchase.

The Easy-Conversion Scam

A program that has truly been tested is fine—as long as you're also buying the specific hardware it was designed for. In the easy-conversion scam, that important consideration gets kicked under the rug. Here the salesman pushes a "proven" programming package even though it's going to be used with a different kind of hardware design. "We can easily convert it," he'll tell you, but let me assure you that conversion is no simple matter. If you go to a different manufacturer—or even a different model from the same manufacturer—you can have lots of problems.

A 12-doctor surgical group on the West Coast found that out. They were told that the software they bought was fully tested and reliable, but not that it was designed for a far larger computer than they required. The firm that sold them the package thought it could be modified to meet their needs. When it turned out to be a more extensive undertaking than anticipated, the company did a makeshift conversion. The new system, however, never worked, and the group was out thousands of dollars.

So when any conversion is involved, get written assurance that the folks doing the conversion will stick with it until the system works to your satisfaction.

In addition to skepticism, there are other precautions you'll be wise to take when you decide to go the computer route in your office.

Run Your Old System in Parallel

Since a shakedown period is inevitable in any computer installation, you can avoid a lot of misery if you continue your manual routine for at least one full cycle after the computer is installed. If you're doing monthly billing, for instance, do it manually, too, for at least a full 30-day period. If your operations are on a quarterly basis, keep the parallel system going for the entire quarter. Check both systems on a random basis to make sure the results correspond.

Monitoring parallel systems during the early stage of your automated system won't prevent your computer from making errors—but it will prevent those errors from fouling up your whole operation. The Midwestern medical group I referred to earlier is a case in point. The six doctors abandoned their manual accounting system as soon as the new computer took over. When the system failed to produce, they had no way of straightening out their accounts because all the billing data were on the computer. Without a manual backup, they couldn't re-create the information that the system had dropped. The doctors put their financial loss for this period at about $11,000 a month.

Check Availability of Service

Have it spelled out in your contract that the firm that has sold you the computer will service the system after it's installed. Ideally, the service office should be located fairly near you so that somebody local can come in every month to check the circuitry and the machinery's moving parts and be readily available to provide remedial maintenance if your terminal or printer breaks down. Also make certain that the company keeps an inventory of backup equipment on hand should your system go completely awry.

Avoid Lock-In Contracts

Suppose you realize, as some of my clients did, that your computer isn't working as you expected, that you've made a bad deal, and you want out. That may be impossible if, say, you've financed your purchase through a third-party leasing arrangement. With this kind of contract, the bank or leasing company buys the computer for you and pays the vendor; you repay the lessor in monthly installments. At the end of the lease, there's a final payment, and then you own the computer outright.

The catch is that if you're not satisfied with the way the computer is working, it's your problem, not the lessor's. You're still stuck with making your monthly payments; all you can do is sue the vendor and hope for a decent settlement.

That's why I advise against these transactions. If you do finance your purchase through a leasing arrangement, have the contract stipulate that the lessor will give no money to the vendor until you say it's okay. That's after you've tried out the computer system and are satisfied it's working properly.

Get Some Expert Advice

It may not be easy for you to check out all the relevant factors I've cited, such as the company's reputation and financial position, the validity of its test results, and its servicing capability. So I have one final suggestion: When in doubt about a company's suitability, consider hiring a professional computer consultant.

Select someone who isn't tied to any particular manufacturer and won't get any commission on whatever system you buy. How can you locate a qualified independent consultant? Word-of-mouth is best. Ask other doctors for recommendations; you'll want a computer expert who's advised medical offices, because he understands doctors' special automation requirements.

Such a consultant will cost you anywhere from $700 to $1,500 a day. You could use him in one of two ways: either to draft the request for proposal—a document specifying your office's needs that goes out to various bidders—and to evaluate the responses, or simply to come in and survey your office and tell you whether the system you're considering is appropriate.

Whether or not you use an outside expert, you should be able to protect yourself from a con job if you stick with a reputable company, take nothing on faith, and don't look for bargains in the computer marketplace. There aren't any.

Thomas K. Christo is a lawyer from North Hampton, New Hampshire.

CASE 3
The Decision at St. Vincent
Healthcare System

AFTER A BRIEF immersion in the computer technology literature, Bill Pugh finally began to collect his thoughts and think
about making the big decision. Inundated with the jargon, hype,
and advertising, his head was spinning. How does one choose the right
system and what does the executive need to know in order to make a
judicious choice? Bill, a corporate vice president of operations for St.
Vincent Healthcare System, a multi-hospital system in the Washington,
DC area, had been recently charged with the task of selecting a MIS
for the corporation. His graduate management education in public
administration provided him with a foundation in management skills
and techniques but, as most managers of his generation, he found
the world of computer technology and MISs fraught with jargon and
computerese. Yet, he had been given the responsibility to choose the
right system for his organization.

The St. Vincent Healthcare System

The St. Vincent Healthcare System is a multi-hospital system with
three acute care hospitals, four nursing homes, two ambulatory health
care centers, a medical laboratory and imaging center, and a home-
health care organization. By most accounts, the St. Vincent Healthcare

Table 3.1 The Decision at St. Vincent Healthcare System

St. Vincent Healthcare System Network Options

Computer Networks	Description
Mainframe computing	Many users connected to one mainframe computer through terminals. Allows users to share resources, but can be very slow.
Work station computing	One computer for each user in the network. Individuals have more power at their fingertips, but the system is only as powerful as its components.
Distributed computing	Many computers for each user, forming a web of specialized services—each desktop computer has access to many specialized systems including parallel computers, database computers, graphics processors, and supercomputers all seamlessly drawn together by a high-speed network.

Table 3.2 The Decision at St. Vincent Healthcare System

St. Vincent Healthcare System Integration Options

Integration Approach	Description
Centralized or sole-vendor approach	Applications are developed with a common design methodology.
Networked "ad hoc" approach	Uses a common connectivity strategy to support multiple application vendors and hardware platforms connecting disparate systems.
Repository or duplicate database approach	Uses a separate system to collect and maintain integrated information/data from all systems in a central data repository so that information is stored in one place.

System was located in an overbedded region. Several local hospitals had recently partnered with larger regional health care systems.

The 1990s brought many changes in health care, and the St. Vincent Healthcare System found that these pressures, combined with the immediate environment, required a rethinking of general operations.

Table 3.3 The Decision at St. Vincent Healthcare System

St. Vincent Healthcare System Terminal System Features

Configuration Characteristics	Options
Terminal portability	__ Desktop computer __ Handheld computer __ Laptop computer __ Personal digital assistant
Microprocessing power	__ Pentium chip __ 486 chip __ 386 chip
Hard disk storage capacity	__ 300MB __ 200MB __ 120MB
Operating memory	__ 16MB __ 8MB __ 4MB
Printers	__ Dot matrix __ Ink jet __ Laser
Fax communication	__ Fax modem
External modem	__ 9600bps __ 2400bps __ 1200bps
Input devices	__ Scanner __ Digitizer
Acquisition	__ Lease __ Own

Mergers and shared service strategies had become common among institutions in the area. Although managed care penetration had been low in recent years, there was a sharp increase in managed care contracts among the area's health care systems. Price competitiveness and cost-consciousness had become the guiding force behind operations. The necessity to have the right information at the right time forced many institutions to look toward high technology. Suddenly, detailed internal analysis and reliable, extensive data became indispensable to operations. Additionally, information sharing within the organization and among the community health networks had become essential. There was also a need for the easy flow of data and information among various operating entities. In the current milieu, clinical departments that were once autonomous would be required to understand the financial and administrative consequences of everyday operations.

Recent statistics indicate that hospital data processing expenditures have risen dramatically over the past several years, and most hospitals and health care systems were looking at information technology not as an expense item, but rather as a value-added necessity for cost savings and efficient management. This change in viewpoint explains the tremendous boom in the health care information systems business. Purchasers or users of such systems were faced with an almost infinite number of vendors, as well as choices of systems, hardware, software, and peripherals. In addition to the vast opportunities for choice, other variables such as initial capital expenditures, maintenance costs, and "hidden" costs needed to be considered. Generally, the more complex the system, the more time and money is involved. The question remains, Does the biggest or best system equate with the system that will get the job done?

Because of the confusing nature of the terminology and the complex nature of the technology, Bill had to carefully consider the potential configuration, network, and integration options. He devised a number of matrices, factoring in the variables he felt were important in making the right decision. The items in each matrix represent respective system characteristics.

Questions for Discussion

1. What criteria should Bill use in making his decision?
2. What are the opportunities and constraints facing Bill in making his decision?
3. Which variables are important in making the final decision? Why?
4. With what jargon should Bill be familiar in order to make his decision?

THINKING SYSTEMATICALLY

THE TYPICAL life cycle of computerized information systems has been described by some experienced observers as a remarkably consistent progression in several stages.[1] The cycle begins with "wild euphoria" when decision makers hear about how much a computer system has done for other organizations and want to acquire one for their own. Visions of instant information and more efficient processes excite beleaguered project heads. Stage two emerges almost immediately after the computer is plugged in. It is marked by "mild concern" when the anticipated payoffs fail to appear or when "bugs" crop up.

"Broad disillusionment" arises in a third stage when users realize that the system fails to meet expectations or, instead, causes new problems. Employee unrest with using the "confounded machines" is a common symptom in this stage, which is followed by the culminating stage, "unmitigated disaster." Such disasters include the failure of the automated billing system to get out the bills, or a printout of a patient record that gets into the wrong hands, producing a privacy lawsuit, or a "crash" which erases a disk with no backup.

This stage, of course, is followed in rapid succession by a search for a perpetrator, punishment of the progressive innocent, and promotion of the obstructionary who had been against computerization all along. In hospitals, in government health offices, and in small and large health care facilities this scenario has been constantly repeated. It is so common that a professional computer consultant with McKinsey and

Company has coined, from his experience, "Golub's Laws of Computerdom," the first of which states: "No major computer project is ever installed on time, within budget, with the same staff that started it, nor does the project do what it is supposed to. . . . It is highly unlikely that yours is going to be the first."[2] Golub does proffer a caveat to this enduring tenet—his laws are not always true, just most of the time.

Stories abound that give evidence of this strange cycle. Many organizations entered the information age with little in the way of long-range plans, no formula for growth, and lots of attitudes similar to "everybody's using computers, we will too."[3] The consequences of this shortsightedness is that many managers find themselves in the unenviable position of having a computerized information system that fails to address the needs of the organization and, perhaps even worse, impedes the efforts of those seeking useful information.

Why is this so? The major reason is a lack of enlightened analysis— a lack of systematic thinking about the entire project, an absence of user involvement and control, a failure to ask the right questions. In brief, this cycle dominates because no one "in-the-know" focuses on what needs to be done to make a computerization project work. Technicians, who frequently are put in charge, are experts about what technically needs to be done, but only user-managers are in a position to know the organization's needs and to have the overall responsibility to make the system work.

Why have managers failed to exert the same kind of control over computer operations that they exercise over other aspects of their organization? One reason is that the technical aura of computers has tended to conceal its broader ramifications. It has thus been difficult for managers to learn how to think about computerization.[4]

The Role of Managers and Users

Managers and computer users have tended to abrogate their proper and necessary role in systematic thinking by falling into traps, the three most common of which are the vendor trap, the hardware trap, and the technician trap.

The vendor trap entails leaving the thinking to the computer manufacturer in the mistaken belief that its experts know what needs to be done to make its computer work well in a particular organization. In reality, employees of the manufacturer seldom have managerial insight and expertise about your agency.

The hardware trap assumes that computer use and integration into the organization immediately follow acquisition. This trap, therefore, leads a manager to focus on purchasing a computer, instead of on meeting organizational needs.

The technician trap places unfair responsibility on and unfounded confidence in the data processing technician or "system analyst" to do the careful thinking needed to make the computer productive. In truth, while a technician can well think through technical needs and implications, only a user-manager can steer a technically sound system toward organizational effectiveness.

Succumbing to these traps is seductively simple. Many managers routinely delegate technology decisions to the computer "wizards." But, the development of computerized information systems affects an entire organization—from strategy to structure. Delegating to wizards does not assure that the information technology effort will work. In fact, it practically guarantees that it won't. The technical experts seldom have a deep enough understanding of where the overall business is going.[5]

The health care professional's role in developing a computerized information system requires involvement, planning, and communication. Managers and system users should be thoroughly involved in the development of computerized systems. Automation requires careful planning and an investment of time as well as attention to the problems that inevitably arise. Managers should ensure that technicians and system users frequently interact so that problems are quickly discovered and resolved.[6] As one veteran of this process puts it: "My best advice is to start planning as soon as you can."[7]

But what specifically constitutes "managerial involvement"? How do managers wisely "plan" the application of computers to their activities? How is communication between technician and user accomplished? How, in short, can managers exercise control over the task of employing computer technology?

One practical answer is to ensure that proper systematic analysis takes place before, during, and after the introduction of computers. This involves identifying objectives, gathering information on how to meet them, formulating alternatives, deciding and implementing the most suitable alternatives, and monitoring what happens. Good systematic analysis is asking all the right questions and getting the best answers possible. Good management is ensuring that all the right questions are asked and that the best answers are sought.

Most challenges and problems of computerization can be anticipated if the relevant questions are posed; most obstacles can be recognized if the development process is systematically monitored; most difficulties can be handled if users and managers systematically observe and learn from actual organizational experience. Systematic thinking is one way health care managers can anticipate, recognize, and address barriers to the successful use of computer technology.

Systematic thinking in managing computers entails attention to the *process*, as well as to the *substance*, of planning, designing, and implementing modern information systems. By substance is meant the series of questions and tentative answers that guide the effort to adopt computers. Process involves developing the computerization effort in systematic phases, carefully monitoring the actual experience as it evolves, and modifying the effort as important new questions are discovered and better tentative answers learned.

The Substance of Systematic Thinking

In terms of substance, most health care organizations have, historically, employed a kind of systematic analysis for computer applications. They have generally raised questions about and addressed matters of system objectives, alternatives, impacts, and development. However, because user-managers historically have not been intimately involved in the analysis, critical nontechnical questions have received cursory treatment at best. In particular, impact analyses have typically been limited to fiscal and technical considerations. The impact of a computer system on personnel and clients, the likelihood of resistance, and the implications for data security and privacy have often been neglected in planning and analysis. Yet, problems in these areas have frequently been the key impediments to effective use of computers. Clearly, systematic thinking on these matters is needed.

The substance of systematic thinking is asking the following types of questions and analyzing the answers:

Specification of Problem
- What is the problem that might benefit from computerization?
- How is the problem area currently handled?
- Why does the problem exist?
- Who is involved in the problem area?
- How severe is the problem for the organization?
- What priority does the problem have in relation to other organizational problems?

Definition of Objectives
- What do we want to accomplish?

- To what extent can we accomplish it?
- By when do we want to achieve the objective?

Development of Alternatives

- How could we accomplish the objective?
- Are there options other than computerization?
- What computerization alternatives exist?
- How have other organizations pursued similar objectives?
- What are the pros and cons of each alternative?

Impact Analysis

Fiscal Impact

- What will the project cost?
- How much will hardware and software cost?
- How much will personnel cost?
- How much will training cost?
- How much will development and implementation cost?
- How much will operating and maintenance cost?
- What savings can be expected?
- What nonquantifiable benefits can be expected?
- What are the cost-benefit implications of the project?

Technical Impact

- What technical expertise will be needed to develop and operate the system? Do we have that expertise? If not, where can we get it? How long will it take to get it?
- How will the system affect other technical systems in the organization? Can they be made mutually supportive?
- What is the "state-of-the-art"? Are pertinent technical developments likely in the near future?

Organizational Impact

- How will the system affect organization structures? Will it change the information flow? In what ways? Will any reorganization be necessary or desirable?
- Will the system increase or decrease anyone's power?
- How might it affect informal structures, such as social groups, within the organization?
- Will the system be used? How do we know?
- How might resistance to the system be expressed?

- Who might be threatened by and resist the system?
- How would system failure affect organizational operation?
- What could be done to minimize or overcome resistance?
- What could be done to minimize the undesired organizational impact?

Personnel Impact

- Will some existing staff no longer be needed?
- How can unneeded staff be prepared for other work in the organization or be placed in another organization?
- What training will be needed? Who will do it? When will it be provided? How much will it cost?
- What new staff will be needed? Can they be recruited? How long will it take to recruit them?

Legal Impact

- What do current privacy and freedom of information laws require?
- Can the system meet these requirements? What will this cost?
- What new laws are likely, and how would they impact the system?
- What legal protection can be built into contracts with vendors?

Security Impact

- What security risks are inherent in the system?
- What security problems have other organizations experienced with similar systems?
- What security protections are available to minimize the risk? How much would they cost?

Social Impact

- How will the system affect the organization's clients?
- How might it affect professional or health care system values?

System Development/Implementation Plan

- In view of the above questions and answers, what activities are required to develop and implement the system?
- Who will do them?
- When will they be accomplished?
- How do they interrelate, and who will coordinate them?
- What resources will be needed, and when will they be needed?

Additional specific questions should be raised to suit the particular applications and organization. Since finding answers can require a good deal of time and money, the extent of efforts employed in finding answers should be determined by the importance of and investment in the project.

It is important to remember that effective management of computers and information systems requires that a broad array of questions be raised and systematically addressed. Management's job is to ensure that the right questions are asked and that there are satisfactory answers. Management must also ensure that questions are continually posed and answers updated as more is learned. That is, managers should ensure that there is a systematic process for developing the substance of systematic thinking.

The Process of Systematic Thinking

A critical aspect of systematic analysis is the timing and frequency of posing the kinds of questions suggested above. The questions are typically asked, and answers developed, once—at the beginning of a computerization project. This is done through a so-called "system study," usually conducted by technicians, consultants, or both, after which computer resources are acquired and a system implemented in accordance with the system study.

There are two serious problems involved with this kind of system study approach. First, even an extraordinary system study can neither anticipate all the problems that might impede a particular computerization effort nor be expected to provide sufficient answers. Some problems will occur unexpectedly or in a different form than initially predicted, and inevitably some answers will prove to be inadequate. Second, the approach permits only marginal user-managerial control in that, once a user-manager commissions a full-scale system study, the project can easily proceed to implementation and use untempered by a practical, nontechnical, user-oriented perspective.

For these reasons, systematic thinking should also entail a phased process of monitoring developments and modifying the project as a computer application is being developed. That is, systematic thinking means not only using existing knowledge and insight, but also learning from your own actual experience with the project and using the knowledge and insight gained from that experience. Many computerized systems are failures because their development is guided solely by a preproject system study with little attention given to what actually happens as the project proceeds, or to a serious review of why it happened. This occurs because no provisions were made for learning as the project unfolded or for using the knowledge gained to modify the system study plan. In effect, the system study tends to be "written in concrete" with no serious review process brought to bear on it.

In contrast, a controlled process of systematic thinking recognizes that a system study is just a guess at what might and should happen and continually monitors that guess, adjusting it as new facts emerge. Such a process can be established and controlled by organizing computerization projects into distinct steps or phases that provide for conscious user-manager review and decision making at the end of each phase.

For example, a computerization project can be organized into eight phases as follows:

1. **Project Initiation Phase:** involves a few people and little money; focuses on initial clarification of the problem, objectives, and alternatives; obtains quick answers to basic questions.

2. **Preliminary Study Phase:** involves more people and money in a more detailed examination of questions; objectives and feasibility of computer options for the organization are probed.

3. **System Study Phase:** involves a significant investment of resources in an in-depth analysis of information needs and the formulation of a specific plan of system development; at this stage the substance of systematic thinking would be thoroughly developed as was previously discussed.

4. **System Design Phase:** the measures planned in the system study phase are actually designed; specialists, for example, design training programs, and users and technicians design output forms.

5. **System Development/Selection Phase:** hardware for implementing the design is tentatively selected; software is developed or identified.

6. **Testing Phase:** a key stage for controlling the project; plans and design are tried to ascertain what really happens when they are implemented; focus is on correcting any inadequate pretest answers and discovering questions not previously asked.

7. **System Installation:** the stage in which the major financial investment is made.

8. **System Evaluation Phase:** an ongoing series of reviews to see if new questions or problems have arisen, if old answers need updating, and if the system requires modification to meet organizational objectives.

The most important aspect of such a process is that at the completion of each phase the user-manager intervenes, reviews the outcome of the phase, and provides direction to either proceed to the next phase, halt the project, or return to a previous stage for additional answers. For example, a preliminary study might be reviewed by a manager who finds that questions on privacy impact and personnel resistance were not raised. The manager could then, at an early stage before development work is begun, direct that the system study address these questions before a decision is made to proceed with system design; important modifications could result.

Figures 4.1 and 4.2 depict such a process in flowchart form.[8] They show the inherently repetitive nature of the process and how the various stages interrelate. The flowcharts stress two important characteristics of such a systematic process: (1) the clear and unambiguous involvement of user-managers in the process, and (2) the continual review and decision making by the user-managers. Notice that at the completion of each stage in such a process a decision is made to continue, to stop the project, or to modify a previous phase.

This kind of a controlled, systematic process is, in effect, a process of asking questions and trying to get better answers as needed. The test phase, for example, can uncover impacts that were not anticipated in the preliminary study or system study phases and that, by being identified and addressed, can prevent serious problems from occurring when the system is fully installed. Specifically, a manager might direct that the system study be expanded to explore a problem (such as user resistance) discovered in the test, and that a second test be conducted before full implementation.[9]

Similarly, the evaluation phase can disclose problems that were not recognized in the system study or test phases and point to modifications that might improve the system's effectiveness. More than a few unproductive uses of computers remain in health care organizations because of a lack of periodic systematic evaluation.

In sum, a process of systematic thinking about computerized information systems can prevent the cycle from "wild euphoria" to "unmitigated disaster" that was described earlier. It can provide a framework for managing computer use, for avoiding an uncontrolled rush to expensive installation, and for steadfastly focusing computer projects on organizational realities and needs.

The substance and process of systematic thinking can and should be applied by health care professionals to the development of new computerized information systems and to the improvement of existing ones. It provides a fundamental framework for managing the technology and information systems that organizations need. The following

Figure 4.1 Process Flowchart—Study and Design

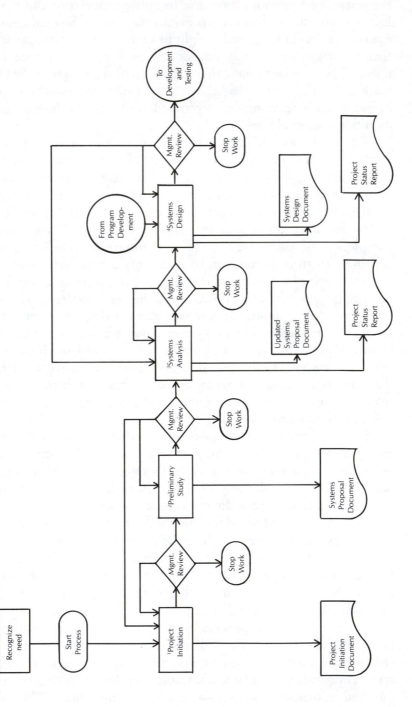

Figure 4.2 Process Flowchart—Development and Installation

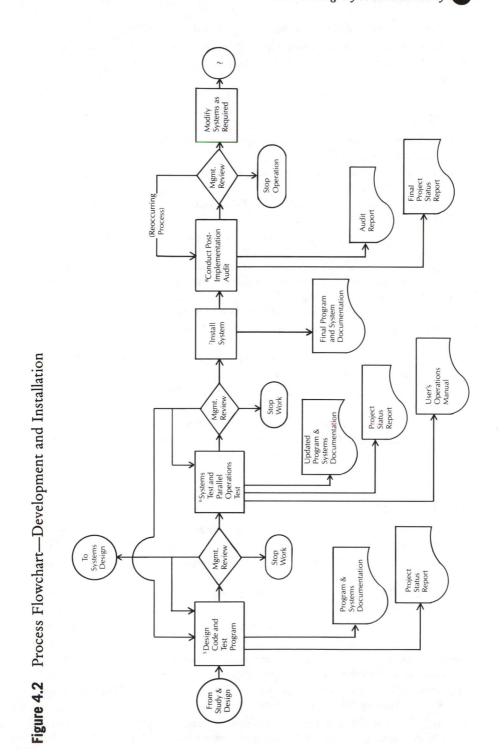

chapters discuss some of the most important and difficult questions of the "substance" of systematic thinking—questions concerning organizational impacts, personnel and resistance, security, privacy, and social ramifications.

Notes

1. J. G. Burch, "Designing Information Systems for People," *Journal of Systems Management*, October 1986, 30–34.
2. J. A. Groobe, "Maximizing Return on EDP Investments," *Data Management*, September 1972, 28–32.
3. M. Smith, "Adventures in Dysfunctional Computer Land," *Nonprofit World*, July–August 1991, 6.
4. The chapter is intended as a framework. It does not get into details of systems design that are important for managers directly in charge of computer projects. Many books are available for insight on these details, most notably C. J. Austin, *Information Systems for Health Services Administration*, 4th Ed. (Ann Arbor, MI: Health Administration Press, 1992).
5. T. H. Davenport, M. Hammer, and T. J. Metsisto, "How Executives Can Shape Their Company's Information Systems," *Harvard Business Review*, March–April 1989, 130–34.
6. J. W. Spence, "End User Computing: The Human Interface," *Journal of Systems Management*, February 1988, 15–23.
7. K. Lumsdon, "The Clinical Connection: Hospitals Work to Design Information Systems that Physicians Will Use," *Hospitals*, 5 May 1993, 16.
8. We are indebted to Harry Smith for his work on these flowcharts.
9. See N. D. Meyer and T. M. Lodahl, "Pilot Projects: A Way to Get Started in Office Automation," *Administrative Management*, February 1980, 36–44, for an excellent discussion of testing.

Selected Readings

Bowden, A. B. "Negotiating a System Purchase: Eight Principles for Protecting Your Institution's Interests." *Healthcare Executive* (January–February 1992): 17–19.

Burch, J. G. "Designing Information Systems for People." *Journal of Systems Management* (October 1986): 30–34.

Correll, R., and S. L. Ummel. "Critical Decisions, Critical Plans: Purchasing Hospital Information Systems." *Healthcare Executive* (January–February 1992): 22–24.

Digiolio, L., and T. Zinn. "Criteria for Success." *Computers in Healthcare* (March 1987): 41–46.

Ginsburg, D. A., and W. Garetta. "Selecting an Automated Patient Accounting System." *Healthcare Financial Management* (May–June 1987): 58–63.

McFarlan, F. W. "The Information Archipelago—Plotting a Course." *Harvard Business Review* (January–February 1983): 145–56.

Meyer, N. D. "The Office Automation Cookbook: Management Strategies for Getting Office Automation Moving." *Sloan Management Review* (Winter 1983): 51–60.

Muller, B. "System Design Without the Camel." *Data Management* (August 1985): 36–39.

Owen, D. "Information Systems Organization—Keeping Pace with the Pressure." *Sloan Management Review* (Spring 1986): 59–69.

Rhoads, J. L. "How To Select a Computer System for Your Long-Term Care Facility." *Nursing Homes* (September–October 1986): 38–41.

Rosenberger, H. R., and K. M. Kaiser. "Strategic Planning for Health Care Management Information Systems." *Health Care Management Review* (Winter 1985): 7–17.

Spitz, B., and B. Stuart. "Selection Guidelines for Health Information Systems." *Business and Health* (October 1986): 34–38.

Tharrington, J. M. "The Science of MIS Planning." *Infosystems* (June 1985): 52–53.

Tozer, E. "Developing Plans for Information Systems." *Long Range Planning* (October 1986): 63–76.

Worthley, J. A. "Computer Technology and Productivity Improvement." *Public Productivity Review* (March 1980): 10–21.

READING

T HE FOLLOWING reading provides additional perspectives on systematic thinking about computer applications. Davenport, Hammer, and Metsisto argue that managers can no longer avoid the process of making decisions concerning information technology. Their down-to-earth approach offers practical guidelines for health care professionals.

How Executives Can Shape Their Company's Information Systems: A Down-to-Earth Approach to Making Important Technical Decisions

Thomas H. Davenport, Michael Hammer, and Tauno J. Metsisto

A big bank headquartered in New York had to make a decision about its information technology. The bank was expanding its London operations and needed a new computer system there. Technical specialists in London were certain that only one particular vendor could meet the requirements. The information-systems people in New York were equally certain that another vendor's system was the best choice.

When, after several months, the technical managers still hadn't chosen a vendor, they took the issue to a senior management policy committee. New York and London each stated its case in terms like "instruction set architectures," "file system performance," and "transaction throughput rates." The policy committee, confused by these technical issues, kept postponing the decision. Meanwhile, the head of the London office complained that the stalemate threatened the unit's growth.

How should the policy committee choose a vendor?

In the past, managers simply delegated technology decisions like this to the in-house computer wizards and attended to other matters. But managers can no longer easily avoid the process of making decisions about information technology (IT). IT affects the entire business—from organizational structure to product market strategies. Delegating such important decisions doesn't ensure that IT investments will further the company's business strategy. In fact, it practically guarantees that they won't. The technical experts just don't have a deep enough understanding of where the overall business is going.

General managers, however, usually don't know much about computers. They may like the idea of using information technology strategically, as companies like American Hospital Supply and American Airlines have done. But they seldom know how to translate their wishes into specific IT investments. They may not even know what questions to ask, and the technical jargon can sound like a foreign language. So they tend to delay IT decisions or avoid them altogether.

Yet the consequences of postponing or mishandling IT decisions can be severe. The company might lose out on important competitive opportunities, it might waste money on relatively unproductive technologies, and it might have to spend heavily to get its IT on the right track later.

One industrial-products company learned this lesson the hard way. As part of its business strategy, senior management eliminated administrative tangles by cutting the number of distributors carrying its products. Meanwhile, it delegated hardware and software selections to the information-systems groups in each division. The IT groups were unaware of what top management was trying to accomplish, and top management was unaware of the decisions each IT group was making. By the time senior management realized that it would be much easier to consolidate the distributors if all divisions were using the same order-processing system, it was too late. The divisions had already bought or built applications that were incompatible. It took the company years to redo the ordering systems so distributors had access to all the products.

A division of a large chemical company learned a similar lesson. Technical managers consulted their product-manager peers and became convinced that a customer data base integrating information from all four product groups would be useful for cross-selling and coordinating customer orders. But neither the technologists nor the product managers knew that senior management planned to move several product groups into different divisions and to sell off others. The senior managers also had no idea that the integrated data base did not allow a product group's information systems to move with the group. The company had to undertake an expensive and disruptive crash project to separate the systems.

Clearly, many companies need a new approach to IT decision making, one that blends the technical knowledge of the computer experts with the vision of senior management.

Simple Truths

We have studied the IT decision-making processes of more than 50 large organizations, many of whose IT efforts were lacking direction. A few companies, however, had articulated their basic philosophies about IT, and they seemed to be using technology more effectively. They expressed these philosophies through a set of IT management principles that summarized how the company would use IT to achieve its goals. Those principles then guided any technology decisions that arose over the next few years. If the decision was in keeping with the principles, it was also in keeping with the corporate strategy.

Principles are simple, direct statements of an organization's basic beliefs about how the company wants to use IT over the long term. By translating the main aspects of a company's business strategy into the language of technology managers, these principles bridge the communication gap between top managers and technical experts. This way, business strategy drives technical strategy, as conventional wisdom says it should.

Think again of the opening example of the bank that was expanding in London. The debate was not about technical issues at all. The tension was between operating-unit autonomy and global consistency. The London office wanted to penetrate a new marketplace as quickly as possible; packaged software on its preferred computer would allow it to be up and running quickly. Headquarters in New York had a different concern: to give top management a complete and instantaneous view of the worldwide business. If the company had established a principle like *"Computing hardware should facilitate global information consistency"* there would have been no conflict. The technical experts in both New York and London would have been working toward the same end, and their decision would have been easy to reach and consistent with the organization's most important goals.

The industrial-products company whose top managers wanted to consolidate distributors would have benefited from a principle like

"All product data should be accessible through a common order-processing system." The IT groups at the divisions would have known from the start that their ordering systems must be compatible, since the principle conveys the important relationship between business strategy and technology.

The chemical company whose information systems couldn't move with the product groups could have used a principle like *"All product groups should be self-sufficient in their information systems capabilities."* This would have ensured that specific technical decisions would not interfere with senior management's need for flexibility.

Sometimes decision makers have trouble sifting through the details to the more enduring connections between IT investments and strategic goals. Principles can help the decision maker keep long-term strategic issues in perspective and give a clear basis for the decision. A marketing manager who needs better market research may select the local area network LAN that can run a certain software package, even though the LAN precludes a later shift to regional marketing. A principle like *"Marketing data and applications should be easily movable to field sites for regional and local market analysis"* would make it easier for the manager to choose the right LAN.

Similarly, a chemical research director wanting to speed product development might choose the star scientist's favorite high-powered workstation—only to discover later that it cannot communicate with other computers in R&D. The statement that *"Research computing should be integrated with computing in development and testing"* would help the research director make a better choice.

The First Move

The "principles" approach to IT begins when someone—generally the head of information systems (IS)—takes the initiative to introduce the idea to the organization and begins to assemble a task force. Senior managers must be involved, so getting their cooperation is often the first hurdle.

The number of people on the task force and the mix of backgrounds varies from company to company. Generally speaking, the key is to gather a handful of people who deeply understand either the business or the technology and who are committed to the process. One good way to assemble such a team is to think of it in two parts: five to ten senior managers, including a senior information-systems person, who know the organization well and can get people throughout the company to endorse the principles later; and a small group of IS managers who will create the initial set of principles.

Before writing the principles, the task force should identify the topics it wants to consider and make plans to interview those senior managers not on the study team. The interviews should draw from senior executives as much information as possible about broad strategic or organizational issues. The idea is not to ask top managers to discuss computers or to reveal company secrets but simply to understand their views on where the business is headed.

Among other things, the interviews should focus on issues of risk, user autonomy, and the role of IT. How much risk is the company able to take? Some organizations are perfectly willing to accept technology-related risk, while others want to avoid it at all costs. As one senior manager at a money-center bank commented, "We will accept any reasonable technology risk that has significant business payoff but that will not compromise our name in the industry."

Some companies believe their users and user-managers can make intelligent decisions about technology, while others prefer central control. Finally, many businesses—though certainly not all—have accepted that IT can play a strategic role rather than simply displace costs. Such basic attitudes toward technology tend to be deep and persistent. The company's technology principles should reflect these attitudes—not try to change them—so the task force must identify them.

The overall direction the business is taking is also an important consideration. A principle supporting common application systems, for example, is inappropriate if the company's strategy involves big acquisitions and divestitures in the near future. In such a turbulent business environment, divisional systems should usually stand alone yet be capable of communicating with those in other divisions.

The team should gather information on the existing systems portfolio to unearth unresolved technology problems and to note if existing systems make proposed principles unrealistic. If, for instance, a company discovers that several dozen LANs are already in use, it would be unwise to draft a principle that discourages LANs and instead favors minicomputers. And the team should scan available and forthcoming technologies. The IT experts probably know the technology landscape, but other participants need to understand it too.

Although the interview and information-gathering process can be time consuming, especially when there are many people to talk to, the bigger problem is scheduling. The task force should be sure to make the rounds quickly so that it finishes the process in weeks, not months. Things tend to move faster if one person takes on the role of expediter. Some companies have completed the whole process—including drafting and refining the principles—in three months.

Once the interviews are done and transcripts of the responses have been distributed to team members, the task force can reconvene to discuss and summarize the results. With a synopsis of the company's business plans, IT problems, and values in hand, the team is ready to tackle the principles. The subgroup of IS managers usually takes over from here to draft an initial set.

Good Principles

While the process of establishing the principles is itself constructive because it forces managers to think things through and make their ideas explicit, the principles are the real goal. If the principles are good, general managers and technical experts will turn to them time after time for clarification and guidance. If, however, the principles are vague, managers will ignore them.

It's not a matter of coming up with the "right" principles. It's more a matter of creating principles that are helpful and appropriate for the particular company and its environment. They should reflect the organization that created them. Most companies need just 20 or 30 principles to capture their approach to technology management. Normally, this approach is deeply rooted in the company's culture, management style, and business strategy, and since those things change slowly, principles should remain valid for a few years. Only when the organization changes its basic business direction or undertakes widespread restructuring would it need to reconsider its principles more often.

The principles themselves should hold clues about the industry and the corporate strategy. If they don't, they may be too general. It is tempting to state principles like *"Data is an asset."* Consensus will be easy to reach. But when isn't data an asset? Such a statement is of no help at all when it comes to decision making. It is a cliché—not a guide for action. If a principle has any power at all, its opposite should also be a meaningful statement. The principle *"We are committed to a single vendor environment"* is contradictory to *"We will select the best technology for each business situation, regardless of vendor."* Either one is a useful guideline.

It helps to divide the work of drafting the initial set of principles by category of IT investments. Most companies' IT decisions fall into one of four areas: hardware and communications infrastructure, applications, data, and organization.

Infrastructure includes the number and types of computers the organization uses, the operating software that runs on them, and the communications networks that allow individuals and computers to talk to each other. *Applications* are the function- or process-specific computer programs the organization uses and also the process by which they are created, maintained, and managed. *Data* are of course all of the company's information. *Organization* is the often overlooked human support for IT, without which departments may receive the technical equipment they need but no help using it. By dividing the technology this way and creating five or six principles for each category, the team can be sure that the guidelines apply to nearly all technology decisions. The following examples illustrate principles for each type of resource.

Managers of an office-products company knew that the business was changing fast and were often frustrated by their inability to get current data. To fix this situation, they came up with the principle that *"IS will develop only real-time applications so that data bases reflect the current state of the business and information is available when needed to affect decisions and actions."*

The executives of an electronics company felt the need for various functions to act more like one company rather than independent operations. They established this principle, which fit into the applications area: *"IS will provide applications that support cross-functional integration of business processes."* This principle made cross-functional systems the priority and empowered IS to manage the complex issues that arise in their implementation.

One insurance company wanted users to choose IT products from the list of approved vendors and equipment. It felt, however, that users might rebel if they were prohibited from making their own selections. Moreover, there was little means to enforce such strict control. The company thought it best to offer a carrot instead of a stick, to offer support instead of threatening control. One of its principles in the infrastructure category captured this philosophy: *"The IS department will maintain a short list of supported products in each technology category. Users may purchase other products at their discretion (subject to spending approval limits), but IS will not support them."*

The IS organization in a different insurance company had responsibility for constructing computer systems, but it was not in a good position to implement the business changes needed to make the systems successful. The user who sponsored the system almost always had ultimate control over the resources and business processes in the department or function. A principle in the organization area put this fact on the record: *"The user-sponsor of a systems project will be responsible for the business success of the system."*

A consumer-products company wanted to make its telecommunications network more efficient. It had one voice-communications network and 24 separate data networks, many of which were incompatible. It wanted the data networks to be compatible not only with each other but also with the voice network. The company established a principle that said, *"We will strive to achieve integration of voice and data communications for purposes of efficiency and increased functionality"*

Fine Tuning

When the smaller groups have finished their work, the entire task force should meet again to resolve any inconsistencies and to agree on the rationale for and implications of each principle. These are also put in writing. Take, for example, the following principle: *"Data created or obtained within the company belongs to the corporation—not to any particular function, unit, or individual. It is available to any user in the company who can demonstrate a need for it."*

The rationale behind it might be: *Data is an important resource and often has greatest value when shared across the corporation. No particular part of the organization should be able to restrict the flow of data except for reasons of corporate information security or the integrity of the data base. To obtain access to data, a potential user generally needs only to request it from the data base custodian.*

The implications would likely include: (1) *Data custodians should respond favorably to reasonable requests for data access;* (2) *the technology infrastructure should make it possible to share data across functions and units;* (3) *IS needs to furnish data custodians with criteria for assessing concern about data security and integrity;* (4) *if the need for access is disputed or if the custodian feels that the security or integrity of the data are threatened, the technology policy committee will resolve the dispute.*

The set of principles, with their rationales and implications, is not a finished product. The task force should present it to senior managers in a workshop setting and encourage everyone to discuss and modify the principles. Although this might seem like an invitation to undo a lot of hard work, more often than not, managers strengthen and refine the principles—they don't tear them apart and try to start from scratch.

The task force should encourage workshop participants to test the principles by applying them to recent decisions or to unresolved issues. One company, for instance, had just decided to bring in an external vendor to manage its telecommunications network. It found this decision consistent with the principle that nonstrategic, utility-oriented aspects of IS would be purchased externally. A company in the financial services industry found, however, that technology investments that business units had recently made on their own were proof that a principle mandating central coordination of investment decisions was not realistic.

Only after senior management has tested and endorsed the principles is the process complete. The task force can then publish and circulate them, and managers can begin to use them. Shortly after it developed its principles, a pharmaceuticals company needed to select its primary data base management software. The principle *"Data base design should emphasize effectiveness in the business environment rather than efficiency in the technical environment"* was the deciding factor in choosing between two of the final software alternatives.

Some companies find it useful to keep narrowing the guidelines for decision making. They can do so by following the principles with a set of models. A model might specify such things as how computers should be linked or how a divisional IS group should be structured. Technology standards make the guidelines even more detailed by stating the particular vendors or equipment the company favors. The standards must conform to the models, and the models must conform to the principles.

Whether or not models and standards accompany them, principles simplify the lives of managers who face one tough technology decision after another and of executives who would otherwise be consulted in each instance. The time and effort spent to discover the common ground between the IT manager and the business manager *puts* the company on firmer ground when it comes to making IT investments that truly reflect business priorities.

Thomas H. Davenport is a senior research associate at the Harvard Business School and is on leave from Index Group, a consulting and research firm, where he was director of research. Michael Hammer is president of Hammer and Company, a consulting and research firm, and he is the research director for the Partnership for Research in Information Systems Management (PRISM). Tauno J. Metsisto is vice president of Index Group and is responsible for the firm's technology architecture practice.

CASE 4
The Consultant's Report

TO: Vice President, Operations
        Eastern Medical Group
FROM: Computer Consulting, Inc.

The following consultant report addresses the pertinent organizational issues that relate to the impending computerization conversion at Eastern Medical Group. This analysis is based upon the perceptions gathered by us during an on-site visit and on information provided to us by your staff.

Organizational Factors Relevant to the System Study

In our initial meeting with your executive board the following facts were discussed:

- Eastern Medical Group, Inc., a multispecialty prepaid group practice has until recently experienced rapid growth, in terms of both patient volume and personnel. The group has 21 permanent full-time physicians, all working on a salary-plus-incentive basis.
- The executive director for the past three years is leaving in six months and a new executive director will be hired to take his place.
- Competition from several other multispecialty group practices and health maintenance organizations has affected the total revenue

(there have been decreases of 5 percent, 10 percent, and 15 percent, respectively, over the last three quarters).

- Expenses have risen steadily over the past two years (6 percent and 9 percent, respectively).
- Turnover in clerical and administrative staff has increased substantially over the past 18 months. Of the 87 nonphysician staff employed 18 months ago, 68 have been replaced by new employees.
- Billing and patient records are decentralized; that is, each physician ("operating unit") bills separately, and accounts receivable are recorded and monitored by each physician's secretary or staff.
- Accounts payable, appointments, internal communication, and other centralized service units are managed by the central office.
- Each physician receives a basic salary plus incentive payments, determined by the number of patients he or she sees. Incentive payments are calculated quarterly and come from the residual that remains after all Eastern Medical Group expenses are paid from patient revenues. The residual has decreased over the past year.
- Eastern Medical Group provides comprehensive medical care for families living in the greater metropolitan area. Although preventive care is emphasized, enrollees are provided with comprehensive medical services including hospitalization, maternity and child care, drugs and medications, a 24-hour emergency service and laboratory and x-ray facilities.
- All information is manually managed at present. The executive committee in charge of planning has contracted with this consulting firm to evaluate the feasibility of implementing a well-designed system that would computerize all medical, socioeconomic, insurance, and administrative data. Out of this, the organization will derive utilization, financial, and comparative data. These kinds of data might be useful in, for example, comparing the Eastern Medical Group patient population with like-sized populations from other groups. Or, data that provide a profile of all physicians in Eastern Medical Group could be used to compare these physicians to groups of physicians elsewhere.
- Every individual in the organization has expressed an eagerness to experiment with a new MIS.

Organizational Objectives of Eastern Medical Group

Consistent with the goal of providing high-quality health care in a cost-effective manner, the objectives are:

- To increase revenue flow through efficiencies in patient billing and receivables management

- To increase accuracy of patient records
- To increase the efficiency of the patient diagnosis and treatment process
- To control resource consumption
- To decrease the number of malpractice suits
- To increase marketing efforts
- To reduce the amount of paperwork
- To increase the efficiency of patient and clinic scheduling.

Analysis of Potential of MIS Conversion at Eastern Medical Group

The problems facing Eastern Medical Group are hardly rare. The inefficient operating methods, inconsistent spending patterns, frequent errors in billing and scheduling, chaotic record keeping and general lack of control are all problems that have a common solution—computerization. Conversion to an automated data processing system can solve all of these problems. Our assessment of your organization is that you should implement a change as soon as possible for the following reasons:

1. The executive committee, physicians, and staff all feel that computerization will improve the efficiency and effectiveness of the organization.
2. There is hardware and software presently available that cannot only fulfill your present needs, but can be installed immediately.
3. Organizations similar to Eastern Medical Group have installed similar computerized MISs and have been generally satisfied.
4. An extensive cost-benefit analysis of Eastern Medical Group indicates that the installation of a computerized MIS will pay for itself in less than three years. The startup costs will therefore be compensated for by the efficiency the system generates.
5. The present level of technical expertise of staff can be enhanced through training to enable them to operate almost any new system.
6. The present organizational structure can be utilized to maintain autonomy over the system, although some technical support is needed.
7. The present physical plant is sufficient to accommodate a computerized MIS.
8. The choice of a hardware and software system will include system design support that will assist the users in articulating the information needs of the organization. The system designers will

be available to define an automated system based on the procedures and functions of the manual system presently in operation.

Recommendations for Implementation

We recommend that the development of a computerized management information system be accomplished in seven incremental phases, each of which will contain two subphases. Furthermore, we recommend the establishment of a core working group, under the authority of a manager of information systems, to facilitate and manage the conversion. This core group will be responsible for the initial design and the training of staff to use the system. The development phases are as follows:

1. **Development of the financial system:** This system will include patient billing and accounts receivable, accounts payable, and general accounting applications.
   a. Familiarization with system, formatting forms, data entry, building master files, and installation of on-line functions.
   b. Training staff for on-line functions.
2. **Development of patient scheduling appointment and registration.**
   a. Familiarization, formatting, data entry, and installation of on-line functions.
   b. Training staff for on-line functions.
3. **Development of order entry/charge capture for ancillary supplies.**
   a. Familiarization, formatting, data entry, and installation of on-line functions.
   b. Training staff for on-line functions.
4. **Development of personnel and payroll system.**
   a. Familiarization, formatting, data entry, and installation of on-line functions.
   b. Training staff for on-line functions.
5. **Development of management reports for monitoring financial condition and efficiency.**
   a. Familiarization, formatting, data entry, and installation of on-line functions.
   b. Training staff for on-line functions.
6. **Development of patient care applications.** These include medical records, medication profiles, and all data pertaining to patients.
   a. Familiarization with system, data entry, building master files, and installation of on-line functions.
   b. Training staff for on-line functions.

7. **Development of interfacing systems for interoperational unit communication.**

   a. Familiarization and installation.

   b. Training staff for implementation.

Each phase will integrate a series of identical stages that will facilitate conversion. These stages are as follows:

1. **Initiation:** clarification of departmental functions and problems
2. **Analysis of needs:** formulation of needs and development of plans for necessary data
3. **System design:** design of output forms
4. **System installation**
5. **System evaluation.**

Questions for Discussion

1. Based on the organizational factors, discuss the justifiability of converting the manual MIS to a computerized MIS at Eastern Medical Group.
2. What further information concerning the organization is needed to justify the conversion?
3. Develop a set of appropriate questions to ask about conversion to a computerized system. Divide the questions according to type and prioritize them.
4. Evaluate the systematic recommendations for installation made by the consultant.
5. What changes do you recommend?
6. Devise a systematic process of conversion in which management intervention, review of outcomes, and management direction are taken into consideration.

MANAGING ORGANIZATIONAL IMPACTS

N REPORTING on the increasing presence of computer terminals in organizations, a *New York Times* reporter observed that "the effect has for the most part been a subtle one, often unnoticed amid the ballyhoo attending the technical innovations." But, she concluded, the impact has been considerable: "The look, sound, and sometimes even the shape of the workplace, after computerization, will never be the same."[1]

This insight has been repeatedly confirmed. For example, in a study that examined the effect of computer technology on the workforce and workplace, Mirvis, Sales, and Hackett found major organizational impacts resulting from computerization,[2] and Morris and Brandon contend that "it is the ability to analyze the full organizational impact of computerization" that will determine the success or failure of reengineering a hospital information system.[3] Most observers agree that computer technology "shakes up the organization for better or worse."[4] Innumerable studies show that productivity,[5] organizational structure,[6] and levels of stress[7] in organizations are affected by computer technology.

These studies and commentators suggest three important lessons for health care professionals. First, the power of computer technology is such that it inevitably has an impact beyond the planned and ostensible area of its application. Second, these organizational impacts have historically been extremely significant for the effectiveness of computer applications. Indeed, they often determine the success or failure of the automation effort. Third, the organizational impacts of computers have routinely been neglected, unanticipated, and not understood—that is, they have not been managed. Both the *Times* reporter and Mirvis and associates point to this phenomenon, the former in discussing the "ballyhoo" focus on the technical aspects, the latter in asserting that the impact of computer technology on people and the workplace is rarely anticipated. As a result the technology fails to bring the increase in productivity that the manager expects.[8] The strategies for computer implementation must, therefore, be clearly understood and carefully constructed.[9]

What can, and usually does, happen when computers are introduced or an existing system is changed? How can managers anticipate what the impacts might be? What can health care professionals do to minimize any disruptive or undesired organizational impacts?

A Framework for Organizational Impacts

Impacts from computerization run the gamut from the obvious to the sublime. Clearly, work methods are often affected, new procedures are established, units are reorganized, and new employees are hired. The office environment is affected by terminals, data processing departments are established, clerical work groups are disestablished, and new jargon is heard. Less obviously, the status and power of units and individuals often change, and work satisfaction and employee morale are affected. How can a manager systematically anticipate and prepare for impacts like these in health care settings?

One way is to use a framework like that developed by Joseph Whorton of the University of Georgia in collaboration with Robert Quinn of the State University of New York at Albany.[10] Their framework consists of a simple matrix which recognizes that there is both a formal and an informal reality to every organization, and that for each there is the individual, the group, and the organization as a whole to consider. Their matrix, thus, can be depicted as shown in Table 5.1.

The formal reality of agencies consists of organization charts, written rules and procedures, work groups, individual job descriptions, and

Table 5.1 Whorton-Quinn Matrix

	Organization	Group	Individual
Formal			
Informal			

so forth. The informal reality is composed of those unwritten, but unmistakable, phenomena of every organization such as "grapevines," power, social groups, individual status, and morale.[11]

The matrix clarifies the six aspects of the agency that computerization might impact:

- Formal organizational structure and processes
- Informal organizational structure and processes
- Formal group structure and processes
- Informal group structure and processes
- Formal individual tasks and processes
- Informal individual structure and processes.

Organization Level—Formal Impacts

At the formal organization level, structures and processes might be affected in a variety of ways. Computerization often entails structural reorganization, such as establishment of a data processing department or expansion of a unit to absorb the computer function. One study has found that computerization typically produces consolidation of departments, reduction in the number of hierarchical levels, and decrease in the control span.[12] Indeed, such restructuring is often a logical result of a pursuit of greater efficiency.

Automation usually has a considerable effect on organizational centralization and decentralization. The impact in this area has been mercurial. During the era of large mainframe computers, information flow was more centralized. With the advent of minicomputers, distributed processing is having a decentralizing effect by dispersing computers, computer personnel, and decision making throughout an organization.

Overall, it is system design, not the computers, that affects centralization and decentralization. For example, even if information processing is centralized in a mainframe computer, decision-making authority can be more decentralized through wider access to the information. On the other hand, a decentralized minicomputer network can be used to reduce decentralized decision making by linking the systems to a central computer with limited access.

In addition, computerization can affect formal procedures. Typically, computers increase both the speed and volume of data collection which, in turn, leads to more standardized operating procedures to deal with speed and volume. Patient flow in a clinic, for example, might be changed to accommodate the system. These procedural changes usually entail tighter controls to ensure data input accuracy. Information flow patterns are the chief procedures that can be affected. Computerization enables both consolidated information processing and wider access to the processed data.

Finally, computerization can have a significant impact on the operating functions of staff departments. The personnel office may find special difficulties in recruiting computer technicians. The legal office may have to deal with privacy legislation. The audit department may find its task complicated by the lack of a written audit trail. In short, computerization may well cause extra work for organizational units.

Organization Level—Informal Impacts

The most telling informal impact is on power in the organization. Computerization tends to shift power from line professionals to staff technicians who know the technology and control information processing. Managers feel this impact when they realize their dependence on the outputs from the computer over which they may have limited control.

This, in turn, can exacerbate department rivalries and create antagonisms among operating units competing for data processing services, as well as between data processing and operating units. In the same vein, the technical jargon can cause communication difficulties within the organization that can nullify the system's potential to meet user needs.

On the other hand, computerization can increase the level of cooperation among organizational units.[13] Standardization of procedures often necessitates analyses of missions and consensus-developing dialogue that can improve organizational harmony.

Group Level—Formal Impacts

Automation can affect work groups in several ways. New work groups might be created and old ones changed to accommodate computerization. Group tasks might also be affected, particularly those associated with data collection. Finally, superior-subordinate relationships may be affected. For example, superiors may be required to quantify worker performance for input to a computerized file.

Group Level—Informal Impacts

In noting the importance of managing change in organization information systems, Joseph Matthews and Robert Smith assert that "any change in the kinds of tasks, form of technology, reporting relationships, and personalities may have a stressful and disruptive (but perhaps unanticipated) impact on the overall performance of the work group."[14] Their point is that formal group impacts inevitably produce latent impacts on the informal group, and that these effects can be serious. In referring to the increased interest in automated clinical systems, Halseth and Paul appreciate this point: they maintain that successful computerization efforts in an organization require a cooperative "partnership" among technical, management, and professional groups.[15] In all organizations informal social groups are a powerful phenomenon. Frequently, these social group realities are the source of considerable satisfaction and are important to group members. Moreover, they typically control the "grapevine"; that is, they are key communication mechanisms, and they establish and maintain group norms of work and productivity. The grapevine structure is so important that, in fact, some Total Quality Management and Continuous Quality Improvement approaches empower and formalize the grapevine structure among work groups and quality teams.

These informal groups can be impacted in a number of ways. First, when formal group structure is changed (by removing or adding members) the social group changes, producing new interactions. This may seriously affect worker satisfaction and alter group norms, resulting in reduced group interactions that affect morale. Group authority and leadership can also be undermined. For example, supervisors who appear to be ignorant of the new systems may discover that their ability to affect the group may be impaired. All of these impacts can, in turn, cause resistance to computerization, a problem so critical that the entire next chapter is devoted to it.

Individual Level—Formal Impacts

At the individual level, the most obvious formal impact is on the nature of individual tasks. New forms might entail less individual discretion and more control over workers; new processes might reduce personal contact and entail worker interaction with an impersonal terminal instead of with another worker. Similarly, a decision maker who previously interacted with several colleagues or subordinates to gather information may obtain it directly from a terminal, thus being able to make decisions faster and with more information, but with less personal contact. On the other hand, the change could ease the individual task and even make the job more fun.

Second, there may be new individuals and new tasks after computerization, and also layoffs or transfers. Technically competent individuals might replace interpersonally competent individuals.

Third, actual experience with computerization indicates that personnel turnover and increased employee absenteeism[16] are fairly common phenomena after automation. Shortages of technical workers have produced a seller's market in which health care organizations have difficulty competing with business organizations that offer higher salaries. Not unexpectedly, a recent survey from the College of Healthcare Information Management Executives revealed that employment turnover for health care chief information officers is very high and appears to be on the rise.[17] Reasons attributed to this high turnover include ambiguity about the position and its expectations, and a poor understanding of the corporate culture by many CIOs.

Individual Level—Informal Aspects

Informal or latent impacts at the individual level have proven to be among the more critical, yet underappreciated and unattended, factors affecting computerization. The formal changes and impacts at all levels obviously do not occur in a vacuum—they inalterably affect the feelings and perceptions of the individuals involved. Reorganization can produce fear and stress just as more standardized tasks can create boredom and a perceived loss of autonomy. Changed tasks and processes can reduce the status and power of individuals, particularly those not schooled in the technology. These individuals, in turn, may feel intimidated by the new technicians. All of these feelings and perceptions can produce resistance to and resentment of the computer which can generate individual actions aimed at undermining the system.[18] On the other hand, individuals could feel greater job satisfaction if computerization eases the physical burden of the job, makes it more rewarding, or offers opportunity for skill development.

The above discussion is merely suggestive of the variety of possible organizational impacts. A tool like the Whorton-Quinn matrix can be useful in triggering insight on the possible impacts of computerization in your own organization. For example, using the matrix, the impacts discussed above are summarized in Table 5.2.

Managerial Implications

The use of computer technology unavoidably involves a variety of possible impacts on both the formal and informal organization. The significance of these impacts for managers is suggested by Sharon First, who notes that "New computer systems or software can become symbols of the unwanted, uncontrollable change in employees' work lives, especially in a period of corporate transition."[19] Indeed,

Table 5.2 Possible Areas of Organizational Impact

	Organization	Group	Individual
Formal or visible	Centralization/ decentralization Departmental tasks Operating procedures Communication network Monitoring mechanism	Work group Structure Tasks Intra-group relationships	Task content Autonomy Recruitment needs Retention
Informal or latent	Power centers Departmental cooperation or rivalry Communication effectiveness	Social group Structure Group norms Attitudes Authority and leadership Morale	Stress Status and power Attitudes Feelings

experience in health care organizations strongly indicates that, left unmanaged, these impacts do derail computerization efforts that are otherwise viable. Successful use of computer technology depends on the ability of managers to understand, anticipate, and manage these organizational impacts.

In addition to identifying areas of organizational impact, health care managers need to understand how these impacts might arise and develop. Several observations are important. First, there is a strong interrelationship among impact areas. For example, a direct impact at the formal organizational level usually produces indirect impacts on both the formal and informal areas of the group and at individual levels; a direct impact at the formal individual level will typically cause indirect impacts at the group and organizational levels. To illustrate, a small change in the individual's task, as in moving a secretary from a typing pool to an isolated word processor, might (1) force the secretarial pool work group to alter its work process; (2) disrupt the secretaries' social group; (3) produce feelings of isolation and boredom in the secretary assigned to the word processor; (4) eventually alter organizational operating procedures to accommodate word processing capabilities; and (5) create new power centers of units having the required skills for word processing. In other words, managers must anticipate the full spectrum of subtle, as well as obvious, impacts.

The degree of impact will undoubtedly vary depending on the nature of the organization and on the computer application. More structured organizations in more stable environments that computerize routine tasks seem to experience less significant organizational impacts than do more complex organizations that introduce computers into more discretionary areas of work. For example, automation of hospital laboratories has produced far milder organizational impacts than has computerization of patient records.[20]

Finally, what can managers do to control or influence the course of these organizational impacts? Two general guidelines are: (1) be as alert to the human systems involved in computerization as to the technical systems; and (2) adapt and sacrifice machine and structural efficiency in favor of social and personnel concerns.

More specifically, managers can plan and implement precise actions to mitigate, enhance, or otherwise control anticipated impacts in each of the six areas discussed above. At the organizational level, managers can consciously determine the amount of decentralization desired and design the change accordingly. They can involve affected department heads to facilitate cooperation, determine where they want power to be distributed and act on that determination, and restrain inclinations to unnecessarily tighten operating procedures.

At the group level, managers can train supervisors before computerization occurs so that the supervisors' authority and status will not be jeopardized; involve group members in discussions of how best to restructure work groups; and intentionally maintain social groups by, for example, not disbanding work groups.

At the individual level, managers need to initiate special recruitment and retention efforts, such as "ego" enticements in place of unavailable financial lures, and provide for ongoing professional development and improvement if they are to acquire and keep good technical people and manage technology resources wisely.[21] They can also provide training before computerization occurs to ease the likelihood of stress or status loss in nontechnical workers, and establish rotating tasks to relieve the boredom of repetitive computer-related tasks. These recommendations are not always easy to put into practice without the requisite organizational development skills. Some managers might, in fact, benefit from outside professional assistance to help implement some of these recommendations.

Conclusion

A key lesson for health care professionals is that unintended organizational impacts are inevitable and, if unattended, can mean the difference between the success or failure of otherwise well-designed information systems. Management of these organizational impacts requires deliberate anticipation, creative and adaptive responses, and a perspective on human and technical realities. Many organizational impacts are predictable and controllable, others can be recognized and influenced. A strategy for effectively managing the change engendered by computerization is crucial for managing modern information systems because organizational impacts can produce resistance which, as the next chapter points out, can result in the failure of the entire computerization effort.

Notes

1. *New York Times*, 23 April 1978, R-6.

2. P. Mirvis, A. Sales, and E. Hackett, "The Implementation and Adoption of New Technology in Organizations: The Impact on Work, People and Culture," *Human Resource Management*, Spring 1991, 113–39.

3. D. Morris and J. Brandon, "Reengineering: More than Meets the Eye," *Computers in Healthcare*, November 1992, 52–54.

4. L. Rogers and R. Farmanfarmian, "Technology Shakes Up the Organization—For Better or Worse," *Working Woman*, November 1986, 100–5.

5. V. Elder, E. Gardner, and S. Ruth, "Gender and Age in Technostress: Effects on White Collar Productivity," *Government Finance Review*, December 1987, 17–26.

6. N. Bailey, "Why the Computer Is Altering Decentralized Management," *International Management*, June 1986, 79.

7. C. M. Ray, T. M. Harris, and J. L. Dye, "Small Business Attitudes toward Computers," *Journal of End User Computing*, Winter 1994, 16–25.

8. S. E. First, "All Systems Go: How to Manage Technological Change," *Working Woman*, April 1990, 47–54.

9. M. Sumner and R. L. Klepper, "The Impact of Information Systems Strategy on End User Computers," *Journal of Systems Management*, October 1987, 12–18.

10. R. E. Quinn and J. A. Whorton, "Computers and Public Administration: Predicting Resistance to Change," Unpublished manuscript, Spring 1978.

11. For unequaled insight on the informal aspects of organizations, see the classic Harvard Business School Background Note by J. R. Fox and P. E. Morrison, "Informal Networks—The Keys to Successful Management"; and R. R. Ritti and G. R. Funkhauser, *The Ropes to Skip and the Ropes to Know* (Columbus, OH: Grid, 1977).

12. K. Rachid, L. Combs, and K. Harper, "Government Workplace Environment: Quality Workplace Environment Program—The Impact of Computers and the Future Environment," *Bureaucrat*, Summer 1990, 17–22.

13. D. Mirvis, A. Sales, and E. Hackett, "The Implementation and Adoption of New Technology in Organizations: The Impact on Work, People and Culture," *Human Resource Management*, Spring 1991, 113–39; C. Foner, M. Noue, X. Luo and J. Kim, "The Impact of Computer Usage on the Perceptions of Hospital Secretaries," *Health Care Supervisor*, September 1991, 27–36.

14. J. R. Matthews and R. J. Smith, "Gauging the Impact of Change," *Datamation* (September 1978): 241.

15. M. Halseth and J. R. Paul, "The Coming Revolution in Information Systems," *Computers in Healthcare*, November 1992, 43, 45.

16. For a representative case in point, see G. W. Dickson, J. K. Simmons, and J. C. Anderson, "Behavioral Reactions to the Introduction of Management Information System at the U.S. Post Office," in *Computers and Management*, ed. D. Sanders (New York: McGraw-Hill, 1974), 410–21.

17. J. Glaser and B. Hersher, "Turnover Rate High for Many Healthcare CIOs," *Health Management Technology*, February 1994, 49–52.

18. T. Reed, "The Frustrations of the Pre-Tech Exec," *Industry Week*, 21 March 1988, 14.

19. First, 47.

20. J. Darnell, "LIS Technologies Must Grow into the 21st Century," *Computers in Healthcare*, September 1993, 41–42.

21. See S. O'Connell, "Five Principles for Managing Technology Resources," *HR Magazine*, January 1994, 35–36.

Selected Readings

Annereu, M. R., J. J. Marsh, and P. Kendrick. "Planning and Implementing a Hospital Information System." *Nursing Administration Quarterly* (Winter 1986): 39–46.

Augustine, F. K., T. J. Surynt, F. A. Dezoort, and D. K. Rosetti. "Organizational Impact of Decision Support Technology: What's Ahead for the 1990's?" *Journal of End User Computing* (Spring 1993): 26–30.

Dorf, B. "How to Install Your New Computer." *Public Relations Journal* (February 1988): 35–36.

Duck, J. D. "Managing Change: The Art of Balancing." *Harvard Business Review* (November–December 1993): 109–18.

Hudgings, C. "Challenges in Information Management for Nursing Practice." *Nursing Administration Quarterly* (Winter 1987): 44–49.

Karon, P. "Having a Champion Is a Key to a System's Success—Installing a Computer System." *PC Week* (19 January 1988): 33–34.

Kortbawi, P. A. "From Manual Charting to Computers: Easing the Transition." *Nursing Management* (November 1993): 89–90.

Metz, E. J. "Managing Change toward a Leading-Edge Information Culture." *Organizational Dynamics* (Autumn 1986): 28–41.

Nurius, P. S., N. Hooyman, and A. E. Nicoll. "Computers in Agencies: A Survey Baseline and Planning Implications." *Journal of Social Service Research* 14, No. 3/4 (1991): 141–55.

Pollalis, Y. A., and I. H. Frieze. "A New Look at Critical Success Factors in Information Technology." *Information Strategy: The Executive's Journal* (Fall 1993): 24–34.

Rivard, S. "Successful Implementation of End-User Computing." *Interfaces* (May–June 1987): 25–34.

Sullivan-Trainor, M. "Three Team Leaders Master a Framework For Managing Change." *Computer World* (2 March 1987): 51–56.

Worthley, J. A., and J. J. Heaphey. "Computer Technology and Public Administration in State Government." *The Bureaucrat* (Fall 1978): 32–37.

READINGS

THE FOLLOWING readings provide concrete illustrations of the concepts in this chapter, as well as some penetrating insights on the nature of organizational impacts in health care. Although both articles focus on the hospital environment, their discussions are equally relevant to other health care settings.

Coralie Farlee provides a comprehensive view that includes specific examples of impact, a different framework from that presented in the chapter for analyzing and anticipating organizational impacts, and concrete suggestions of the kinds of accommodations that can be made to deal with organizational impact. Her framework uses the concepts of formalization, specialization, standardization, and stratification developed by Hage and Aiken, and her analysis offers some major insights on the process of managing change.

Judith Miller introduces a dimension that is often overlooked in information system technology implementation: the implicit organizational culture and norms. This reading suggests that the performance of any technology cannot be separated from the social structure and organizational characteristics of an organization. Taking these issues into consideration is the first step in relating the new technology to organizational effectiveness.

Both Miller and Farlee stress the importance of participation, education, and training in controlling organizational impacts, and both allude to the resistance nemesis that is probed in the next chapter.

The Computer as a Focus of Organizational Change in the Hospital

Coralie Farlee

Administrators and other organization heads often decide to adopt Hospital Information Systems (HIS) in order to achieve greater control over the work of health professionals in the care delivery setting. Sometimes, such information systems are introduced in order to achieve organizational change. Whether introduced as a catalyst for change or for improved control over care delivery, the HIS produces changes rarely anticipated.

Often, the health care administrator contracts for an automated system designed to support certain patient care functions. Rarely is the system assessed for its probable impact on the hospital as an organization (that is, its subunits and organizational structure).

This article is designed to help nursing administrators and others assess the potential impact of technological innovations introduced in health care organizations. The organizational changes often accompanying the introduction of hospital (or medical) information systems will be examined and discussed.

Hospital Information Systems: Functional Characteristics

The most sophisticated computer-based hospital information systems establish patient files in computer memory and make provisions for adding information into these files in an on-line, real-time basis, that is, as successive events occur. The most basic system sorts data entered and disseminates the information to departments throughout the hospital in the form needed and at designated time intervals. Lists, records, and reports can be assembled at scheduled times or on call. Some systems also possess other functions, such as patient billing (linked to the accounting department), or results reporting (linked to a laboratory system).

Input alternatives are of two major types, involving either (1) nursing personnel transcription or physicians' orders, or (2) direct physician input. The latter type usually requires input via the cathode ray tube on whose TV-like screen the physician or a person designated by the physician is presented with questions or choices for the sequence of decisions to be made in creating, extending, or canceling orders for patient care. Some hospital information systems propose to eliminate the patient's medical records file and other written records except for those documents that require patient signatures.

Reprinted with permission from *Journal of Nursing Administration* (Feb. 1978). © 1978 J. B. Lippincott Company.

Whatever system is adopted, the major consequence of this technological change for the workers involved (physicians, nursing staff, pharmacists, dieticians, etc.) is to reduce the flexibility and options involved in decision making and to increase the standardization of the work.

The hospital (organizational and occupational) functions to be performed by the computer are specified in various ways. Typically, this sort of technological change is begun by documenting elements of information required or currently received by various units of the organization. Rules and procedures are derived to specify the elements of information and to structure the manner in which the information is to be entered into the computer terminal. Checks for missing data and for entries that exceed specified limits are programmed into the controls of the information system.

Cautions about certain combinations of information may be included (for example, drug incompatibilities, allergic reactions, or scheduling of meals versus lab tests). As the nursing staff or physician interacts with the terminal, it indicates deficiencies of information in the messages they are attempting to enter and, in such situations, will ask for re-entry or correction or confirmation of the input data.

Usually, rules are specified about who can enter information, who can have access to different levels of information, and what types of data elements should be entered at which points in time.

Among computerized hospital information systems, there is wide variation in the extent to which job functions will be formalized, or standardized. The extent of change depends largely on whether it is assumed that physicians will input directly to the computer terminal, or whether the nursing staff will continue to be responsible, as on a completely manual system, for transcription, interpretation, and, often, completion of physicians' orders. Increased job formalization (to be more fully described) is a byproduct of the procedural standardization required by a computerized system. A specific example of job formalization might be the requirement that medications be administered to all patients on all nursing stations within a half hour. Thus the computer system would expect all medications to be "confirmed" as "given" to patients by that time. If confirmations were not entered in the terminal by one half hour after the time of the ordered administration, reminder messages would be generated. This simplistic procedure allows for no difference in size of nursing units or in patient needs between geriatric, newborn, general medical, or surgical nursing units.

Other organizational changes generally accompany the increased standardization of job functions, rules, and procedures: new jobs or occupational specialties are often added. These jobs bring computer personnel into the organization, and may include new personnel located at nursing stations whose major function is to enter information, and not patient care or other medical or health-related work. During the process of change, the relative status of various departments and of occupational roles may be clarified—(by the priorities assigned and resources allocated)—even more precisely than many would have desired.

Theories of Organizational Change Relevant to Technological Change

A series of studies of technological change have reported a variety of outcomes relative to effects on the organization and the extent of workers' perceived control over work tasks.[1] While studies of automation in industry must be applied with caution to the clinical setting, Blauner's studies of the effect of technological change in various types of industries does set the tone for examining the *functional* change involved in technological change.[2] Changes of functions must be examined in order to assess more clearly the extent of change in worker control.

The most comprehensive yet comprehensible theoretical construct in which to view complex organizational change is that developed by Jerald Hage and Michael Aiken.[3] This paradigm details eight organizational variables, four of which describe the means (or processes) by which organizations operate and four of which describe the *objectives* (goals or outputs) that organizations expect to achieve. Following is a list of the eight organizational variables, each of which is defined.

Means

Formalization The number of rules that define how a job is to be performed; the relative flexibility permitted within jobs.

Centralization The organizational level at which decisions are made; the number of occupations allowed to participate in decision making.

Complexity, or specialization The number of occupational specialties or disciplines in an organization; the variety of levels of education or training among personnel.

Stratification The differences in status among jobs as measured by differential power, income, or prestige; the rate of mobility between status levels in the organization (for example, the number of nurses who become nurse administrators, hospital administrators, or physicians).

Objectives

Productivity The number of units produced per unit of time (such as patient days per year).

Efficiency The average cost per unit of output (such as cost per patient day) and the manner in which resources are utilized.

Adaptability The organization's rate of change and ability to change (often indicated by the number of new programs or new techniques introduced and accepted, or by the amount of time required to introduce change and bring about its acceptance).

Efficient and productive organizations are found to result from high-level decision making; extensive standardization of rules and procedures; rigid stratification; and low task specialization within jobs requiring only minimal skills, education, or training. This sort of static organization is also characterized by a low level of satisfaction among employees and consumers.

But hospitals, like educational institutions and other "people processing" systems, have generally been characterized by a concern with the quality of their output or service—concern that their patients are well cared for. They have also been noted for the diversity of medical and organizational specializations and their concern with innovation.

Recent financial pressures and demands for service are forcing hospitals to reconsider their priorities: efficiency (cost per unit of output) and productivity (effectiveness) are being defined as more relevant organizational goals than previously. Health care administrators hope these new objectives can be achieved without a deleterious effect on patient care and without reducing satisfaction among employees or consumers.

Hospital information systems have been promoted as one mechanism for improving efficiency and productivity. In the following section, we will discuss the four previously defined means of achieving organizational objectives in the context of the HIS.

Hospital Information Systems and Means of Achieving Organizational Objectives

The four means variables are presented in the order of the extent of change they would probably undergo as a result of the introduction of an HIS.

Formalization

The major effects of the introduction of an HIS are likely to be an increase in the number of rules and procedures, more formal or specific requirements for job incumbents, and more direct enforcement of these requirements through the automated system. Any change that increases formalization, or rule enforcement, tends to encounter opposition. The main characteristics of HIS—its provision of greater structure for codification of segments of jobs and its imposition of scheduling requirements and restrictions on many roles—reduces the flexibility and autonomy characteristic of professions.

The essential task, then, is to examine the variation among hospital information systems' software in terms of specification of procedures. Procedural requirements contribute in various ways to increase formalization. These requirements include:

- Specification of the type of personnel able to enter or access information in particular locations. (Access to patient records is often controlled via coded badges or ID numbers.)
- Requirement that each order be complete, with all basic components uniquely identified, before the order can be entered and processed.
- Requirement that all orders be entered in advance (thereby decreasing flexibility to provide emergency medical care or procedures).
- Use of standardized formats for requests, order options, diagnoses, observations.
- Security requirement restricting modification of orders once entered (thereby limiting cancellations, refund options and billing updates).
- Use of schedules, lists, reminders.

Centralization

Decisions about change made at the highest organizational level—such as by boards of governors or federal agency administrators—are likely to be met with resistance by employees. Centralized, high-level decision making is often associated with an absence of channels of communication between organizational levels and limited access to decision-making channels. Consequently, when new ideas are suggested at the organization's lower levels, their approval (and implementation) may take a long time. In addition, if employees recognize that certain procedures and assumptions in packaged software systems are inappropriate for the specific organizational environment, their comments and suggestions will reach a limited audience of decision makers.

The decision to adopt an HIS should be made with the participation of nursing, medical, and administrative personnel. Following implementation of the system, their continued involvement in decision making can be ensured by designating a competent full-time staff member as HIS project director and by the formation of a users' committee to help make technical decisions on operational problems. (This delegation of decision making cannot be a substitute for commitment and support of the hospital management.) The users' committee should include representatives of nursing, medicine, pharmacy, laboratory, and other important hospital units.

Most suggestions to introduce HIS will not originate at the lowest levels. However, it is important to ensure that subordinates and users are free to participate in the selection of a system from the many available and, after its implementation, to suggest necessary modifications.

Specialization

Program change often introduces new occupations or skill clusters into the organization. If persons are recruited from outside, it is unlikely that they will be familiar with the organization's unique characteristics; consequently, existing staff may offer resistance to the program change—in part as a reaction to the introduction of the new roles and new personnel. If individuals from within the organization are selected for retraining, they may never become fully aware of the innovation's implications and potentials, for they may have a limited perspective and may remain oriented to the former status quo.

With the introduction of HIS, it is almost inevitable that increased specialization will occur. An organization may choose either or both of the above options for filling the new specialty positions. Vendor specialists may be introduced into the organization—in addition to or instead of recruiting matching specialties for the regular hospital staff. The hospital may have to integrate such new occupations as a data processing (DP) head and programming staff, DP nurses, DP clerical workers, HIS project officers, and others in liaison capacities to the medical staff, hospital departments, employees, and vendors.

Recruitment of competent in-house computer staff is not without its problems, of course. Programming for HIS requires sophisticated people who support efficient utilization of the computer technology through selection of appropriate trade-offs and alternatives in software procedures. If computer personnel are not added to the organization, the change in occupational specialization will be slight, but the decision not to add such personnel is based on the assumption that the HIS software and procedures are compatible with the organization's structure and goals, and that changes in the vendor's product and hospital procedures will be minimal.

Stratification: The Increased Structuring of Roles

The more that program change is accompanied by increased clarification of status differences in an organization, the greater the likelihood of dissatisfaction with the change, since high stratification tends to increase rigidity and reduce communication and interaction between levels of occupations and organizational units.

Hospitals are work settings where the occupational mix and the rights and obligations of occupations are governed by state and professional licensing agreements. The introduction of badges or regulations specifying which job occupants can perform which tasks results not only in the development of rules within jobs (formalization), but also in a clearer specification of which roles and which organizational units (e.g., nursing department, x-ray department) can have access to particular kinds of information or can perform certain tasks. This clarification of the hierarchy of access to information results in a more precise exposure of the differential rights, obligations, and distribution of rewards (status) among jobs and departments.

When new occupations are introduced (specialization) with the HIS, the hospital has several options regarding departmental and hierarchical placement of the new personnel. The occupants of the new roles can be inserted into existing departments, or else new tasks can be added to old roles. In either case, the location of HIS-related tasks is generally clearly specified or easily assumed. This occurs, for example, when data processing is added to the finance and accounting department on the rationale that data processing serves the financial interests of the organization. Their status is also clear when DP personnel are introduced at a nursing station on the assumption that they work for the head nurse and do tasks similar to those of clerical workers.

On the other hand, if a new HIS department is created, at staff level, the status of HIS versus other departments may not be clearly defined. The HIS department can receive and consider requests from the finance and accounting department, from nursing, laboratory, dietary, and other departments, as well as from members of the administrative staff and physicians. This structure also permits a loose definition of the status of HIS staff or liaison personnel in other parts of the hospital; it may, for example, permit a colleague-type relationship to develop between the head nurse and the DP person taking on unit manager tasks.

Progress of Change

Low formalization, low centralization, high specialization, and low stratification are most conducive to employee acceptance of and accommodation to the sort of technological change introduced by the HIS.

It is also important that the time schedule of the system's introduction not deviate substantially from the expectations of those affected and that the change assume a steady though not necessarily rapid rate. Optimally, there should be a realistic implementation schedule agreed to by all major parties involved; this schedule along with the objectives for the HIS should be published, and the schedule adhered to as far as possible. If there is a deviation from the schedule or from announced objectives without the full participation and consent of those affected, interest will lag and confidence in the new system will wane. It is also important that users of the system know that the change has occurred, that is, when the parallel, or test, phase on particular segments is completed and that the information in the automated system is to be relied on.

Acceptance of Innovations: Socialization Models

A number of sociologists have developed models of the process by which new norms of behavior are internalized. These socialization models are presented here with a view to managing behavioral change in conjunction with technological change in organizations.

Talcott Parsons has outlined four major stages of socialization.[4]

Stage 1

In this, the "permissiveness" stage, crucial inputs from the socializing (or change) agent are *information about the change and expected new behavior and opportunities to learn* the new behavior. Lowered rewards for, and decreased satisfaction with, the prior behavior and achievements should provide some incentive to take on the desired new behavior.

Stage 2

In this, the "support" stage, the inputs from stage 1—information about the change and opportunities to learn new behavior—continue to be offered, but *external rewards for the new behavior* are given and *confidence in performance of the new behavior* is encouraged. The latter two elements should, theoretically, produce increased internal satisfaction with performance of new behavior. (The disorganization generated at the first stage will decrease as the sense of accomplishment increases with improved performance of the new behavior.)

Stage 3

In this, the "denial of reciprocity" stage, the inputs from stage 1—information about the expected new behavior and opportunities for learning it—are still offered, but *external rewards are decreased*, while the new patterns of behavior are internalized. Rewards for the new behavior come from internal, rather than external, sources.

Stage 4

During the final stage, external rewards, gratification, self-rewards, and satisfaction for performance of the new task are all increased, while information about performance and opportunities for performing the behavior are maintained.

By the time stage 4 is reached, the target of change should have given up the old behavior because it is no longer rewarded (the costs of doing it are too high). It is assumed that the new behavior expected by the change agent has been adapted.

Bredemeier and Stephenson have summarized and elaborated upon Parsons' scheme.[5] Their model indicates that to achieve the desired change, the change agent should reduce rewards for prior behavior by reducing approval from the original reference group (that is, those whose opinions matter a lot); changing the definition of the original reference group so that their sanctions are no longer so important; increasing the interaction between change agents and change targets; providing opportunities for self-approval resulting from correct performance of the new behavior; and giving opportunities for pleasure for performance of the new behavior or for giving up the old behavior. Then change agents should increase rewards for the new behavior by providing a period of anticipatory socialization (where change targets are eagerly awaiting the change and its consequences); providing contingent rewards; deferring gratification for new behavior; and reducing feelings of relative deprivation. Further, the change target should be provided with a clear definition of his or her status and with consistent expectations from the change agents. Change agents should also allow for flexibility in learning, furnish adequate role models for the new behavior, and provide facilities for learning the new behavior.

The literature recommends that change agents in organizations gain the confidence of the change targets, for only when agents are trusted will their efforts at providing rewards for new behavior and negative sanctions for old be meaningful.[6] Often, change agents do not have a prior or stable base in the organization, and thus they must compete with existing reference groups in the resocialization effort. If this is, indeed, the case, efforts to reduce the importance of previous reference groups will be more difficult.

Relevance of Socialization Models for Hospital Information Systems

Most of the literature on behavioral change is derived from theories based on groups having little power, such as the young minorities or the handicapped.[7] However, in the case of HIS, the change targets hold a stable and powerful position in the organization, whereas the change agents are in a more tentative position. Nursing staff and physicians must learn new procedures that involve changes in task structures and in certain role expectations. Both groups are powerful and may resist change initiated by personnel whom they consider to be peripheral to circumstances surrounding the delivery of health care. Thus, in order to be effective, the change agents should be in occupational roles that traditionally have some leverage with the group whose behavior is being affected. It is not realistic to expect that clerical workers or nurses can have a large impact on physicians. Nurses put in the role of change agents for the purpose of changing physicians' order writing practices are not likely to have the necessary leverage (they are not and will not become the important reference group needed) and they are likely to experience status inconsistency. Likewise, it is improbable that data processing staff will have an impact on the decision making and health care practice of either physicians or nursing staff. However, some software packages incorporate significant behavioral change and attempts at social control of the health professionals. It is thus extremely important that nursing administrators be actively involved in this technological change, for it is likely to have a major impact on the nursing staff.

It is important to examine the functional implications of any specific hospital information system being explored. If new occupations are to be introduced into the hospital, if older writing and other aspects of the practice of nursing and medicine are to be affected, hospital and nursing administrators should be aware of the probable restructuring of roles that will follow introduction of an HIS. If extensive formalization (reduction of flexibility) is to occur with respect to major job functions of health professionals, negative "unanticipated" consequences are likely.

When program change is attempted, it is followed by an effort to gain employee conformity, or compliance, with new procedures and behaviors required by the change. In this effort it is important to provide hospital personnel with accurate knowledge of the change;

facilities and resources that will help them learn the new behaviors and procedures; rewards for conforming behavior; and negative sanctions for inappropriate behavior. Inappropriate behavior includes both irrelevant prior behavior and deviant or innovative behavior that may develop in response to the technology being introduced.

Change agents should be significant to others who are involved in communicating their expectations about the new behavior and should develop meaningful rewards for conformity and appropriate and negative sanctions for deviance.

Selecting Hospital Information Systems

Hospital information systems are said to produce increased formalization, centralization, and stratification, all of which should result in increased efficiency and productivity. However, organization theory hypothesizes that these factors are inversely related to employee satisfaction and accommodation to change. Furthermore, sociological theory postulates that abrupt and extensive attempts to achieve increased efficiency, often effected via increased job structuring (formalization), will not necessarily result in improved productivity and effectiveness. This hypothesis is supported by the results of a study conducted by the author to observe the implementation in one hospital on HIS medications application.[8]

Administrators, including nursing administrators, must make a crucial decision when weighing the various approaches to HIS. In order to achieve the optimum effect on organizational and unit productivity and effectiveness, a moderate increase in organizational centralization, job formalization, and occupational stratification is recommended. The following guidelines should be helpful in this effort.

1. Permit only a moderate increase in job standardization. This can be achieved by ensuring that:
   - health professionals have unrestricted access to patient data in order to carry out their functions of ordering, charting, and carrying out treatment plans
   - orders can be entered and accessed in a manner as similar to the present (manual) procedures as is feasible. Some standardization between nursing units may still be felt necessary, since there can be wide variation in treatment plans and individual physician ordering patterns by type of patient diagnosis (and thus by type of nursing station).
   - there is flexibility in the technological system to accommodate organizational and health professionals' needs for lists, schedules, and ordering patterns.

2. Insist on sufficient participation in decision making by relevant sections of the organization. The increase in centralization can be moderated by ensuring
   - participation by health practitioners in decisions about applications, changes, vendor's role, etc.
   - participation by unit and department administrative staff in committees and decisions affected by the HIS.
3. Soften the effects of increased occupational stratification, which is often an unintended consequence of the introduction of an HIS, by
   - incorporating any change agent roles (e.g., DP nurse, HIS physician) within the organization or by selecting as change agents health professionals who are opinion leaders with a political base and constituency who support the change and will effectively communicate the need for new behaviors and routines.
   - providing flexible options regarding access to patient record so that, for example, nurse aides, occupational therapists, are *not* prevented access to diagnostic and treatment information available to practically *anyone* looking through a manual, or paper, record.

In the initial phases, at least, the factors contributing most to successful implementation of the HIS are the organizational variables *formalization* and *centralization*. The author suggests that the HIS would be most likely to win acceptance in a hospital setting under the following conditions: (1) the HIS is not permitted to change the physician's role extensively or place excessive restrictions on the nurse or other health practitioners (formalization); (2) all occupations, departments, and users are allowed to participate in decision making about the system and its modifications (centralization); (3) excessive changes in hierarchical stratification of occupations are not introduced (stratification); and (4) the progress of change is definite, continuous, visible, and in conformity with the advance plans and schedule.

A Caveat

Frequently, reality does not turn out to be the way theories predict it will be. And schemes such as the one proposed above do not always encompass all the factors that bear upon decisions.

Vendors of HIS offer a variety of approaches to the same applications, and so a hospital's HIS committee may select the approach it favors.[9] Some hospital organization heads are fairly knowledgeable about the various alternatives, objectives, and probable effects of HIS.

Members of the organization could, therefore, be more effectively involved in decision making about the HIS, even those with service or "turnkey" (software) arrangements.

In some instances, decision makers (with some assistance from federal or state governments and insurance companies) may determine that the HIS that *does* attempt to provide the *most in standardization and control* over particular roles and/or the one that has the *most effect on restructuring* the roles is the right system for their organization.[10] A hospital may select one particular HIS approach and philosophy precisely because it wishes to achieve more conformity to policies and procedures.

The above presentation should not be interpreted to mean that the system that attempts to achieve more administrative control over the documentation-related activities of all types of health practitioners should not be attempted. Rather, the intent here is to point to the potential risks and outcomes involved in such an attempt and to outline possible unanticipated consequences for the organization.

When decision makers are aware of the risks and alternatives inherent in the various hospital information systems being promoted, they can make informed decisions regarding the selection, adoption, and implementation of one of them. It is hoped that knowledge of these factors can help make decision makers and implementors, including physicians and nursing administrators, aware of those areas in which reorientation and education programs are most necessary.

References and Notes

1. See, for example, the following studies: Karsh, B. and Siegman, J. Functions of ignorance in introducing automation. *Social Problems*, Vol. 12, No. 2, 1964, pp. 141–50; Friedmann, G. *The Anatomy of Work, Labor, Leisure and the Implications of Automation*, translated by Wyatt Rawson. New York: The Free Press of Glencoe, 1961, pp. xiv–xv; chapter VII and p. 50.

2. Blauner, R. *Alienation and Freedom: The Factory Worker and His Industry*. Chicago: The University of Chicago Press, Phoenix Edition, 1967, p. 170.

3. Hage, J. An axiomatic theory of organizations. *Administrative Science Quarterly*, Vol. 10, no. 3, 1965, pp. 289–320; Hage, J. and Aiken, M. *Social Change in Complex Organizations*. New York: Random House, 1970.

4. Parsons, T. and Bales, R. F. *Family Socialization and Interaction Process*. Glencoe, Ill.: Free Press, 1955, pp. 234–37; Parsons, T., et al. *Working Papers in the Theory of Action*. New York: Free Press, 1953.

5. Bredemeier, H. C. and Stephenson, R. H. *The Analysis of Social Systems*. New York: Holt, Rinehart and Winston, 1962, chapter 4.

6. Bennis, W. G., et al. (eds.). *The Planning of Change, Readings in the Applied Behavioral Sciences*. New York: Holt, Rinehart and Winston, 1961.

7. See, for example, Goslin, D. (ed.). *Handbook of Socialization Theory and Research*. Chicago: Rand McNally and Company, 1969, chapters 25–29.

8. Goldstein, B. and Farlee, C. *Hospital Organization and Computer Technology: The Challenge of Change*. New Brunswick, N.J.: Health Care Systems Research, 1972. Copies of the final report are available from the Social and Economic Analysis Division of the Health Resources Administration, NHCSR, DHEW, and are on file with the Hospital Information Systems Sharing Group.

9. The Hospital Information Systems Sharing Group is composed of several vendors with HIS software and various hospitals that are implementing different HIS packages with various structured assumptions and varied organizational consequences.

10. The TRI-service Medical Information System (TRIMIS) is planned for introduction in "all" Department of Defense hospitals over the next five to ten years on the assumption that one standardized system *can* be implemented throughout all DOD hospitals and clinics.

Coralie Farlee is senior staff associate with the Association of Medical Colleges.

The Hidden Dimension in Information Systems Technology

Judith A. Miller

When a hospital decides to adopt or change its information systems technology, those involved in the decision tend to believe that what they are buying is simply a set of software routines and reports. Management expects that the most significant improvements in the hospital's overall organizational effectiveness will be derived from the type of hardware and software chosen; the particular package from the particular vendor. What the hospital in reality is buying, along with the software of choice is a massive program of organizational change, a change so broad as to encompass everything from job descriptions to risk-taking norms to the basic issues of power, authority and decision making style. The extent to which these organizational factors are explicitly addressed as part of both the initial planning and implementation processes, will influence the success of the installation and the degree to which the new technology contributes to the hospital's overall effectiveness as an organization.

Though systems technology has grown from its initial focus on financial reporting systems to include sophisticated clinical applications, the approaches to planning and implementation still come from the "controlling" models of management of the 1960s and '70s, rather than the "resourcing" models of the '80s. Briefly stated, the controlling model is the familiar top-down hierarchy in which each level of management circumscribes and limits the scope of each lower level, reserving the broader functions for itself. The focus is on making sure that what is supposed to get done does get done, and that people do what they are supposed to do. The resourcing model is easily visualized by inverting the normal hierarchical diagram so that the lowest level is at the top and the CEO is at the bottom. In this model, management's role is one of supporting and providing resources for those people for whom they are responsible. By coordinating and facilitating the availability (people, materials, and dollars), each employee is needed to accomplish their goals and performance objectives within the overall organizational mission. It is broadening rather than a constricting model, in which the interrelationships of people and of tasks are resources as valuable as raw materials and dollars.

In the controlling model, the information system exclusively focused on the content of the system—the data elements collected, the kinds of reports produced, the formats of the various screens and so on.

While these are critical concerns, the process of organizational change is also important. If considered at all, the organizational issues are usually misunderstood and dismissed. They are viewed as something to be tolerated, as disruptions to normal functioning that will die down sooner (hopefully) or later, or that will go away if ignored. The hospital rarely views this period of time, the process of systems planning and implementation, as a dynamic opportunity for achieving positive change in its life as an organization.

Some of the issues endemic to the introduction of new technology include:

- *Readiness of management, as well as other hospital personnel, to accept the new technology and accompanying changes.* What is the impact of the lack of commitment and ownership on the planning and implementation process? How can a sense of commitment be built among all personnel, including those who were opposed to the project?

- *Manifestations of resistance and rejection of change.* What kinds of behaviors are demonstrated by those people who oppose the installation but were powerless to prevent it? What kinds of behaviors are the normal and natural reactions to change, even among those supportive of the change? How can resistance be responded to in a positive, developmentally helpful way?

- *Centralized vs. decentralized, controlling vs. resourcing management models.* In a hospital in which no one has any real authority to make a decision except the CEO or CFO, and departmental managers are afraid to accept responsibility (and may not, in reality, be encouraged to do so), how is the myriad of necessary, detailed operational decisions obtained? What kind of changes in the authority structure can be made to facilitate decision making by those who have the expertise, regardless of formal position?

- *Ownership of data and the inherent power in controlling information flows.* When an individual has been the exclusive source of data or a report, his/her sense of self-esteem and importance to the organization can be threatened when the data is maintained by the system and equally available to all users. How can the installation and development process be undermined by a person whose power is so threatened? How can employees' needs for self-esteem in the light of changing role definitions be addressed in a positive way for both the project and individual?

- *Team-oriented problem solving vs. blaming and fault-finding.* How willing and skilled are individuals, across departmental lines, to compromise and collaborate in resolving issues around work flow, data definitions, and departmental responsibilities? Do the organizational norms support this kind of problem solving or is defensiveness and the protection of turf subtly or overtly promoted? What kinds of team-building and communications skills training may be required to facilitate the implementation process?

- *Risk-taking behavior and the reward and punishment system.* Are mistakes considered to be part of the price of doing business or is an unattainable standard of perfection the expectation? Are creative suggestions met with encouragement or are they subject to ridicule? To what degree is management open to constructive, supportive criticism? To what degree does management surround itself with and reward those who are "yes-men?" What kinds of risk-taking norms will assist managers and employees alike in coping with the learning curve involved in any new system's installation?

- *Full integration of the new technology into the work environment.* Many hospital personnel tend to believe that once "the computer comes," their work procedures will be basically unchanged, except that there will be a computer involved somehow. What is the most effective way to stimulate the total rethinking workflow, so that the new system may become the crux of its operation, rather than just an appendage?

Just as these organizational issues and characteristics are impacted by the new technology, they also heavily influence the planning and implementation process itself.

It is well recognized that the hospital is a complex organizational entity. Highly stratified and bureaucratic, it is layered with many detailed policies and procedures that define nearly all activities and interrelationships. Departmental management can be more concerned with matters of turf and the maintenance of control and prerogative, at the expense of achieving overarching hospital-wide goals. The hospital is also an organization in which key powers, such as the medical staff, may not have formal structural position but exert enormous influence within and upon that structure.

The performance of any information systems technology cannot be separated from the context, the organizational culture, in which it is expected to function. The "garbage in, garbage out" phenomenon applies not just to data, but equally to environmental and cultural influences. A new information system will not correct existing management or personnel problems. On the contrary, they will be exacerbated, becoming increasingly dysfunctional at a very critical time. Most current systems, being highly integrated from a design and technological perspective, function most effectively in a consciously-interdependent, team-oriented, problem-focused environment. This is one in which decision making is located at the "lowest" appropriate level, risk-taking is positively regarded, trust levels are high, and collaborative problem solving is the norm. When the interdependency of technology and organizational context is denied or ignored, the hospital will experience problems. Phrases such as "The data on this report is meaningless," "It doesn't do what they said it would," "It takes twice as many people to do the job as it used to," "Nobody likes to use the system," begin to be heard. Any attempted articulation of the specific reasons for the dissatisfaction is often difficult and vague. When expressed, symptoms rather than underlying problems are the focus. Correctives are sought for the symptoms rather than the problems, which only creates further problems. The hospital, frustrated and dissatisfied, begins the search for a new system, a new vendor, a new panacea.

But the search for panaceas is expensive, both in terms of tangible hardware and software conversion costs, as well as productivity and morale. In today's highly competitive, cost-conscious climate, hospital management must turn its attention to this hidden dimension of information systems technology. Management must begin to look closely at the culture and norms in the hospital in light of its overall performance objectives for the new technology. Unless this is done, hospitals will continue to cycle from system to system, panacea to panacea, with little to show for all the time, energy, and dollars involved. Concurrent with the development of a request for proposal (RFP), should be an assessment of the hospital's structure organizational processes relative to the scope of the technological change being planned. As the selection process proceeds, compare its assumptions and norms with those of the proposed systems, to determine areas of congruence as well as difference. From these assessments, strategies can then be developed that will facilitate the planning and implementation of both the chosen technology and the organizational change effort. With recognition and attention, the hidden dimension can become, instead of an ambush, an opportunity through which the new technology can serve as a catalyst for total organizational growth.

Judith Miller is a Senior Systems Analyst with the Information Management Services Division of Travenol Healthcare Information Services.

CASE 5
The Survey

C ARL GRAHAM had felt increasingly disenchanted with the way things were going. Ironing out interpersonal, interdepartmental and organizational problems had taken up most of his time recently. This seemed uncharacteristic for Valley View Hospital, because it always had the reputation as a smooth-running operation. His tenure as chief executive officer of this 235 bed, acute-care community hospital could be characterized, at least up to this point, as productive, with a minimum of major problems. Upgrading the physical plant, developing innovative new programs, and increasing the average occupancy rate had been among his latest accomplishments at Valley View. His most recent accomplishment had been installing a computerized hospital information system. Accompanying the new technological change was a restructuring of the organization. Figure 5.1 shows a simplified organization chart of Valley View before the implementation of the new MIS. Figure 5.2 shows a simplified chart of Valley View after the implementation.

It was obvious that the source of the recent problems had been directly associated with the new changes, although it was difficult for Carl to pinpoint precisely what those problems were. A physician friend of Carl's, after having been told about the recent troubles, commented that it sounded as if the recent troubles were "symptoms." She suggested that the hospital needed a "work-up" and that probably one of the best ways to give it one was to elicit anonymous feedback from

Figure 5.1 Organization Chart, Preimplementation of MIS

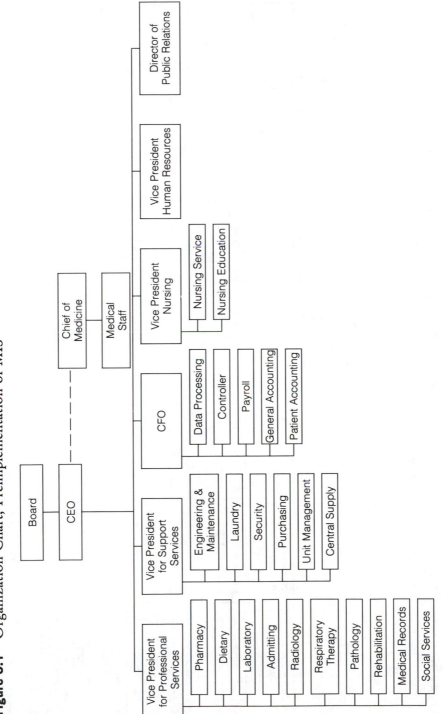

Figure 5.2 Organization Chart, Postimplementation of MIS

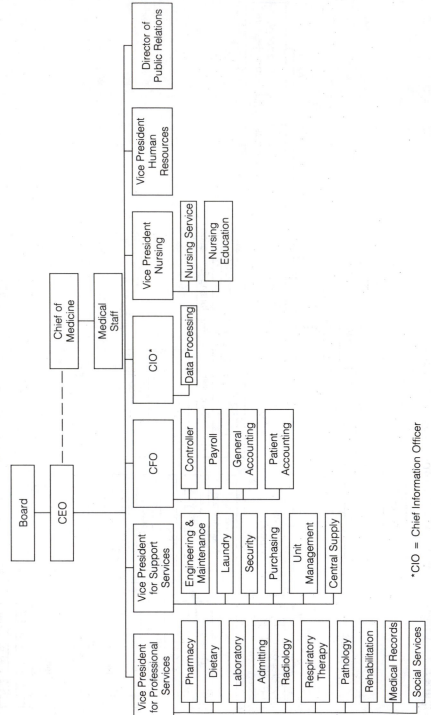

*CIO = Chief Information Officer

the staff and patients of the hospital. Carl put this advice into operation by conducting a written survey, asking recipients to comment, either positively or negatively, on their reactions and experiences relating to the system. Some responses were as expected; others were mystifying.

The Responses

Since you put in this new system there have been many new faces in the hospital and I'm unsure of their jobs. I know they're not doctors, nurses, or administrators. What do they do?

This new "information" department is everywhere. Do all departments report to them, or are they here to service all departments?

I'm basically happy with the new system. As a nurse, it's important for me to spend as much time as possible with patients, and the new portable nursing unit terminal has helped to do that. But, by adding this new "thing" you've eliminated the ward clerks. I think that's a mistake because a machine can't take the place of a person. My ward clerk not only helped with the paperwork, but helped in so many other ways (by answering the telephone, talking with patients and families, and so on).

I've been a secretary for 20 years and I thought I could never learn to use the computer, but I did! I was frightened at first, but I've finally learned. Now that I have gained this new skill I think I should get a raise in pay. I've looked in the classified section of the newspaper and I think I could made more money somewhere else now that I have this new skill.

I'm going to sue the hospital. This job has given me an ulcer. I'm afraid I will be fired if I don't learn how to use the computer. And besides, I hear that sitting in front of a computer monitor all day will make you sick.

Are we a "people processing" institution or a "data processing" institution? Since this new system was put in, I see less of my coworkers, spend less time talking with people, and have no one around to help me get through the day. Computers are boring!

As a manager, it's gratifying to know that this hospital has finally arrived in the twentieth century. I can now work with standardized operating procedures that can't be changed quickly by someone's whim. I'm also no longer burdened by always having to make routine decisions. The computer does it for me now.

This new system is like military school. It has a lot of rules and it is merciless. Before, I could change something in my department if I wanted to; now I have to ask these new guys in information services, or the system won't do what I want it to. I have no flexibility to do what I want. Who's running my department, them or me?

Since the computer, I've had more people call in sick and leave their job. I've spent most of my time trying to hire people in my department who can use a computer.

Why does nursing always come first? It seems as if they get all the training and help when something goes wrong with the computer. When the computer crashed last week, we ran our department just fine, but we heard nursing screaming all day. Everyone in my department refuses to touch the computer and learn the new system; they're always dumping work on me and taking me away from my own work. The new microcomputer in my bosses' office is just collecting dust. He thinks that working on the computer is for secretaries.

I don't like the idea of having patient records on the computer. Can anyone just look at them anytime they want?

Last time I was a patient in this hospital I waited nearly four hours to be admitted. This time I was in and out of admitting in 20 minutes. But you keep sending my ex-wife's hospital bills to my home. I've told the admitting office to send them to her home and they're still being sent to me. What's the matter with that damn computer of yours?

I think the maintenance department should be responsible for ordering, storing, and installing the paper in the printer in our department. Why should we have to mess with the printer? We're not mechanics.

Scrap it!

Questions for Discussion

1. Classify the comments into organizational, group, and individual issues.

2. What were the intended and unintended organizational impacts of the new system at Valley View Hospital?
3. Are the "symptoms" of organizational malaise at Valley View treatable? Why or why not?
4. Could Carl have predicted or averted the various impacts on the organization that were articulated in the responses?
5. Develop a strategy for Carl to effectively manage the change caused by the computerization effort.

MANAGING RESISTANCE

PERHAPS THE single most prevalent, yet underappreciated, negative phenomenon accompanying computerization is user resistance. Both professionals and office workers have consistently tended to challenge the use of computers in their organizations. Because managers often have failed to deal with staff resistance, many technically sound computer applications have been inordinately troubled, or have failed altogether. Shoshona Zuboff, a social psychologist at Harvard Business School has been studying resistance to computerized information technologies for a number of years, and reports that resistance is not isolated, but rather is endemic and " . . . an implied threat to the whole structure of authority."[1]

In recent years this phenomenon has become a focus of research attention. Charles Eberle, a noted information technology specialist consistently finds that " . . . with new technologies . . . resistance is enormous."[2] A survey by Richard Walton of the Harvard Business School supports this contention. Of a large sample of organizations with serious commitments to information technologies, he found middle managers to be major barriers to change.[3] Prompted by evidence of severe resistance to computers at one hospital, researcher Alan Dowling surveyed a randomly selected sample of 40 public and private hospitals. He estimated that staff resistance to and interference with computerized information systems had occurred in nearly half the hospitals that have attempted to implement such systems. Furthermore, he found that "interference can have significant consequences in terms of cost, lost earnings, organizational disruption, and poor quality of care."[4] The magnitude of the problem is nationwide, and it can have an enormous effect on corporate America's drive to reengineer itself. Recent polls show that while 70 percent of large U.S. companies claim to be reengineering their information technology systems, nearly one quarter of these reengineering projects are failing. Experts attribute much of this failure to staff resistance.[5]

Both the Dowling study and the recent poll reveal that the problem is much more widespread and serious than most managers realize. In fact, although Dowling reported that hospital managers generally thought resistance was rare or unique to their hospital, resistance to computerization efforts appears to be the rule, rather than the exception, and it extends from front-line workers to clinicians, and even to top executives. This is illustrated by the wide range of professional journals that emphasize the drawbacks of computerization. Articles such as: "Can a Computer Tell How Good a Doctor You Are?" (*Medical Economics*),[6] "Are Information Systems Your Friend or Foe?" (*Chief Executive*),[7] "Nursing Views Computers as Both Friends and Foes" (*Hospitals*),[8] and "How Soon Will You Be At The Mercy of a Hospital Computer?" (*Medical Economics*),[9] appear to express pervasive resentment by a wide range of health professionals.

Based on his experience as a consultant in private business, Roger Hallock concludes that "many computer systems barely live up to half their potential" because of top management resistance,[10] a conclusion consistent with a *Fortune* magazine article that asserts "information technology cannot reshape an organization unless the organization finds some way to make workers comfortable with computers."[11] These reports all indicate a need for health care professionals to deal with resistance effectively if computerized information systems are to work.

Recognizing Resistance

Recognition of the nature of resistance has frequently been impeded by its subtlety. Resistance consists of any number of acts, deliberate or subconscious, that interfere with the effective implementation or use of a computerized application. The range of such acts runs the gamut from clear, direct, active behavior—such as physical abuse of equipment—to subtle, indirect, and passive forms, such as simple nonuse of a carefully designed system.

Physical sabotage of computer equipment has occurred. Terminals have been smashed, paper clips inserted into scanners, and wires pulled on printers. However, studies more frequently find extensive use of much more subtle, clever, and indirect forms of resistance.

Chief among these is absenteeism of some form, including increased truancy from work, but also lateness, work slowdowns, and nonavailability while at work.

"Bad-mouthing" the system is another common form: "This system stinks. I told you it wouldn't work!" "The terminals are always down. They're a danger to patient care." Comments like these are at least occasionally heard during most computerization efforts. Sometimes they are based on totally fabricated woes, sometimes they blow up minor and anticipated problems, sometimes they are based on intentionally faulty use of the system, such as repeatedly hitting the wrong key on a terminal and then claiming that the system does not work or is too difficult to use.

Nonuse of an installed computer system is a fourth frequently encountered form of resistance. Unwilling to depend on the expensive computer system, workers have continued using old systems, and resisting supervisors have influenced unit employees to not use the computer.

Perhaps the most serious form of resistance is data tampering, which can consist of withholding data or inputting errors. For example, case workers incompletely fill out automated forms on clients, or users intentionally input incorrect data or a wrong code in order to upset the system or arouse complaints.

Who are the resisters? The preponderance of studies find that resistance is found in all levels of the organization.[12] Dowling concluded that each form of resistance "can be used by almost any key staff member at any time during implementation."[13] Indeed, the evidence suggests that professionals, whose tasks are more discretionary than routine, may be the more frequent and effective resisters.[14] This can be understood by examining possible causes of resistance.

Why Resistance to Computers?

There are at least seven possible explanations for resistance to computerization. A basic reason may be the economic determinant. Despite evidence to the contrary, computers are associated with layoffs and unemployment.[15] James Manuso, a specialist in reactions to computers, claims this to be the key cause: "First, of course, is people's fear that they're going to lose their jobs, that some machine is going to come in and do the work instead."[16] Indeed, labor unions often reinforce this perception in vehemently resisting automation during contract negotiations.[17] The computer is viewed as a timesaving and laborsaving device that decreases the need for labor and middle managers. However, research shows that automation does not usually cause job losses; instead, job displacement (e.g., transfer) is a frequent result. Zuboff notes that while executives typically try to justify computer systems by showing how they would eliminate jobs, few managers face the fact that the jobs cut—or redefined—might be their own. Her most recent work shows that organizations that have gone the furthest in using computerized information technologies tend to have only about half the managerial layers as their rivals.[18]

Perhaps the most common cause of resistance, however, is psychological. Computers can easily be ego-threatening. Proud professionals who know very little about computer technology may fear a loss of prestige and status in the organization if computers are used. Secretaries who control file cabinets may resist computers because computers would deprive them of the power to dispense information from the files. Supervisors might resist out of fear that a computer would do the scheduling function that previously was a source of power for them.

Third, computers might be resisted for social reasons. Plans to disperse various members of work groups to isolated terminals or word processors might encounter resistance. It may well be that the prime satisfaction some workers derive from their job is the chance it provides to talk with coworkers. Removing this social benefit can prompt strong dissatisfaction. Additionally, resistance could be caused by a socially acceptable attitude of enmity toward machines. Resisting computers might simply be viewed as "the thing to do."

Fourth, there may be intellectual reasons. Professionals who hold high human values, such as health care and human services workers, may have ideological barriers to accepting anything that might produce less human contact or deprive them of some personal and professional freedom. As one commentator puts it: "Some feel that computers dehumanize the care of patients . . . computerization reflects an increase in technical quality at the expense of humanness (i.e., 'high tech' without 'high touch.')"[19]

Fifth, there may well be historical reasons for resistance to computers, such as a previous bad experience with a computerization effort.

Sixth, organizational causes may be discerned. For example, computers might be resisted because some individuals see little connection between what the machine does and what role they have in the organization. Just as it is unusual to enter any modern organization that has no personal computers, it is equally unusual to enter the office of a chief executive and find a well worn PC. In her book *Leadership and the Computer*, Mary E. Boone says that, "The problem is that many executives don't know that computers are capable of extending their creative and leadership abilities."[20] Similarly, many practitioners in human service organizations perceive that computers are irrelevant to the practice of their profession.[21]

Finally, operational reasons can be identified. As one observer notes, "People love innovation, but hate change."[22] If we subscribe to the notion that technology means ongoing operational adjustment, the increasing application of computers suggests an inevitable operational upset. This aversion to change may simply be that people are obliged to think, work, and interact differently, consequences often associated with computerization.

Obviously there may be other reasons for resistance. It is not easy to determine why an individual or a group in an organization resist the use of computers; however, basic fears of job loss, failure, and change are common in general. The important point is that understandable, though subtle, human needs probably underlie the most overt, as well as the discreet, expressions of resistance to computerization. With an understanding of how and why computers might be resisted, managers can develop the means for dealing with the phenomenon.

Dealing with Resistance

The fundamental guideline for managing resistance to computerization is to focus on the user. Research has documented that computerized information systems are more likely to be accepted if they are responsive to the needs of the users, and if users participate in the development and implementation of the system.[23] As Michael Ginzberg put it: "Being a change agent requires that management . . . really comes to understand the user; that he keeps the user involved through the entire project, making sure the user understands where the project is going and contributes substantially to setting this direction."[24]

This tenet seems to be echoed by all analysts of resistance. For example, *Output* magazine offered the following recipe "for managers who want to introduce technology without fear":[25]

- Consult your staff from the beginning when you're considering the feasibility of new systems.
- Make it clear from your actions that the interests and requirements of the users are being taken fully into account in the design of new systems.
- Explain as clearly and honestly as possible the consequences of these developments, and plan with the staff how problems can be overcome.

Several specific steps can help professionals manage resistance to computers. First, a strategy for minimizing resistance before it occurs, as well as for detecting and addressing it during implementation, should be developed. For this, Dowling's study is useful. In the cases of resistance which he examined in hospitals, Dowling found that "appraisal of the pre-system environment and a priori diagnosis of the system's effects on the staff would have alerted management to impending problems."[26] Dowling recommends using feedback mechanisms for detecting staff reaction and identifying resistance-inducing factors as major elements of an effective strategy.

Second, managers should focus on the causes of resistance. Education and training well ahead of implementation can alleviate threats to egos by equipping staff with the knowledge needed to maintain their status and power. Studies consistently show that there is a significant relationship between education and training and users' attitudes toward computers and technology innovations.[27]

Deliberate efforts to maintain existing social groups can help alleviate the social causes of resistance. And a policy of avoiding layoffs, even when computerization makes staff reductions possible, is needed to temper the economic fear of job loss. Studies indicate that a single layoff can abet this fear. Such alternatives as attrition or reassignment, though perhaps more expensive in the short term, have proven to be far less costly overall.

Third, professionals can take specific measures to sell the computerization effort, much like a marketing professional sells a product. For this to be effective, the benefits of using computers have to be identified, highlighted, and explained. Using orientation workshops well before computerization, presenting examples of favorable computerization in other, similar organizations, and demonstrating strong top management support are some good methods. Particularly important is clarification of the organizational and personal advantages of using computers.

A fourth necessary aspect of managing resistance is user involvement from the earliest stage of the computerization effort through the design, implementation, and evaluation of the system. It is true that this participation takes time, and that nontechnical users can frustrate technical designers; however, if we have learned any lesson from our experience with computers it is that technically sound systems are useless unless people use them. Past experience clearly dictates user involvement in system development.

Keeping organizational staff informed is also important. Few factors create more fear and resistance than mystery and surprise. Making a computerization plan a closely guarded secret is a major mistake in automation efforts.

Finally, managing resistance is aided both by giving time and timing. Rapidly introducing computers in health care organizations has nearly always failed or produced serious problems. A go-slowly approach in which employment of the technology evolves in stages as users become more comfortable with it is more time consuming, but also more cost-effective and successful. Time and exposure do heal fears and antagonisms. In the same vein, timing the introduction of computers with a perceived need for change and improvement can help. Automating a process or activity that already appears to work well can understandably inspire cynicism toward, if not outright rejection of, computerization plans.

In addition, a range of specific resistance-countering techniques should be undertaken. One such example is the use of "ergonomics." With the user in mind, ergonomics refers to the design of equipment and workspace that fits each employee, assures comfort, reduces strain, and avoids injury. The designers of telephone technology, for example, went to great pains to develop a handset, dial tilt, and so forth that would be both easy and comfortable to use. Until recently, widespread efforts in this area had been rare with computers. There is a growing set of theories that links regular use of computer terminals with eyestrain, migraine headaches, nausea, and back pain—conditions that could well cause anyone to resist.[28] More recently, questions have arisen because of persistent worries that video display terminals pose a variety of health risks from cataracts to muscle strain to miscarriages.[29] Many manufacturers now commonly take into consideration terminals and workstations with ergonomic features which, although more expensive, should be part of an overall user-focused strategy. Computer-related periodicals now customarily publish articles that deal specifically with user safety and comfort.[30]

Some organizations have sold employees on computers by introducing the system with games on the terminals. They have found this to be an effective means both for overcoming fear and for training users on terminal and system operations.[31] Others employ error-detection devices to monitor forms of resistance, such as inaccurate inputting and data withholding.[32] Still other organizations suggest the need to induce a feeling of naturalness in user interface design. Nonkeyboard interfaces such as pen-based computers and systems that recognize voice, handwriting, and gestures that substitute for keystroke commands are alleged to make computers more transparent to users.[33] In terms of receptivity, recent studies in nursing show that educational preparation, length of service in the nursing profession and specialization make a demonstrable difference in nurses' attitudes toward computerization.[34]

Of course, when all else fails, managers can order cooperation and use of the computer system, and threaten to fire resisters. Although most studies have found this approach to be counterproductive, some analyses suggest that it can work in certain cases.[35] When employed, however, it is more likely to work in combination with other approaches. In one notable case, a computer system was mandated by a state government for a drug-monitoring program at hospitals. Intended to identify the extent of long-term drug use in the treatment of psychiatric patients, the system was resisted by doctors, nurses, and pharmacists. Doctors felt that the program would be used to make qualitative judgments about the care they were providing, as well as place artificial constraints on their future ability to prescribe medication. Nursing departments expressed concern over the additional workload they would incur by having to fill out more and different medication forms. Pharmacists resisted because it would entail a major change in their processing, distribution, and dosage preparation systems.

Management met this resistance with fairly firm methods. Using a top-down approach, managers first met with hospital administrators and explained the nature of the program. Hospitals were informed that failure to cooperate and install a successful system would result in reduced funding and staff and the transfer of clients to other facilities. The hospital administrators conveyed this order to doctors, nurses, and pharmacists.

At the same time, knowing that resistance was strong, the system managers tried to reduce some of the hostility by offering users alternative solutions to various problems in the system. They agreed to intervene only if decisions were not made within certain time frames. Additionally, great emphasis was placed on adequate staff training to reduce the problems of learning to use the system.

Resistance from nurses was reduced by adapting the new system for use with the old drug-reporting forms. This eliminated increased work and training sessions. Doctors were presented with some benefits in the form of drug information services that would help them in prescribing drugs and dosages.

The greatest impact was on the pharmacists. Computerization in the pharmacy often required a complete revision of departmental policy and procedures. The system managers made it clear that the new system would increase the pharmacists' efficiency and control over inventories and distribution procedures. They also emphasized that the pharmacists' status would be greatly increased because the new program would expand their participation and impact in the process of developing therapeutic drug regimens.

The program has now been operating for a number of years, and managers report that initial studies demonstrate that they are getting accurate and complete information from the system. Properly managing resistance does work.

Notes

1. *New York Times*, 7 February 1988, B-1.
2. Ibid, B-1.
3. Ibid, B-1.
4. A. F. Dowling, "Do Hospital Staff Interfere with Computer System Implementation?" *Health Care Management Review*, Fall 1980, 23.
5. R. Cafasso, "Rethinking Re-engineering," *Computerworld*, 15 March 1993, 102–5.
6. *Medical Economics*, "Can a Computer Tell How Good a Doctor You Are?" 24 January 1994, 136.
7. D. Friend, "Are Information Systems Your Friend or Foe?" *Chief Executive*, Summer 1986, 26–27.
8. C. L. Packer, "Nursing Views Computers as Both Friends and Foes," *Hospitals*, November 1986, 20.
9. S. Brown, "How Soon Will You Be At The Mercy of a Hospital Computer?" *Medical Economics*, 2 March 1987, 160–63.
10. R. I. Hallock, "With Computers, Administrative Attitude Is the Key to Success," *Administrative Management*, March 1979, 80.
11. D. Kirkpatrick, "Making it all Worker-Friendly," *Fortune*, 128, no. 7 1993, 44–53.
12. See C. Dunbar and J. Yound, "Expensive Iron Doesn't Equal High Technology," *Computers in Healthcare*, December 1992, 16–20. M. Dostert, "Candy From Strangers," *Computerworld*, 29 March 1993, 89–92. E. Mutschler and R. Hoefer, "Factors Affecting the Use of Computer Technology in Human Service Organizations," *Administration in Social Work*, 14, no. 1 1990, 87–101.
13. Dowling, "Do Hospital Staff Interfere with Computer System Implementation?" 29.
14. See E. Gardner, "Physician Resistance Major Obstacle to Expert Systems," *Modern Healthcare*, 12 February 1990, 43.
15. See S. H. Applebaum, "Computerphobia: Training Managers to Reduce the Fears and Love the Machines," *Industrial and Commercial Training*, 22, no. 6 1990, 9–16.
16. J. Manuso, quoted in P. Hodges, "Fear of Automation," *Output*, August 1980, 34.
17. See *Business Week*, 26 March 1979, 94–95, for a report on Labor's reaction.
18. *New York Times*, 7 February 1988, B-1.
19. E. A. McConnell, S. Summers O'Shea, and K. T. Kirchoff, "R.N. Attitudes Toward Computers," *Nursing Management*, July 1989, 39.
20. M. E. Boone, *Leadership and the Computer* (Rockilin, CA: Prima Publishing, 1993).

21. J. I. Semke and P. S. Nurius, "Information Structure, Information Technology, and the Human Services Organizational Environment," *Social Work*, July 1991, 354.

22. Quoted in *Hospitals & Health Networks*, 20 July 1993, 44.

23. Mutschler and Hoefer, 90.

24. M. J. Ginzberg, "Steps toward More Effective Implementation of MS and MIS," *Interface*, May 1978, 61–62.

25. Hodges, "Fear of Automation," 39.

26. Dowling, "Do Hospital Staff Interfere with Computer System Implementation?" 32.

27. R. Dean and J. Shorter, "Preparing Your Networking Information Systems in Healthcare Organizations," *Health Care Supervisor*, September 1991, 58–62. Applebaum, 9–16.

28. B. E. Lesin, "Safety Tips for PC Users," *Human Resources Professional*, January–February 1994, 19–21.

29. R. R. King, "Health Effects of Visual Display Terminals," *Nursing Management*, October 1991, 61–64.

30. See M. Heller "Positioned for Success," *Windows Magazine*, November 1993, 171–83.

31. J. Leo, "Coping with Computers," *Discover*, December 1980, 97.

32. Dowling, "Do Hospital Staff Interfere with Computer System Implementation?" 32.

33. H. W. Ryan, "The Human Metaphor," *Information Systems Management*, Winter 1992, 72–75.

34. A. Brodt and J. Strong, "Nurses Attitudes toward Computerization in a Midwestern Community Hospital," *Computers in Nursing*, March–April 1986, 82–86.

35. Notably C. B. Schewe, "The Management Information System User: An Exploratory Behavioral Analysis," *Academy of Management Journal*, December 1976, 577–90.

Selected Readings

Benham, H., M. Delaney, and A. Luzi. "Structured Techniques for Successful End User Spreadsheets." *Journal of End User Computing* (Spring 1993): 18–25.

Duck, J. D. "Managing Change: The Art of Balancing." *Harvard Business Review* (November–December 1993): 109–18.

Gibson, S. "Managing Computer Resistance." *Computers in Nursing* (September–October 1986): 201–4.

Karon, P. "Coping With Reluctant Users: Managers Need Strategies to Keep Users Computing." *PC Week* (3 March 1987): 41–42.

Ryan, H. W. "The Human Metaphor." *Information Systems Management* (Winter 1992): 72–75.

Schewe, C. D. "The Management Information User: A Behavioral Analysis." *Academy of Management Journal* (December 1976): 577–990.

Tushman, M. L., and P. Anderson. "Technological Discontinuities and Organizations' Environment." *Administrative Science Quarterly* (Spring 1986): 439–65.

Vegoda, P. R., and E. Vanacore. "Hospital Information Systems—Friend or Foe? A Management Perspective." *Journal of Medical Systems* (February 1986): 11–23.

READING

IN A HUMOROUS and practical reading, Dianne Horgan and Rebecca Simeon apply some sophisticated theories to the managerial challenges of dealing with resistance to computerization. Their emphasis on identifying types of people in the organization, and analyzing their relationships, contributes significantly to managerial knowledge.

Computers and People—Casting the Players

Dianne D. Horgan and Rebecca J. Simeon

> Identifying the types of people in an organization and analyzing their relationships can make the computer adaptation process more predictable and therefore easier to manage.

People, rather than organizational structure or technology, are the key to understanding adaptation to change in small organizations. In our work with small organizations, we consistently find that the influence of the individual workers on the overall success of an effort to bring about change is much stronger than it would be in large organizations. (A big frog in a small pond can create very large ripples.) Also, we have found that the research on managing change in large organizations does not provide much guidance to managers of small organizations.

Recently we studied how individuals adapt to computers in small organizations. In our experience, successful adaptation in the small

Reprinted with permission from *Business* (October–December). Georgia State University Business Press, College of Business Administration. © 1988.

organization is a very individual matter. Because the small organization can rarely provide extensive support, people who adapt well do so because of their personal characteristics. In our study, we first looked at how individuals adapted to personal computers; then we examined a few diverse computer installations. We found that despite large differences among organizations, the patterns of success or failure in computer use were consistent.

Initially, we thought that expectations were a key to predicting success in learning to use computers and that failure was often related to unrealistic expectations. Before looking at adaptation within organizations, we examined the expectations of individuals about to purchase microcomputers. We then followed up to determine which ones became satisfied computer users.

When faculty and staff at a large university had an opportunity to purchase microcomputers for their personal use at significant discounts, many people seriously considered purchasing computers for their own use for the first time. This gave us an opportunity to look at the role expectations play in determining successful adaptation at the individual level. We conducted a survey to discover the level of knowledge people had about computers and their expectations about how they would adapt to their computers. Of all the questionnaires distributed to faculty and professional staff, 944 were returned. Of those, 39% said they were probably going to purchase a computer in the next year.

In the initial survey, 37% of the potential buyers thought they could solve their own problems, and 31% expected to rely on their colleagues for help. Only 16% indicated that they would seek expert assistance. The less knowledgeable the intended buyer, the more likely he or she was to expect help from experts and from manuals.

A year later, we interviewed the potential buyers and found that 32% had actually purchased machines. The more experienced and knowledgeable the potential buyers, the more likely they were to have made the purchase. Two-thirds of the buyers were very pleased with their computers and reported positive experiences with them during the first year. All of the successful adaptors had relied primarily on themselves for training, and all had expected to do so. Of the one-third who reported dissatisfaction with their computers ("not worth the trouble," "too hard to use"), all indicated practically no prior knowledge about computers and that they had difficulty in getting help. Interestingly, the poor adaptors had taken training workshops and computer courses. The poor adaptors had expected the learning process to be much easier. This unfulfilled expectation seemed the largest factor in their dissatisfaction.

These results convinced us of the importance of good preparation and training: people with little prior experience had false expectations and considerable difficulty adapting to their computers. In particular, they expected experts to help them rather than relying mostly on themselves. We believed that these same variables would be important in organizations undergoing computer changes.

The second study was designed to discover more about the individual characteristics of the good and the poor adaptors, and how others in an organization help or hinder the adaptation process. We were particularly interested in describing those characteristics in terms of knowledge and expectations. We examined how four very different organizations adapted to a major computer installation. We were involved with these organizations in ongoing consulting projects, and we knew the individuals involved. Across diverse organizations, we saw the same patterns of behavior and the same resulting problems. In all cases, the people problems outweighed the technical problems, but the bulk of the planning had focused on the technology. First we will describe the organizations, then we will describe the "types" of people we found. We will use concepts from expectancy theory,[1] open systems theory,[2] and social information processing theory[3] to describe the individuals and to test predictions about outcomes.

Expectancy theory predicts the effort and intensity an individual will put forth in situations where behaviors are somewhat under voluntary control, such as successful adaptation to computers. Basically, expectancy theory says that an individual's level of motivation is a function of (1) the expectations of success (which may or may not be realistic), (2) the perceived value of the expected outcomes (will it be worthwhile to learn the system?), and (3) whether the individual believes that successful performance will lead to attainment of goals. The level of motivation, then, depends on subjective expectations. Reality may have little to do with it. From this theoretical perspective, the success or failure of adaptation to computers can be related to the motivation of the individuals involved. And this motivation will depend largely on individual expectations.

Expectancy theory leads to several predictions:

- Persons with low expectation for success or with low expectation that successful performance will lead to reward will likely be poor adaptors to change.
- Because one's motivation changes as a result of experience, motivation can change dramatically when confronted with unexpected success or failure. Therefore, for some people, the initial motivational level is not a good predictor of a later motivational level.

In *open systems theory*, the concepts of boundaries and relationships are crucial. Boundaries regulate the flow of inputs and outputs in the system. Boundaries may be concrete and formal, as when groups are housed in different buildings. Or, boundaries may be informal, such as those based on status differences. Boundaries differ in their degree of permeability from zero (a closed system), to fully permeable, representing no system at all, where everyone interacts freely with everyone else. Between these two extremes is an optional level of permeability in which the system best grows and expands. Relationships provide integration and stability within the system. Relationships vary in their degree of mutuality, that is the extent to which relevant information is exchanged between members of the relationship. In terms of adapting to change and learning a new computer system, mutual relationships are highly desirable.

Several predictions follow from this theoretical viewpoint:

- When boundaries are optimally permeable and relationships are mutual, adaptation to change is easier than in a more closed system.
- Since closed organizations tend to remain so, and because change is difficult in a closed system, change agents that span boundaries are necessary for adaptation.
- When boundaries or relationships change, the adaptation process will be affected in predictable ways. For example, moves toward a more closed system will negatively affect the process.

The final theoretical perspective we will consider is the *social information theory*, which claims that job attitudes derive from the communicative activities of employees rather than from the employees' internal needs or drives. In this view, job attitudes are determined by the environmental characteristics of the task, the social information available, and the individual's own behaviors. This view contrasts sharply with motivational theories (such as one which claims that people are motivated by their internal needs for self-development). According to this theory, social information influences people's attitudes by helping them interpret complex cues and by focusing their attention on certain cues that lead to their interpretation of the environment. Therefore, we can predict that those who have received negative social information will feel more stress and anxiety about an upcoming change. On the other hand, those who obtain positive social information will probably have more positive attitudes toward change.

Taken together, these theories, suggest that expectations are subjective and at least partially result from social information. The sharing of social information varies according to how open or closed the system is. Adaptation to change can be enhanced by decreasing boundaries and/or by spanning them and by increasing positive communication.

The Organizations

A Retail Chain

Corporate headquarters for a 15-store aftermarket autoparts chain (we will call "Retail") had recently computerized their accounting system. This change had been extremely stressful on both workers and management. At the beginning of our study, management was preparing for another computer installation, this time in the merchandising area. The workers in the merchandising area had received a good deal of negative information from other workers, who had gone through the difficult change in accounting. Merchandise personnel reported feeling anxious about the installation and also had low expectations for a quick, smooth transition. This confirmed the findings of an earlier study, which found that prior information was more important than new information in shaping employees' attitudes.[4]

We interviewed employees in depth prior to the installation. At that time, we gathered background information about their education, prior experience with computers, job history, their expectations, fears, and anticipated problems and benefits. We also asked them about the relationships within their area and their learning style. A copy of the interview guide is presented in [Exhibit 6.1]. As the training and installation proceeded, we visited the company and talked with selected employees. We also asked supervisors to monitor performance and let us know how each person was progressing. We kept track, too, of unusual incidents. For example, the power company accidentally cut a cable resulting in several days of downtime. After the system was established, we returned to interview everyone to find out whether or not their expectations had been met.

A Small College

This college (we will call "College") had a few microcomputers that were used for instruction. When our study began, the college was planning to add computers for administrative purposes. Payroll had been done by the state, and memory typewriters and manual bookkeeping were the norm. Funding came from a federal grant. Employees had little prior information about computers and were suspicious about anything administered and seemingly controlled by the federal government.

As part of another project, one of us was on campus at least weekly during the transition. Each person involved with the transition was

Exhibit 6.1 Sample Interview Guide

INTERVIEW GUIDE

Name _____ Date _____

I. General discussion of progress

How are you doing?

What's been hardest/easiest?

Has it been easier/harder than you expected?

What events have created problems?

What resources of yours have been most helpful? (Experience, ability to follow directions, general intelligence, personality factors, ability to laugh at myself, and so forth.)

What personal characteristics have made it harder?

II. Others

Who's been helpful to you? How? How did their help differ? What did they do?

Who in your work group do you think is doing especially well? Why?

Who do you think is having the most problems? Why?

What kind of support/help/interference have you received from central office? From the stores?

III. Your job

How was your job changed?

What problems did you expect? What ones happened?

If you could start over, what would you suggest?

interviewed several times, and supervisors provided information on their employees' progress.

A Small Consulting Firm

This firm ("Consulting") of seven professionals and three clerks upgraded their word processing and computer system. Previously, the clerks had exclusive use of the microcomputers, all bookkeeping was done manually, and any statistical work was done externally. The upgrade involved both new machines and new software. It was assumed that professionals as well as clerks would use the machines. The change, therefore, involved a new system for the clerks and a first exposure to computers for most of the professionals.

One of us was asked to provide technical advice and some training for this project. Consulting was visited at least once a week during the transition, and a significant amount of time was spent with each employee discussing attitudes toward the system and perceived progress. Here, too, we had access to supervisors' evaluations of each person's progress.

A Private Practice

This firm ("Practice") consisted of one professional, a secretary/ bookkeeper, and a receptionist. They were converting from a memory typewriter and manual bookkeeping to a microcomputer for word processing and bookkeeping. The secretary had no prior experience with computers, but held naive (and incorrect) beliefs about the operation. The professional's prior information was from advertisements and outputs. However, he had no personal experience with computers.

We were called into Practice after the professional became convinced that his secretary/bookkeeper would never learn the system. We had been involved with the company on other projects and knew the individuals. Here, too, we had frequent and close contact with the staff.

Changes in Work Role and Social Structure

Structural changes resulting from these computer installations varied tremendously. At Retail, about a dozen women worked in merchandising as clerks. They shared a range of tasks, including tagging merchandise, calling stores to track orders, managing inventory, and keeping records of transfer of merchandise. Women traded jobs at will and helped each other out as necessary. The merchandise area was physically separate from other functions—entry was by special key only. Not only were there physical boundaries such as locked doors, but the job tasks differed from those in other departments in the same building (accounting, personnel, and advertising). As a result of the interdependency of the interchangeable workers and the physical and task isolation, group cohesion was high. The prior negative information they had, therefore, was homogeneous—all negative stories were shared knowledge.

This group was isolated from other groups (physically as well as socially), but had very close and mutually dependent relations within their group. According to the open systems theory, such a condition is in danger of greater pathology and is not likely to adapt to change. The introduction of the computer system drastically changed the social order. Because of the software and the need for security, jobs were no longer interchangeable—they had to be more clearly differentiated and defined. Some reduction in intragroup mutuality was inevitable. A new social order had to emerge. Some changes in communication with external groups also occurred. Previously, when clerks called stores to locate lost merchandise, the stores had the upper hand—the clerks had no way to verify or challenge the store's report. With the computer, they had correct information about inventory, which gave them a more equal relationship. Thus, while internal mutuality was reduced, external mutuality was increased. Their range of influence and interaction was increasing.

At Consulting, the social changes were from more differentiated work roles to less differentiated ones, but these changes were between groups rather than within one specific group. At Consulting, the lines between professionals and clerks had been very clear. Professionals handed the clerks handwritten materials or dictated tapes. Only clericals typed. When management realized that time and money could be saved by having professionals produce some of their own work at a word processor, some clerks saw it as an invasion of their space, while some professionals saw it as a loss of status. Here, too, there was an increase in external mutuality—professionals had to ask clerks for help. As at Retail, these new, more equal relationships were initially threatening. Prior knowledge and attitudes about computers varied among the whole staff, unlike the situation at Retail. This created a correspondingly wider range of individual problems.

At College, there was a lack of understanding of what changes would result. Some people feared being replaced by the computers. The general level of knowledge about computers was quite low, except for one computer instructor. While top administrators saw the computers as a wonderful gift from the federal government (one that would probably increase their status), the people who would actually use the machines saw them as another symptom of government interference and control. Thus, the already somewhat impermeable boundaries between these groups was heightened by the change.

At Practice, both the secretary's and the professional's attitudes were clouded by misconceptions. The secretary saw the new computer as a slightly improved memory typewriter that was harder to use. The professional saw it as Madison Avenue would want him to. But here, too, the potential for difficult adaptation to change is evidenced by the low expectations of the secretary and the impermeable boundaries between the professional and the secretary.

The Players

Throughout this group of diverse organizations and social situations, we found a relatively small set of roles or types. These roles can be characterized in terms of individual expectations and beliefs. Using the expectancy theory and open systems theory, we can predict how each type of person, or role, will react under specified conditions. A brief discussion follows, describing each type prior to their experience with the new system. People, through experience, can and do shift from one type to another, and we have indicated who might develop into whom.

Love Strucks

Three of the four organizations had presidents and several high-level executives in this category. These individuals had overly high expectations for the success of the transition, but their expectations were not based on a good knowledge of computers and were thus often not realistic—hence the name "Love Struck." Much like a love-struck suitor, they were blind to inadequacies, but they were passionate in their promotion of the new computer system. If the boundaries between them and the other employees are rather impermeable, then their overly optimistic expectations may not be brought into line with reality early in the change process.

People in this group varied in terms of their level of involvement with the computers. At one extreme was the boss who knew just enough to be dangerous. He often started a comment with "I read an article. . . ." At the other extreme were people with equally high expectations and enthusiasm who wanted to maintain their distance from the machines.

The Warm Mama

We found that small organizations desperately need a Warm Mama, although he or she might cause problems later. A Warm Mama has high expectations for him- or herself and for others. The Warm Mama becomes a guru and dominates the informal social structure. A Warm Mama is someone who played a dominant social role before the introduction of computers.

The Warm Mama at Retail was a clerk with some experience and considerable talent with computers. Prior to the computer installation, she was a source of support and help to other workers. Her role expanded as the transition continued, until other workers as well as her supervisor believed her to be totally indispensable. Consulting also had a Warm Mama, one of the professionals with some experience and some talent. Both Warm Mamas had their roles develop around them. The Warm Mamas in these two organizations were not hired as computer experts, but they emerged as the person "to go to for help." The Warm Mama receives great personal satisfaction from her fellow workers' success and from the appreciation and recognition she receives. She (or he) penetrates boundaries and increases the mutuality of relationships.

College and Practice lacked a Warm Mama. One of the effects was the lack of a liaison person to communicate with upper management. Hence the boundary remained impermeable, resulting in unrealistic expectations and very frustrated employees who were unable to meet goals. When the bosses' expectations were not met, they were understandably frustrated and felt that they had been misled by salespeople or let down by members of their staff.

Another very important function of the Warm Mama was training. While large organizations often have formal training, small organizations typically have less. Furthermore, workers are not used to classroom-type instruction and often feel much more comfortable with one-on-one or small group training from a Warm Mama. The Warm Mama already has warm social ties with others in the group, which appears to greatly facilitate learning.

The Warm Mama's best qualities may, however, lead to the serious problem of overdependency. At both Consulting and Retail, the Warm Mamas had difficulties "letting go." The power and satisfaction that came from having everyone dependent on them (higher as well as lower in the hierarchy) was difficult to relinquish. As in studies of leadership in evolving organizations, we found that "solutions breed new problems."[5] Just as the bold entrepreneur may be an ideal leader in the early stages of a company and a serious problem after the company grows, a Warm Mama can save the company during a major change but stifle development of employees later. At both Retail and Consulting, there were times when Warm Mama's influence far exceeded the individual formal status.

The Cold Mama

These people tended to have high expectations for their own success at learning the new system, but rather low expectations for others. The Cold Mamas we saw were characterized by their coworkers as "cold computer types." (In contrast, co-workers used terms like "my savior" to refer to Warm Mamas.) The Cold Mamas at College and Retail gave co-workers the feeling they believed themselves to be superior and that other workers could only learn small parts of the larger task. While Cold Mamas had the necessary knowledge, they lacked the existing social relations of the Warm Mama. They erected boundaries. A Cold Mama, new to an organization, might be able to establish those relationships and become a Warm Mama. In general, however, Cold

Mamas have more formal training than Warm Mamas; hence, they may resent the Warm Mama.

Slack-takers

In Retail, College, and Consulting we saw Slack-takers. Like Warm Mamas, these people have high expectations for both their own success and for the success of others. Their expectations, like the Love Strucks, are often overly optimistic. They lack the warmth and personal relationships characteristic of Warm Mamas. Warm Mamas are maternal—they want their co-workers to succeed; the Slack-takers' role is limited to the computer—they want the system to succeed. At College, for example, a high-level administrator became very interested in the new system. Without the experience (and perhaps the talent) of the Warm Mama, however, he was not able to learn as quickly as he had expected. He had envisioned himself as filling the gap: in short, he planned to become (overnight) the Warm Mama. After something of an identity crisis and a good amount of time, he was able to take up much of the slack. As one might expect, Cold Mama deeply resented the Slack-taker, with no formal training invading the territory. But without a Warm Mama and with a slow-off-the-starting-block Slack-taker, College experienced a very long and disruptive transition.

The Warm Mama may also fear that the Slack-taker will steal some of his or her thunder. Much as some real mothers resent the affection a child may have for a babysitter, the Warm Mama is jealous of co-workers' loyalties and the boss's dependency.

Slack-takers, if their expectations do not become more realistic, may create other problems—they may become drug-store cowboys. At Consulting, a vice president saw himself as a Slack-taker. When he was not able to be as helpful as he liked, he devoted himself to suggesting alternative software and alternative ways of doing things, which greatly confused the staff. Slack-takers often try to span boundaries. If they are ill-informed, this may create even more unrealistic expectations among bosses. Slack-takers can become Warm Mamas when their knowledge increases enough for their leadership to be based on expertise. We observed this both at Retail and at Consulting.

Pessimists

These people have negative expectations and attitudes. If, however, they become convinced of the eventual success of the system, they come around and may become Slack-takers. At Retail, there were a large number of Pessimists, due no doubt to the wealth of prior negative information. The conversion of the Pessimists took time and was largely due to the efforts of the Warm Mama. Warm Mama at Consulting was also the primary force in convincing the Pessimists there. At Practice, the secretary was a Pessimist. Because the professional's expectations were unrealistic, he was unable to give her the positive experience that would convert her. Consequently, her computer went untouched for over a year, until a college student intern—Slack-taker—was able to change the secretary's expectations and attitudes. With a different secretary the situation might have been totally different.

Serious Resisters

Consulting had several secretaries who, in general, were not very adaptive and were extremely hostile about having to learn a new system. Their expectations were for complete failure of the system, and their behavior (usually passive aggressive) was calculated to see that their expectations were met. Luckily, these Serious Resisters were not opinion leaders. At Retail, there was at least one Serious Resister who caused some serious problems. Another function of Warm Mamas is to control the negative influence of Serious Resisters. At both Consulting and College, when the Love Struck bosses tried to counteract the Serious Resisters, they were met with skepticism. As a result, other workers became convinced that the Serious Resisters were more correct in their expectations than were the bosses. Serious Resisters and Pessimists have unrealistically low expectations and Love Struck bosses have unrealistically high expectations. To communicate, they need a Warm Mama or a Slack-taker as a go-between. (Cold Mamas engender too many negative feelings to be effective as go-betweens.)

Self-Developers

These people often have unrealistically high expectations for themselves. A Self-developer believes that learning some new computer skills will result in self-development that will, in turn, result in improved job opportunities. To this group, new computer skills are the way out of a current rut. They expect their status to improve dramatically as a result of the about-to-be-achieved competencies. At Retail, there were several ambitious young women who saw the new system as an opportunity. If, like many medium-sized organizations, Retail cannot offer them substantial advancement quickly, they will become negative influences. At Consulting, one young man who had considerable mechanical ability was earmarked by the Love Struck boss as someone who would "naturally" be good with computers (since they are machines). The anointed immediately envisioned the new, more powerful role he would have within the organization. Later, when it was clear that his mechanical ability did not generalize to skill with software, he became openly hostile to both the Warm Mama and the Slack-taker.

Short-Term Goalers

These people are enthusiastic about anything that will make their lives easier, but they are unlikely to focus on long-term goals. They have fairly high expectations and, typically, very little knowledge about computers. They tend to underestimate the time necessary for a new system to be up and running effectively. They are open initially (unlike Pessimists), but need some positive experiences and realistic reorienting of expectations to avoid developing negative attitudes. These people do well with a Warm Mama. They will have serious problems, however, with a Love Struck boss and no intervening Warm Mama or Slack-taker. At College, several clerical and bookkeeping employees were heavily influenced by the president and the head of finance (both Love Strucks). Naturally they were extremely discouraged when the "dream" did not materialize. They then evolved into Serious Resisters. Had they been exposed more to a Warm Mama, they might have become Rational People.

Rational People

There are individuals whose expectations are fairly realistic and who are not trying to change their status through the computer. At the beginning of a transition, we found very few such people. Almost everyone was unrealistic about their abilities or those of others, about the length of time necessary for success, or about the likelihood of success. By the time a transition period was complete, most workers had moved to this state. As a result of his prior experience with a computer installation in accounting, the president of Retail was considerably more realistic in his expectations than the presidents of the other three organizations. At many organizations, people who do not reach this state will be terminated or will leave out of frustration.

Exhibit [6.2] summarizes these types in terms of their expectations, knowledge, and other characteristics. But how can we get people to the rational state? In all cases, we see that the positive or negative outcome depends on what happens when the person's initial expectations are or are not met. This often depends on the social and communicative relationships the person has. In Exhibit [6.3] people variables (on the left) filter through the subjective expectations and perceptions and, together with environmental variables (on the right), affect outcomes (in the center). The primary outcomes can be classified as the level of adaptation of the users and the changes in the group structures. Some

Exhibit 6.2 Summary of Types of Reactions to Computers

Type		Pitfalls/Prognosis
Love Struck Expectations: of self: ††† of others: ††† Knowledge: Low	*"Computers! Great! This will solve ALL our problems . . ."*	If the boss is Love Struck, may impose unrealistic expectations on workers and create high stress. If they become more realistic and knowledgeable, may become a Slack-taker or even a Warm Mama.
Warm Mama Expectations: of self: †† of others: †† Knowledge: Quick learners	*"This computer is my 'Little Baby.'"*	May jealously guard control of the system. May develop too much power for the position. Can become a Rational Person if the new system does not stay his or her baby.
Cold Mama Expectations: of self: ††† of others: -- Knowledge: High	*"I understand more about the computer than anyone else here!"*	Because Cold Mamas lack rapport with other workers, they are often resented for their knowledge and can engender animosities.
Slack-Taker Expectations: of self: ††† of others: † Knowledge: Varies	*"I'll have this computer thing working in no time at all . . ."*	Slack-takers want to help and may become frustrated if their efforts don't work. With positive experiences, can become Warm Mamas. The Slack-tacker tries to acquire knowledge rapidly which may create frustration.
Pessimist Expectations: of self: -- of others: -- Knowledge: Low	*"Computers! Oh well, there goes my job . . ."*	If Pessimists have positive experiences and gain knowledge, they may become Slack-takers. If they have negative experiences, they may become Serious Resisters.

Continued

Exhibit 6.2 Continued

Type		Pitfalls/Prognosis
Serious Resister Expectations: of self: -- of others: --- Knowledge: Low	*"Say 'No' to Computers!"*	Often opinion leaders, Serious Resisters spell trouble. They may sabotage efforts. Organizations need a strong Warm Mama to control this group. Determined not to learn more.
Self-Developer Expectations: of self: †† of others: - Knowledge: Low to moderate	*"The computer will be great . . . for my career."*	The Self-developer sees the new system as a way for self-improvement, which can be very motivating, but if the organization cannot provide the desired rewards, the Self-developer can become a Serious Resister. If the Self-developer has the ability, he or she may become a Slack-taker.
Short-Term Goalers Expectations: of self: †† of others: †† Knowledge: Low to moderate	*"The computer will make everything so easy . . ."*	The Short-term Goaler expects the transition to be easy and is enthusiastic in the beginning. If not nurtured and well trained, can become a Serious Resister or Pessimist.
Rational People Expectations: of self: † of others: † Knowledge: Moderate to high	*"Why is everyone acting so strange about the computer?"*	Rational People have realistic expectations. Well-trained and well-supported Warm Mamas and Slack-takers are best candidates for Rational People. Pessimists, Love Strucks, Self-developers, and Short-term Goalers may develop into Rational People. Cold Mamas who are able to develop rapport may become Rational People. Serious Resisters are unlikely to develop into Rational people.

KEY: ††† Extremely high   - Somewhat low
      †† High   -- Low
      † Somewhat high   --- Extremely low

Exhibit 6.3 People Variables

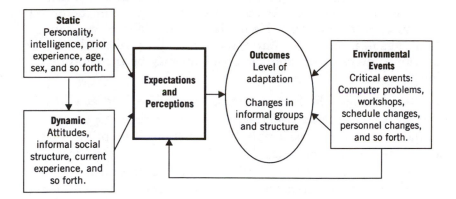

aspects of people variables are more static, such as the personality, intelligence, and prior experience. These characteristics affect the more dynamic characteristics, such as attitudes, and the informal social structure. Both the dynamic and static characteristics lead to the subjective perceptions and expectations that have the most direct influence on outcomes.

The environment directly affects outcomes in ways that cannot be controlled (computer problems, unforeseen complications) and in ways that can be controlled (schedule changes, workshops, extra training, and so forth). Environmental events can also affect outcomes indirectly through subjective expectations and perceptions. Assuming, then, that current employees are not to be replaced, the adaptation process can be controlled by focusing on ways to affect expectations/perceptions. Several general strategies are suggested here:

- We can deal with the expectations that existed *prior* to the change. One research team found that this had a positive effect. At Retail, considerable effort went into preparing people for the change by offering workshops on change and stress and supplying information about the change. While these steps appear to have had some positive effect, it is striking that despite the fact that everyone received the same information, some people (Pessimists and Resisters) reported that they had been underinformed, while others (Slack-takers and Self-developers) felt that they had been well informed. Expectations are highly subjective and supplying the information does not ensure uniform results.
- We can deal with the person when the expectations are not met. Here is where the value of Warm Mamas was evident. With Warm

Mamas, people seem to reach the Rational stage sooner and with less trauma to the organization. At Retail, external consultants also served this purpose. As outsiders with no place in the power structure, they were often able to clarify and calibrate expectations. If an organization lacks a Warm Mama or a Slack-taker who can be developed quickly, an external consultant may be the appropriate intervention.

At Retail (where the first two steps were taken) and at Consulting (where step two was undertaken), the time required to reach a comfortable state was considerably less than at College or at Practice (where neither were done). Retail and Consulting, however, were not free of problems. Both had to deal with the overdependence on the Warm Mamas and the structuring of the organization to reflect new levels of skills and to satisfy the workers' new needs.

• We can correct misperceptions. Good downward communication and good education can help employees perceive the changes accurately. For example, in all organizations we saw people who perceived their progress to be slow. In fact, they were progressing at a normal rate. Here better feedback and accurate information can help.

Exhibit 6.2 suggests other possibilities that we did not observe. While informal social structure was a powerful influence, it was not used to foster learning. Team building and other efforts at building strong group support and efforts to maintain established work teams could be effective in developing positive and realistic expectations. Groups could be formed to ensure that Serious Resisters, for example, do not dominate.

Another possibility is to preselect Warm Mamas. Interviews and tests could identify those with the interest, motivation, and talent to take that role. In the organizations we studied, leaders focused on the technology and overlooked the importance of the social network. Training one's own Warm Mama may be more cost-effective than hiring a Cold Mama. Also, many aspects of the environment are controllable and are thus prime targets for intervention. Careful analysis of the effects of the change may help planners anticipate problems. Disruptions of the informal structure and of work groups are serious and should be dealt with early in the transition.

Conclusion

Identifying the types of people in an organization and analyzing their relationships (both intragroup and intergroup) can make the computer adaptation process more predictable and therefore easier to manage. Expectancy theory, open systems theory, and social information theory provide useful frameworks. Successful adaptation to change may be enhanced through the use of prior information and/or external consultants.

Notes

1. Edward E. Lawler, *Motivation in Organizations* (Monterey, California: Brooks/Cole, 1973); John P. Campbell and Richard D. Pritchard, "Motivation Theory in Industrial and Organizational Psychology," *Handbook of Industrial and Organizational Psychology*. ed. Marvin D. Dunnette (New York: Wiley 1983), 63.

2. C. P. Alderfer, "Change Processes in Organizations," *Handbook of Industrial and Organizational Psychology*, ed. Marvin D. Dunnette (New York: Wiley 1983), 1591; Daniel Katz and Robert L. Kahn, *The Social Psychology of Organizations* (New York: Wiley 1966).

3. Gerald R. Salancik and Jeffrey Pfeffer, "A Social Information Processing Approach to Job Attitudes and Task Design," *Administrative Science Quarterly*, 23 (1978): 224.

4. K. I. Miller and P. R. Monge, "Social Information and Employee Anxiety About Organizational Change," *Human Communication Research* 11 (1983): 365.

5. Larry E. Greiner, "Evolution and Revolution as Organizations Grow," *Harvard Business Review* (July/August 1972).

6. Miller and Monge, "Social Information."

Dr. Horgan is Assistant Professor of Education and Ms. Simeon is a doctoral student in Industrial/Organizational Psychology at Memphis State University in Tennessee.

CASE 6
Smiling Acres Nursing Center

BOB SHERMAN'S desk was piled high with paperwork, and it seemed unlikely that this last workday before a long-awaited summer vacation would come to an end. After reflecting upon the situation that had developed since the new computer system had come on the scene, he decided that he just couldn't go away at such a critical time.

As the administrator of Smiling Acres, a 280-bed skilled nursing facility, he just returned from a staff meeting where it seemed likely that unionization among the professional staff and the nonprofessional staff would take place. How did it get to this point? People in the facility seemed to have changed. He remembers from his graduate school days that the kind of behavior that seems to have developed was what the psychologists called "dysfunctional." His assistant administrator, Mike White, laughingly referred to the staff's condition as "techno-stress." Mike followed Bob into his office and collapsed on the chair and said, "I don't think we'll be able to turn this around. We've tried everything to convince them that their life will be easier with the new system. Now they're retaliating by organizing. They'll never accept the new system and they'll never listen to us."

Bob thought about the different approaches that had been taken to get the system off the ground. Recognizing that change was difficult, attempts were made to soften the blow. He had regular preimplementation meetings, invited wide participation, encouraged involvement, initiated education and information programs, and sought to persuade the staff that the benefits would outweigh the initial inconveniences. An in-house newsletter and a hot line to the director of data processing were the latest innovations, along with regular postimplementation meetings. With this dysfunctional behavior still so prevalent, he wondered whether coercion would be a better approach in solving this "people problem." Thinking that a solution might lie in analyzing people's behavior, Bob resolved to try and understand what had happened over the past year by examining his daily diary. He had learned that by recording and summarizing the events of the day, he could better organize the following day's work. He proceeded to look at his notes taken over the past year.

Bob's Notes

August 2

The computerization committee has decided on the hardware, software, and peripherals. I'm pleased that there was little argument about which way to go. Mike was appointed to spearhead the Committee.

August 3

Lillian, the director of nursing, informed me she thought the computer committee was rushing implementation. I told her I would ask the committee to revise the conversion schedule to extend the easing in period.

August 5

The rumors are rampant! Mike tells me that some people think they'll lose their jobs, others say that computers always break down; still others maintain that computers hinder patient care. Some people are ridiculous.

August 14

I held a general staff meeting to squelch the rumors. It went well, although attendance could have been better. The usual complement of cynics for this kind of gathering seemed to be subdued.

August 28

The first preimplementation meeting for department heads was held today. Some gave me the impression that this was just one more burden they had to bear. Lillian appointed her assistant, Dorothy, to represent the nursing department at this meeting. She seems pretty savvy. The

Director of Medical Records asked me after the meeting why Lillian hadn't attended.

September 8

In the employee dining room today Mike overheard the dietary staff complain that they were going to have to learn how to type and they were going to have to memorize the new computer manuals that were delivered to each department.

September 9

I called Joe, the Director of Dietary, to my office to explain what Mike had overheard. He thought it was simply idle gossip, but expressed a fear that the new codes for inputting would be confusing.

September 18

The second preimplementation meeting was held today. Dorothy, Lillian's assistant, announced in the meeting that her husband's firm had implemented computers last year. According to her, their computer system is always down, and people were laid off after implementation. She wanted to know if the same thing would happen to us. I told her that it wouldn't happen at Smiling Acres.

September 27

Another staff meeting was held today to help allay fears. The younger staff members seem to be taking this better than the older staff members. A small group of people (I'm not sure which department) announced they would resign if they were forced to learn. I'm not sure they will ever trust me or computers.

October 1

The director of social services resigned today. She mentioned " . . . impending changes that may compromise issues of privacy and quality of care . . ." as one of the reasons for her leaving.

October 16

The hardware is finally here! Installation begins today.

October 17

Some of the hardware was damaged overnight. I hope I can get the vendor to credit the loss.

January 3

Training of staff and inputting of data has taken longer than expected. According to Mike, the biggest problem has been the fact that everyone has different degrees of skills and potential for understanding. The fiscal systems went "live" first, but nursing is still not completed. I don't know when nursing will be tied into the system.

January 12

The department of public health visited the facility today. Apparently, a patient's family sent a letter to the department complaining of chronic staff shortages. Lillian blames the time and energy the staff has spent on the computerization effort for these shortages.

January 30

The system is finally "on-line."

February 20

Mike blames the inputting errors for all the bugs in the system. Patient billing still isn't right, and dietary sent a hot fudge sundae to a diabetic patient today. Dietary blames nursing and nursing blames dietary.

February 26

The dietary department went back to their old manual system. They said it was just a "short cut." I insisted they use the new system.

March 3

In the department head meeting today, I mentioned the fact that the increased overtime must stop. It's doubled in the past year. The operating budget just can't take it, and I'm getting pressure from the Finance Committee of the Board. All the department heads want to take their vacation in June.

March 23

Our entire month's billing to Medicaid for last month was disallowed. Patient days were not entered and wrong ID codes appeared on the billing sheet.

April 14

Nursing staff held a meeting today and decided on a work slowdown for next week. They call it the "white flu." Half of the patients' nursing care plans were erased from the system today. Mike's not sure what happened, but I called the software vendor.

May 11

All management reports for April are missing. The controller said it was no great loss because people didn't look at them anyway.

May 30

I need a vacation.

Questions for Discussion

1. What forms of resistance were evident at Smiling Acres?
2. Discuss possible explanations for the resistance that occurred at Smiling Acres.
3. Evaluate Bob's responses to what occured at Smiling Acres and appraise his methods of managing resistance.
4. What should Bob do now?
5. Develop a strategy with which Bob can overcome resistance effectively.

MAINTAINING SECURITY

A FEW YEARS ago Louis Charbonneau wrote a novel about an intruder who electronically penetrates the computer system of a municipality in the northeast United States. Titled *Intruder*, the book tells about a threat to "crash" the computer system and put government services into chaos unless a $5 million dollar ransom is paid. Fiction, right? Wrong! Recently some eighth graders at New York's Dalton School penetrated the computer system of major corporations in Canada, disrupting the operation of one system and actually seizing control of another, destroying some data in the process—all from a small terminal in their Upper Eastside school.

The growth of personal computer use has dramatically increased the number of people who are familiar with systems and who can manipulate them. Additionally, new communication technology allows access to systems by phone with relative ease. In one company, for example, it was found that employees had set up one computer with a modem connected to a telephone line. With a phone call they could connect their personal computers at home to the office network. No password was required and software on the computer linked to the telephone allowed anyone to call in to read, delete or change data or software on the entire computer network.[1]

Most experts agree that breaking into the computer systems of nearly all government and health care organizations, as well as corporations, is both technically feasible and much less complicated than most of us realize. Take, for example, the case of two young "hackers" who were charged by the government with using a home computer to break into data systems at a Federal Court and at the Boeing Company. According to the U.S. Attorney prosecuting the case, the motive appeared to be simply, "the challenge of breaking into the computers . . . hackers have a name for it called 'network navigating.' "[2]

Warning that the nation's computers are not secure, the National Academy of Sciences recently reported that the government's critical computer systems are extremely vulnerable to abuse, and that "there is reason to believe our luck will soon run out."[3] At a recent congressional hearing on this subject, Congressman Robert Toricelli blasted those responsible by asserting that "Our economy, our traffic control system, the IRS and the entire Social Security program depend upon computer systems that are at risk because federal agencies have failed to put simple computer security controls in place."[4]

Studies by the Inspector General of the U.S. Department of Health and Human Services acknowledge the rapid growth and profitability of computer abuse. Theft and abuse by computer appears to be more lucrative, much safer, and to carry less punishment than many other criminal activities.[5] To compound the seriousness of the situation, one source predicts that computer crime will increase more rapidly than controls that detect and thwart crime.[6] With the increase in computer literacy, this trend has the potential for creating serious management issues for all health care organizations.

Legions of horror stories about computer security breakdowns have been chronicled. Virtually every week another computer scandal comes to light. Almost everyone has heard of the Cornell graduate student who released the "Cornell Worm," a rogue program that went out of control and stalled thousands of computers connected to the Internet, a network of business, government, and military computers. Or the trial of the "Legion of Doom" hackers accused of stealing secrets from BellSouth Corporation.[7] These stories are by no means limited to the United States. A pair of British computer hackers, who boast they can "tap into anything," even America's defense network, challenged British authorities and the FBI to catch them. Claiming that it is easy to breach almost any computer system, they have tapped into Fort Knox, Fort Leavenworth, and the Pentagon. Especially disconcerting to the British authorities is their claim that they have Queen Elizabeth's unlisted phone number![8]

Yet, despite the apparent extent and severity of the problem, little seems to be done about it. According to *Newsday*,[9] most computer systems users do not have safeguards and, of those that do, many do not bother to use them. In health care, this sentiment is substantiated by Dennis Van Auken, Vice President of Source Data Systems, who says that "Until recently, many healthcare institutions simply have not paid attention to security."[10] In reflecting upon this problem, Jeff Schiller, who looks after a network of computers called Project Athena at the Massachusetts Institute of Technology, comments that computer vulnerability is common because "people who use computers generally don't worry about security."[11]

The result is that those traditionally charged with the responsibility for protecting and maintaining the resources of an organization often have very little understanding of the degree of exposure and vulnerability they have. One commentator goes so far as to say that, if managers really understood the liability and risks to the assets of an organization (and their professional reputations), they might shut down all networks and data centers.[12] Indeed, the highly respected Research Foundation of the Financial Executive Institute defines the increasing reliance on poorly understood and managed computer information systems as the "Achilles heel" of modern organizations.[13] Those health care managers who are cognizant of the security problem, are "in an endless arms race pitting new systems of security against new weapons of intrusion."[14]

The Nature of the Security Problem

Computer security is the very practical administrative and technical matter of protecting the organization's data and equipment. It is a critical problem, since billions a year are stolen by computer tampering, most of which is never detected or reported. However, this is only the financial aspect—it does not include computer security breakdowns that do not entail direct financial loss.

The problem has five major components, the first of which involves the physical security of computer equipment. Some time ago the computer system of a Vermont firm was destroyed by fire,[15] a disaster which has struck the Pentagon's computer, some hospitals, and numerous other organizations. Some systems have been physically sabotaged, others flooded, many vandalized. As costly as these vulnerabilities can be, they are perhaps the easiest to guard against. Many sophisticated measures are available, since the challenge of protecting the physical equipment of computer systems is essentially the same as protecting any equipment.

Loss of data is less easily protected by traditional security measures. A classic case a few years ago involved a firm in Chicago that stored its accounts receivable file on a computer tape. Every Monday the appropriate tape was taken from the tape library and used to process bills. One Monday morning no bills were produced: several hundred thousand dollars in receivables were at stake, and the company did not have a duplicate record. What happened? The tape, stored on the bottom shelf in the new tape library, was accidentally erased by the magnetic coil in a new heavy-duty vacuum cleaner. The point is clear: stored data can be lost.

A third component of the problem is data manipulation. Changing data stored on computer systems without leaving any trace of tampering is a fairly simple matter. At a New York college, for example, a "D" student received a Phi Beta Kappa key and was named to the Dean's list on the basis of a computerized transcript that showed all "As." The student had a friend in the college computer center who, for a small fee, was willing to raise "Ds" to "As." Three years after the student graduated the ploy was accidentally discovered by a physics professor who noticed a discrepancy between his handwritten grade sheet and the transcript printout.

There is also the problem of unauthorized access to computer systems. A *Saturday Review* report illustrates the scope of the vulnerability:

> At 19, Jerry Schneider was president of his own thriving electronic equipment business, Creative Systems Enterprises. The "creative" aspect of the business was that the equipment he sold belonged to the Pacific Bell Telephone Company. Posing as a magazine reporter, Schneider toured Pacific Bell's computer installation; he asked a lot of questions and pocketed a handful of discarded punch cards. Armed with this information, his basic high school knowledge of computers, and a touch-tone telephone, the teenager keyed into Pacific Bell's inventory and supply computer and robbed the company blind.[16]

Finally, there is the problem of misuse of both equipment and data by authorized and unauthorized users. Incidents include using the organization's computers to run personal businesses. In one case, two employees established their own company on $2 million of time on a large government computer in San Jose, California. More serious is the misuse of sensitive data. Examples include the use of sensitive personal information by criminal justice or health care workers to embarrass, bribe, or otherwise harm individuals.

The most recent computer security problem that could potentially halt the flow of information is the lethal presence of "computer viruses."[17] Viruses are snippets of computer code that are deliberately introduced into a computer system by way of a software program "down-loaded"—received and captured electronically—from another computer. Some viruses have even turned up in commercial software packages. The most common destructive virus infects a disk and scrambles or erases files. Other viruses are used to open "trap doors" in a computer system, allowing an individual to gain information or exploit the system. Common terms associated with viruses are "trojan horse" and "logic bomb." A trojan horse is an unauthorized set of instructions in a computer program hidden from the user which directs the computer to perform certain functions. A logic bomb is an unauthorized computer program designed to be executed at a designated time or when certain conditions occur. Put in place by a trojan horse, the unauthorized program will cause the "bomb" to detonate, and any number of malicious acts might occur (e.g., removal of a terminated employee's name from a personnel file, erasing a payroll file, or issuing a big check to the perpetrator).

Many industry experts agree that these viruses are bound to change the way we think about computer systems. As a result, some organizations are beginning to instruct their employees in the practice of "safe computing."[18] These computer security problems are so widespread that most organizations have probably been affected. Security breaches affect the availability, integrity, or confidentiality of information systems. A major cause of the problem is computer users' ignorance of the particular security vulnerabilities that come with automation.

How Computer Security Is Different

Protecting computerized information systems is far different and more difficult a challenge than protecting a file cabinet with diamonds, gold, and organizational secrets. While criminal acts are the same as they have always been—fraud, theft, larceny, embezzlement, extortion, sabotage, espionage—computers have created a unique environment. Access codes, passwords, and encryption all work, but none is a foolproof defense. Walter Kleinschrod notes that "crooks constantly 'think security' because security is their business. Business people only rarely think security because 'thinking business' is their business."[19]

Whereas traditional security procedures deal with visible, physical items, computer security involves protecting invisible property. Once data is stored in a computer, or on a tape or disk, they are imperceptible to the human eye. We cannot see whether data has been removed, or directly notice whether changes have been made. There are no jimmied locks on file drawers, no missing folders to alert us to a break-in, no erasure marks on the paper. Moreover, an intruder can instruct a computer to erase any invisible electronic evidence of a system invasion.

Second, the remote access capability of computers means that intruders can invade an organization's computers from the privacy of their own home—or from another organization's computer, or even from a phone booth—using a portable terminal. Dead bolt locks on doors provide little protection.

Third, computers involve strange forms and codes so that even a visible indication of data manipulation, such as an unauthorized change in software, might go undetected. Nontechnical users can look at the printout of their own application program and not notice a change.

A fourth, and perhaps the most significant, security factor is technical personnel—the computer experts who are, as Kleinschrod observes, "in almost total situations of trust." Many of them, he insists, "know how to do anything to a computer without being detected."[20]

Finally, the sheer scope of computerization affects security. Computers can and do store more information than was ever stored in manual systems. Moreover, much of this information is integrated or networked so that a violator can obtain a variety of data at once. In addition, unauthorized manipulation of computerized data can affect hundreds of users.

Aggravating these computer-related conditions are social, legal, and organizational realities. The challenge to "beat the machine" gives some social acceptance to efforts to break into computers. Take for example the aforementioned young "hackers" using a home computer to break into data systems with the motive simply being the challenge of breaking into computers.[21] Or the second generation hackers known as "cyberpunks" who roam the electronic pathways of cyberspace and break into systems for the sheer joy of damaging, destroying, or capitalizing on the data they find.[22]

Our legal system has lagged behind technological realities so that prosecuting computer criminals is difficult. Legal sanctions are ineffective because prosecutors have been unable to document the theft since the stolen data is invisible and physically breaking and entering is unnecessary. Legislation intended to proscribe using government computer systems in an unauthorized manner, the 1987 Computer Security Act, appears to do little good. A recent congressional study found that a number of government agencies have simply failed to implement procedures mandated by this legislation.[23]

Some organizations lie about the status of information security in their organizations. One of the most common rationales for denying security problems is the "principle of secure image," which holds that if an organization is perceived as vulnerable, it invites attack and exploitation. Operating on this principle, many organizations choose not to disclose that they have been victimized by breaches of security for fear that disclosure would invite similar breaches, loss of confidence, and investigations into the adequacy of supervision.[24]

Organizationally, the efficiency and speed of computers can prompt users to avoid efficiency-limiting procedures, such as security measures, which clearly impede operations. End users of the technology want user friendliness and do not always understand the nature of security threats, potential methods of abuse, or the value of some of the information resources they are manipulating, and often resist anything that they perceive as delaying their work.[25] A typical pattern involves the security measure of access codes for terminals. To save time, users will often write the access code on a strip of paper taped to the machine, thus undermining security. Other common behaviors include the sharing of passwords indiscriminately, unattended but logged on computer terminals, and improper disposal of printed reports.

In sum, securing computerized information systems is a different task from securing the organization's valuables. It is thus clear that managing the security of computer systems requires some creative action.

What Health Care Professionals Can Do

Managing the security of computers is a technical and administrative task that requires creative user-manager action.[26] It cannot be left to the technician. Managers must be guided in this effort by a sober awareness that there is no such thing as a completely secure computer available today, and that more security means more cost and less efficiency. Therefore, the first issue is to decide how much security is needed.

Probably the most effective action managers can take is to organize the information they collect and maintain, because poorly organized information systems are easier to breach. Organizing information for security is a three-step process of (1) reviewing data needs, (2) eliminating unneeded data, and (3) classifying needed data into security-related categories such as routine, sensitive, and critical.

Many organizations maintain sensitive data that is not needed; eliminating it immediately reduces the problem. Since it is estimated that only 10 percent of an organization's required information is highly sensitive or critical, and since security measures are expensive and sometimes cumbersome, classifying information can be important. For example, once sensitive information has been identified and classified, it can be stored on a small, dedicated, highly secure system for security.

Managers can also assess vulnerabilities and risks in order to decide how much security is needed. How attractive and valuable is the data? Who can be hurt and how badly? What is the probability of an intrusion? How vulnerable is the system and what are its major vulnerabilities? What could be the legal or replacement costs of a security breakdown?

Nearly all studies have shown that the greatest vulnerability is the insider—the technician who has access and knows the system and its security measures. Therefore, a third measure for managers is to devise a careful personnel strategy to counter a dishonest, disgruntled, or careless employee. This may entail special recruitment procedures, such as more extensive background checks; organizational separation of duties, such as not allowing programmers to operate terminals; special attention to technician morale; and continual security training for users and technicians as part of a "security consciousness" effort.

In addition, managers can install a range of technical measures such as fire safety devices to protect the physical hardware: access codes, programming instructions that shut the computer down when anything unusual happens, and encryption of data. The technology can indeed be used to protect itself. Many organizations program terminals to automatically record the user, the information input, and the terminal used in the transaction. Still others restrict access to certain files and processes. In effect, through creative programming, a computer can be instructed to be its own watchdog, to immediately alert a manager when anything unusual or suspicious occurs.

Similarly, managers can take a range of administrative measures from restricted physical access to the computer facility, to the use of burn bags for discarded papers, to identity checks of all visitors. Ideas on possible administrative and technical procedures are catalogued in various manuals such as Leibholz and Wilson's *The Users Guide to Computer Fraud* and John M. Carroll's *Computer Security*.

Finally, nothing can better disclose the effectiveness of security measures than trying to break into the system. Some organizations hire former computer criminals to do this, others use legitimate "computer busters," such as the System Development Corporation in California, whose business is to break into computer systems and thus disclose weaknesses. In addition, all organizations are well advised to conduct a periodic audit of their computer security system.

In short, information security requires a package of measures. The problem is considerable, and its resolution depends on the understanding and action of user-managers as well as technicians. In health care, in particular, attention to this reality is critical.

Notes

1. D. Charles, "Can We Stop the Databank Robbers?" *New Scientist*, 26 January 1991, 24.

2. *New York Times*, 15 November 1992, 5.

3. *New York Times*, 6 December 1990, 26.

4. E. Newlin, "A Better Way Is Needed to Keep Computer Systems Under Lock and Key," *The Business Journal of New Jersey*, September 1990, 17.

5. R. Knotts and T. Richards, "Computer Security: Who's Minding the Store?" *The Academy of Management Executive*, vol. 3, no. 1 1989, 63–66.

6. Ibid, 63.

7. Newlin, 17.

8. L. C. Levy, "The Crime of the Future Has Arrived," *Newsday*, 18 February 1980, 7.

9. R. Hard, "Keeping Data Secure within Hospitals," *Hospitals*, 20 October 1992, 50.

10. *New York Daily News*, 7 February 1994, 4.

11. Charles, 24.

12. K. Weiss, "One Time Passwords: The Key to Secure Systems," *Datacenter Manager*, September–October 1990, 42.

13. *New York Times*, 10 June 1980, D-13.

14. W. A. Kleinschrod, "Thinking Like A Crook," *Administrative Management*, January 1987, 62.

15. D. Williams, "When the Computer Goes Up in Smoke," *Output*, August 1980, 27–33.

16. J. T. DeWeese, "The Trojan Horse Caper," *Saturday Review*, 15 November 1975, 10.

17. C. C. Sanford, "Computer Viruses: Symptoms, Remedies, and Preventive Measures," *Journal of Computer Information Systems*, Spring 1993, 67.

18. *Time*, 11 April 1988, 52.

19. Kleinschrod, 62.

20. Ibid, 48.

21. *New York Times*, 15 November 1992.

22. J. Caniglia, "Cyberpunks Hate You," *Utne Reader*, July–August 1993, 88–96.

23. Newlin, 17.

24. C. C. Wood, "Lying About Information Security," *Computer World*, 10 February 1992, 2.

25. Weiss, 42.

26. A. Radding, "Plans for a Safer System—Strategic System Security," *Computer Decision*, 6 April 1987, 38–41.

Selected Readings

Angel, J., and A. Evans. "Data Protection and the Subject of Access." *Personnel Management* (October 1987): 52–56.

Ball, M. "To Catch A Thief: Lessons in Systems Security." *Computerworld* (14 December 1987): 75–78.

Berton, L. "Low-Tech Steps Can Help Guard Computer Data." *Wall Street Journal* (28 December 1987): 15W.

Brooks, G., T. Semenuk, and V. Vaughn. "Controlling Information: Who, What, How." *Computers in Healthcare* (January 1988): 16–21.

Carter, K. "Information Systems Security—Top Priority for Medical Records." *Modern Healthcare* (22 November 1985): 82.

Diamond, S. "Computer Disruption: Planning for the Worst." *High Technology* (7 May 1987): 54–56.

Findlay, G. "Data Security: Reducing the Risks." *Accountant's Magazine* (June 1987): 57–60.

Hicks, S. M. "PC Security: Implementing a Corporate Program." *Credit and Financial Management* (January 1987): 28.

Hitt, J., and P. Tough. "Terminal Delinquents." *Esquire* (December 1990): 174–219.

Hoffman, M. N. "Managing Computer Security." *Healthcare Financial Management* (May 1987): 101.

Krema, J. "Preventive Measures to Ensure PC Data Security." *Office* (March 1988): 37–39.

Martinott, R., and J. Winton. "Getting a Lock on Computer Security." *Chemical Week* (28 October 1987): 26–32.

McMenamy, E. "On the Trail of A Hidden Threat—Data Security." *Infosystems* (December 1986): 38–40.

Nakagawa, R. "Network Security: Control versus Convenience." *Datacenter* (September–October 1990): 33–35.

Peterson, I. "Computing a Bit of Security." *Science News* (16 January 1988): 38.

Schweitzer, J. "Tangible Losses: How to Shape an Information Policy that Won't Let Data Slip through Your Fingers." *Computerworld* (18 January 1988): 75–80.

Sweet, F. "How to Build A Security Chain—Data Processing Security Measures." *Datamation* (1 February 1987): 34–44.

READINGS

THE COMPUTER security focus of this chapter is explored in more depth in the accompanying readings. Jack Hitt and Paul Tough in their *Esquire* article provide hard core consciousness of the extent of the computer security challenge. Stuart Madnick's essay is still among the most comprehensive and detailed treatments of managerial approaches to this challenge.

Terminal Delinquents

Jack Hitt and Paul Tough

> Once, they stole hubcaps and shot out streetlights. Now they're stealing your social security number and shooting out your credit rating. A layman's guide to computer high jinks.

On a muggy Friday night, we putter about the entrance to the Chelsea Hotel in New York City, nervously chatting about nothing in particular, pacing, thumping a dead coffee cup, waiting. A massive sun—garishly orange, unnaturally close—tries to wash this skeezy neighborhood with its maudlin rays, but this is Manhattan, the Chelsea, where Nancy Spungen asked Sid Vicious to stab her to death; no way. It moves on, down the runway of Twenty-third Street to the Hudson River, like all the traffic on this block, unnoticed. We are here to meet Kool and Ikon,* reputedly two of the most talented computer hackers this side of Newark. They had agreed to reveal the secrets of their craft, but only if we chose a place such as the Chelsea, where our work would be untraceable.

The film-noir tactics are necessary these days because hackers are on the lam. During the last few months a federal sweep of computer hackers, known as Operation Sun Devil, targeted the country's hacker elite. Last spring, Secret Service agents raided the homes of scores of kids, seizing not only computers but every piece of electronic equipment in sight, down to answering machines, cassette recorders, even soldering irons. These searches had all the subtlety of SWAT raids: six armed agents—guns drawn—to take one teenager into custody. In one Manhattan bust, a fourteen-year-old boy stepped from the shower into the sights of an agent's shotgun. In all, the government has seized twenty-seven thousand computer disks from forty suspected hackers. Two of them are to meet us tonight.

Hacking, as most of us know it, means breaking into private computer systems. More broadly, hacking is about solving problems, getting around obstacles, clearing the way. It involves not only the technical methods of skirting computer security, but also convincing the people who run the machines to divulge their passwords. Here at the Chelsea, the obstacle we're circumventing is the U.S. Secret Service.

Until recently, hacking was done in the comfort of one's bedroom, plugged into Mom and Dad's home phone. But a government wiretap can do a lot to change old habits. Now many hackers carry mobile computer rigs that attach to any phone—whether it's a pay phone on the street or the room phone in a hotel.

According to the media kit issued by the Secret Service, the boys we are scheduled to meet pose a clear and present danger to the security of both the government and the American people: "The conceivable criminal violations of this operation have serious implications for the health and welfare of all individuals, corporations, and United States government agencies relying on computers and telephones to communicate." In other words, for "the health and welfare" of us all.

But when the boys finally arrive and the four of us stand in the lobby of the Chelsea, chatting, we find that they are courteous, even deferential. It is difficult to see them as the new Communists, the new menace, the enemy within. And if it is hard to see them as the government's clichés, it is equally difficult to see them as the media's, which has chosen adjectives from a different page of the thesaurus, depicting hackers either as a group of buck-toothed dweebs or the lazy sons of the white middle class whose loathing of their parents is so intense that they wreak their Freudian revenge upon the aptly named Ma Bell.

The most recent poster boy for computer subversion is Robert Morris Jr., a former Cornell graduate student convicted earlier this year of releasing a virus that disabled nearly six thousand computers nationwide. Morris's father was the head of the National Computer Security Center, the government's computer-security agency, and the media delighted in painting Morris Jr. as the spoiled son of privilege ruining his father's good name. The Ivy League student stared out from a thousand newspaper photos, pale and owl-like in his glasses. No longer would the government be forced to denounce phantoms; computer hacking now had a face and a name.

But these boys are teenagers—nearly ten years younger than Morris—olive skinned, descended from Mediterranean stock. Home is a working-class urban neighborhood in New Jersey. They could never consider graduate school at Cornell; they're thinking about Passaic County Community College.

Though handsome, they possess the awkwardness of youth—they are seventeen and eighteen years old—so with a little imagination, we could certainly write them up as geeks. Their clothes are standard issue for peer-pressured teens: baggy jeans, no belt, low-top sneaks, long-sleeved T-shirt. No pocket protector, but no hair sculpted into a Dairy Queen offering, either; just careless teenage hair. They are similar in appearance—medium height and lanky. Ikon is the shorter of the two and tends to be the more serious. His jokes are often put-downs, mocking the stupidity of those around him. Kool's humor is more playful, even lewd; he's constantly checking out the girls.

Their language is urban, toughened by *dems* and *dozes;* and youthful, brimming with uhs, *likes,* and *you knows.* But take out that oral punctuation, and the syntax is textbook correct. Their conversations are surprisingly sophisticated in their understanding not only of the complex workings of the computer but of the caprices of the human heart as well.

Under false names and paying in cash, we check into our cheap room, space just big enough for the four of us, painted white every year for half a century and furnished with flimsy items stained the color of cocoa. We quickly redecorate, hauling the desk next to the bed, and pulling up the chair so that we can all sit and see. We set their portable laptop computer on the desk and string a tangle of wires among the computer, various electronic gadgets, and the hotel telephone. Ikon's fingers fly across both the phone's keypad and the computer's keyboard with blinding speed.

Eeeep. We have connected. We are here to learn how to do this, but for now we just stare into the shimmering green screen. In a matter of minutes we are deep in the heart of the telephone company's computers. It appears that Ma Bell has been expecting us; the screen suddenly displays a boxed note, unambiguous in its meaning:

WARNING

Access to this computer and to the computer data and computer materials accessible by use of this computer is restricted to those whose access has been authorized by NYNEX or its subsidiary companies. This computer, computer data, and computer materials may only be used for approved business purposes of NYNEX or its subsidiary companies. Use by unauthorized individuals or use for unauthorized purposes is a violation of Federal and/or State Laws.

Kool asks Jack for his home telephone number. More light-speed hand movements. The room is still with concentration, interrupted occasionally by an incomprehensible chatter of acronyms and a strange, bureaucratic-sounding shorthand. Suddenly, a series of numeric patterns blooms on the screen. It looks like this:

```
M00 TR01 555 0000
0000
LEN 10 121 306
001 000 000 000 000 000 4
000 000 000 000 000 000 000 000
0 0 0 0
0 0 0 0 0
```

"Doesn't mean much to you, does it Jack?" asks Ikon. "This is what a phone number really looks like. The LEN is your line-equipment number. It's the actual hardware, the only thing that matters. Your phone number is just scratch-pad nonsense. I could change it right now, if I wanted to. It could be anything at all."

More clacking on the keyboard, and a new image appears.

```
M 01 TR75 1 DN 555 0000 00000002
PIC 222 TTC
```

Ikon makes a few changes, and the configuration looks like this:

```
M 12 TR75 1 DN 555 0000 00000003
PIC 288 TWC TTC
```

Jack has just been granted three-way calling (TWC) and has switched his long-distance carrier from MCI (222) to AT&T (288). At such profound digital levels, these changes will escape the NYNEX business office. Consequently, Jack will never be billed.

This deep into the system, many other things are possible, from the simple, such as finding an unlisted phone number with an address or a name, to the sinister, such as monitoring the conversation of anyone we choose by quietly dropping in on the phone line like an operator, undetected. All of it is rather simple, they insist, once you understand the structure of the system. If you're not *stupid* (the ultimate hacker put-down), if you apply common sense to the system, hacking is a piece of cake.

The image of the powerful and reckless hacker, capable of rooting around in our most-secret computer systems, unleashing crippling computer viruses, disrupting phone service, crashing hospital computers, and changing school records, is the one most often affirmed by law-enforcement officials and the daily media. This is not only because it easily suits the respective purposes of these institutions—whip up public loathing so the little sons of bitches can be arrested; sell newspapers—but also because it is largely true. This representation fails, however, because it doesn't answer the most obvious question: If hackers really have the knowledge to do such things, why haven't they used it? Why aren't we living in a constant nightmare of paralyzed phone systems and crashing computer banks? To answer this question, we have spent the last year getting to know more than a dozen of the best hackers in America. Over time, we won their trust and were admitted into their ranks. We apprenticed ourselves to them so that we could learn what damage they really *can* do and why they don't do it.

Hacking, at its most mechanical, requires that you arrange an electronic conversation between your humble laptop (Radio Shack, $800) and a huge computer—brimming with information—inside some corporate headquarters, government agency, or university. The conversation takes place in a very human way—using a telephone. The laptop uses a modem (Radio Shack, $150) to translate the digital pulses of a computer into the hisses and beeps that travel over regular phone lines.

In the comfort of your home, a modem can be plugged directly into the back of the telephone. When you're using plugless phones, like hotel phones and pay phones, one more step is required. An acoustic coupler (Laptop Shop, $150), tightly strapped to the phone receiver, allows the computer to fire audio tones directly through the handset, the way we do when we speak.

Just like people, computers have phone numbers, known as "dial-ups." When you call a computer, its own modem hears the tones coming through the phone line and translates your hisses and beeps back into the electronic pulses the computer can understand. You're connected. The hacking can begin.

Exhibit 7.1 A Hacker's Primer

Here's What You'll Need

A. Acoustic Coupler: Sleek suction cups fit over the earpiece and mouthpiece of your phone. Portable and sturdy, these are perfect for home or the road. $150.

B. Modem: Although many top-of-the-line laptops come with a modem built in, the budget hacker will need an external modem to connect the computer to the acoustic coupler. $150.

C. Laptop: When the situation demands prudence, the cautious hacker uses a portable laptop for work outside of the home. $750–$2,000.

D. NBC Cap: No hacker can do without this handsome and versatile social-engineering prop. Perfect for those late nights at the Empire State Building. $10.

E. Jolt Cola: *The* soft drink of elite hackers has "all the sugar and twice the caffeine." One can will keep you hacking until dawn. $.60.

There are thousands of systems to hack, and dozens of hackers for each one. For Kool and Ikon, though, there's only one game in town—the phone company.

Hacking Ma Bell dates back to the late Sixties, when phone hackers, then dubbed "phone phreaks," discovered that the entire AT&T phone system could be controlled by whistling tones at various frequencies directly into a phone. One notorious hacking pioneer, John Draper, made the farcical discovery that the toy whistle in a box of Cap'n Crunch perfectly mimicked the 2,600-hertz tone that engaged a long-distance line, enabling him to make free calls anywhere in the world. Draper assumed the cereal's name as his *nom de haque,* and he and his generation spent years deciphering the meanings of different tones. The perfection of the "blue box"—a portable device that duplicated the tones needed to master the phone system—became the ultimate mission.

With the advent of long-distance calling cards, which are easily filchable, hackers today take free long-distance calls for granted. What interests Captain Crunch's descendants are the computers that control and link our phones. Soon after the Captain Crunch era, AT&T was broken up into a network of "baby Bells" (regional phone systems). These are now the main event. Kool and Ikon hack NYNEX, which handles phone service for all of New York and New England.

The first stop for your phone line, after it snakes out of your house, is a local switching center. This "switch" directly controls all the phones in your neighborhood. A switch performs the same service as Lily Tomlin's cranky operator, Ernestine, who would plug your phone jack into the line that you were calling. Today, your switch makes that connection electronically, and does it for as many as 150,000 phones.

Each neighborhood switch is controlled by its own huge computer; these computers are the essential targets of the phone-company hacker. If you can access the computer for a switch, you can control every phone it does. You can turn those phones on and off, reroute calls, and change numbers.

When this knowledge grows boring, the explorer can investigate the dozens of NYNEX's more complicated computer systems, each containing hundreds of new passageways and strange domains. For the advanced hacker, one of the more attractive is the infelicitously named NYNEX Packet Switched Network, or NPSN. Its beauty is its strength: The system allows you to enter each of the more than one thousand switches in New York and New England. Even more appealing, it allows you to ricochet off onto regional maintenance systems such as COSMOS and MIZAR. Among its many talents, COSMOS sends out instructions to create and kill phone numbers. The local MIZAR actually does the work. Since COSMOS keeps the records and MIZAR doesn't, most hacking done on a MIZAR is undetectable. MIZARs are a hacker favorite.

In order to get into any computer, you need a dialup number, an account name (or "login"), and a password. Most people encounter the basics of this process every time they approach an automatic-teller machine. Knowing where to find an ATM is your dialup; placing your card with its black magnetic strip in the slot is like entering your account; punching in your personal identification number is like typing your password. The secret of obtaining these three keys for breaking into a phone-company computer—or any computer—is simple, our tutors explain, and can be learned as easily over a banana split in an air-conditioned diner as over a computer screen. We abandon our sweltering room at the Chelsea and head to the local joint. On the plate-glass window of the restaurant we notice a decal that boasts, INSIDE: A PUBLIC PHONE YOU CAN DEPEND ON.

Over burgers and ice cream, we learn that there are several mechanical ways of learning accounts and passwords, but that there's an easier way, known as social engineering. Basically, social engineering is bull[__]ing—calling someone who has access to a system and convincing them that you are a legitimate user who needs a dialup number, an account, and a password.

For the adventurer, social engineering may seem like cheating. Getting a password *can* be done by purely technical hacking means: programming a computer to try thousands of passwords. But to these guys (and even to their apprentices after a few weeks), this method is as irritating as playing the first levels of a video game after you've mastered them. You want to whiz right past such tedium to the more interesting levels. Getting a password is not hacking. It is a pain in the ass.

Social-engineering a used-car dealer (see [Exhibit 7.2]) is easy, even if you don't know what you're doing (because he doesn't, either—although his natural suspicion as a civilian often means you don't get past the hellos). Social-engineering a computer specialist with high-level access is easy only if you do know what you're doing. The professional needs to hear a few bits of jargon, just enough artfully expressed codes to make him feel that he is talking to a member of the guild. Both forms are surprisingly successful.

"Sometimes," says Kool, "it's so *simple*. I used to have contests with my friends to see how few words we could use to get a password. Once I called up and said, 'Hi, I'm from the social-engineering center and I need your password,' and they gave it to me! I swear, sometimes I think I could call up and say, 'Hi, I'm in a diner, eating a banana split. Give me your password.'"

Like its mechanical counterpart, social engineering is half business and half pleasure. It is a social game that allows the accomplished hacker to show off his knowledge of systems, his mastery of jargon, and especially his ability to manipulate people. It not only allows the hacker to get information; it also has the comic attractions of the old-fashioned prank phone call—fooling an adult, improvisation, cruelty.

In the months we spent with the hackers, the best performance in a social-engineering role was by a hacker named Oddjob. With him and three other guys we pulled a hacking all-nighter in the financial district, visiting pay phones in the hallway of the World Trade Center, outside the bathrooms of the Vista Hotel, and in the lobby of the international headquarters of American Express.

Oddjob's magnum opus takes place along the south wall of the phone bank leading to the Vista's bathrooms. We bolshevize six chairs from the women's powder room and attach our computer to a pay phone. Throughout the night, the hackers compliment one another

Exhibit 7.2   Here's How You Do It: Social Engineering

Social engineering in practice can be staggeringly easy. One good session, for instance, is all a hacker needs to break into TRW, the company that houses the credit files on 170 million Americans. Like to check your neighbor's credit rating? Here's how:

Call information in a faraway town and ask for a used-car dealership. Say you get Louie's Used Cars. Call and ask for the finance department. Whoever answers the phone will be the one who uses the TRW account at Louie's to check on the credit worthiness of customers. Now lay on the bull[___] as Kool says, "in your best Joe Isuzu voice." Here's one riff that works only too frequently: "Hi, my name is Gary Jenkins with Compuline. We're doing a few repairs on the TRW lines in your area. Have you been having any trouble with your terminal?"

Now, who among us has not had trouble with a computer? Your friend at Louie's will likely greet you enthusiastically, thanking God you called. So proceed: "Okay, we need to check the line. Could you start up your system and talk me through this? First of all, what dialup are you using?" He'll then give you his local dialup for TRW. Write it down.

"Yeah, that's what I thought. Okay, when you first get in, what do you type?" The ten-character sequence he gives you is his account. There's no password; this is all you need. Write it down. Tell him you'll check out the problem and call back. Thank him for his help. Always be courteous; you may need to call again.

Now that you have a dialup and an account, you can call TRW from anywhere. All you need is a person's name and address to uncover his or her social security number, credit numbers, and credit history.

on the sheer genius of the place: chairs, a dozen phones, a computer with coupler, a snack bar down the hall, and—on a nasty, humid city night—air conditioning.

At the rarefied level these four have reached, an evening's work often revolves around the links between networks in the NYNEX system. On this night, one of our links is down; a password has been changed. Oddjob begs for a chance to social-engineer something, anything. His method, he explains, is to sound like a regular person, to assume the accents of those who do the day-to-day keypunching and processing—the heavy lifting of the information age. He has a considerable repertoire. . . . Tonight's composition will be performed in the key of Flatbush.

Oddjob paces furiously on his lilliputian stage, tethered to the pay phone by the irritatingly short steel line, firing suggestions to the crowd on whom to call, taking in ideas. Part of the thrill of social engineering is clearly the improvisation of it all. But it's improvisation with a competitive edge. You show your machismo by waiting until the last possible second to prepare yourself. The moment after dialing, before the phone is answered, a true hacker will suddenly request vital information: "Where should I say I'm calling from?" "Who do I ask for?" or even "Where am I calling?" Oddjob is feigning such recklessness when the phone is answered. He opens by establishing his credentials in thick Brooklynese:

"Yeah, hoi deh. Dis is Tucker calling from Pearl Street operations. Yeah, hi. You guys havin' trouble gettin' into NPSN deh? You guys are goin' through a packett switch, right? Yeah, when you go into COSMOS. Okay, 'cause dat's where the problems are—ya day guy reported it. Okay, what do you use for the packet switch when you first connect—do you have your own code?"

She does have her own code; unfortunately, she is not about to give it to him. She tells him to solve his problem by checking the manual. So Oddjob loudly flips through the pages of a nearby phone book, pretending to read from its pages, and finally, frustrated, heaves the phone book toward the wall, with a crash. But it's done in a way that says: *Geez, aren't these manuals frustrating? We, the folks who do all the work, are supposed to make sense of these?* She's beginning to cotton to him and reveals that the first part of the code is the user's initials. Oddjob cranks up the charm and moves in for the kill.

"Okay, so what do you put in? GWT? Are those your initials? What's your name? Gail? That's a nice name. Mine? Tucker. Yeah, that's my last name. I don't like my first name because it sounds really dumb. No, I'm not telling. *Noooooooo.* I'm not gonna tell you. *Oooooohh.* You really want to know? Okay, it's . . . Edmonton. Oh, come on, Edmonton is *not* distinguished, it's silly. They used to kid me in school. Yeah. Heh, heh. Anyway, just so I can get to the right system, would you walk me through it?" She does, and he gets most of the information he wants.

By 4:00 a.m. we had been thrown out of the Vista and were spread out across the waxy, marble lobby of American Express headquarters, listening to Oddjob con another sucker on the phone. Kool was trying out a few breakdancing moves. The evening had been devoted almost exclusively to social engineering; we hardly used the laptop at all.

As the edge of the horizon began to lighten and the two of us had said goodnight to the hackers and were walking home, we realized that the entire evening had provoked an eerie deja vu. As teenagers, we had both survived many of these Friday nights; trying halfheartedly to get into trouble, sitting around with the guys, waiting for something to happen. It's no accident that there are no hackers older than about twenty-one; serious hacking requires the kind of tireless devotion that only teenagers possess.

As with all teenage pursuits, hacking doesn't last forever. For most hackers, manipulating technology in imaginative ways is nothing more than rebellion. They learn high-tech pranks, such as changing the outgoing message on their algebra teacher's home answering machine, or they figure out how to chat with other hackers around the country for free. But these amateurs lack the patience and resolve to ascend to the levels our companions have attained. They fool around for six months or a year, get bored, and quit.

Like any group of teenagers with a common pursuit, serious hackers have nothing but contempt for amateurs. And when a fellow pro moves on, they treat it almost as betrayal, scorning the traitor as having "faded away into society." They can't imagine it happening to them.

Hackers are a group that has always existed in teenage society. They are not the genius nerds seen on TV. Nerds, by definition, are prosaic. They lack the creativity, the badass guts needed to hack. Nerds, in fact, are the ones who grow up and get hacked. Real hackers are the rebellious brains: the video-game addicts, the crystal-radio connoisseurs, the Dungeons & Dragons freaks. They are the guys who understand, even love, the way systems work: They don't just take things apart and put them back together—they make them do something else, something *better*. Where we see only a machine's function, they see its potential. This is, of course, the noble and essential trait of the inventor. But hackers warp it with teenage anarchic creativity: Edison with attitude.

Consider the fax machine. We look at it; we see a document-delivery device. One hacker we met, Kaos, looked at the same machine and immediately saw the Black Loop of Death. Here's how it works: Photocopy your middle finger displaying the international sign of obscene derision. Make two more copies. Tape these three pages together. Choose a target fax machine. Wait until nighttime, when you know it will be unattended, and dial it up. Begin to feed your long document into your fax machine. When the first page begins to emerge below, tape it to the end of the last page. Ecce. This three-page loop will continuously feed your image all night long. In the morning, your victim will find an empty fax machine, surrounded by two thousand copies of your finger, flipping the bird.

Ikon and Kool have been hacking the NYNEX phone system for about six years. Although much of their work has been done alone, they have each been in dozens of informal partnerships and groups, which tend to form quickly and dissolve just as fast. In the early Eighties, some of the best hackers in the country formed the Legion of Doom, which, despite its wicked name, basically served as a conduit for information. The quest to understand NYNEX is a far-flung, collective enterprise, like the space program, only run by teenagers—experiments aren't done in scrubbed laboratories but in hotel lobbies; information isn't exchanged at symposia in Geneva but at hastily called meetings in peculiar locations. One such meeting has been institutionalized: first Friday of every month, Manhattan Citicorp building at Fifty-third and Lexington at—where else?—the pay phones.

Although the channels hackers use to communicate are highly sophisticated, the way information travels is similar to the way knowledge is passed on in an oral tradition. Teleconferences are held on "bridges"—illicit phone links; technical information is exchanged on private computer bulletin-board systems run out of hackers' bedrooms; samizdat magazines are distributed with names like *Phrack* and *2600*. The latter name is an homage to Captain Crunch's 2,600-hertz tone, a tacit recognition that this oral tradition stretches back decades.

"Even though hippies were blue-boxing for all it was worth in the Sixties," explains Ikon, born the year Captain Crunch went to jail, "they didn't really understand what they were doing. In the Nineties, we're on a search for technical knowledge; what *we're* doing is figuring out how the phone system really *works*."

Once you understand the architecture of the system, all sorts of opportunities present themselves. Consider those telephone hybrids found beside most automatic-teller machines—the ones that connect you immediately with a bank employee. We see a way of getting help; a hacker sees unlimited free long-distance phone calls. Here's how:

When you pick up that phone, you hear a moment of silence before the automatic dialer beeps out the seven tones that call the bank's service center. That silence represents an open phone line, waiting to be told what to do. So instead of waiting for the automatic dialer, click the phone's hook ten times in rapid succession. This action perfectly imitates the ten spluttering pulses of the last hole on the rotary dial— the operator. When the seven tones sound, they are ignored; you've already seized control of the phone line. Wait a moment and the operator will answer. Explain that you're having trouble reaching a certain number in the Gobi Desert; could she dial it for you? Piece of cake.

Yet if technology giveth, it also taketh away. One hot Friday night in July, we get the call to pick up the boys at Penn Station. They are

Exhibit 7.3 Here's What Happens if You Get Caught

In the past, hacking was done with little concern for legal ramifications. But these days, as the federal government mops up a three-year investigation of computer hackers known as Operation Sun Devil, the conversation at hacker get-togethers is as likely to concern jail time as the intricacies of newly discovered systems.

Sun Devil has cast a wide net, snaring not only hackers but fanning out to nab even those suspected of *associating* with hackers. Craig Neidorf, publisher of the hacker magazine *Phrack*, was indicted in February for printing a document that had been hacked out of a BellSouth computer. The government based its case on BellSouth's claim that the purloined text was worth $79,449. When a BellSouth employee reluctantly admitted on the witness stand that the document was available from a catalogue for just $13, the case against Neidorf collapsed. Neidorf was left to figure out how to pay his $100,000 legal bill, and his magazine is defunct.

As more cases come to trial, angry prosecutors are seeking severe penalties for the perpetrators of what they describe as an "astronomical" crime wave. But when the judges hand down the sentences to those accused of unlawful curiosity, they might reflect on the parable of the two Steves. Among the earliest hackers, Steve Jobs and Steve Wozniak built their own "blue boxes"—the small, illegal devices designed to let you make free long-distance phone calls. Not only did they use them to call the pope, they also peddled them door-to-door in the Berkeley dorms. In 1976 Wozniak and Jobs applied the lessons of the blue box to more complicated circuitry and, from a garage in California, started Apple Computer.

bringing along some friends and a full agenda. Tonight, we're informed, will hold many lessons for us. When we meet, Ikon gravely explains the situation: "We seem to have lost our resources." It appears that NYNEX is starting to change passwords on them, and the one dialup into NPSN that was still working is now disabled. It just rings and rings. We will be starting practically from scratch.

We walk east on Thirty-fourth Street toward the Empire State Building. We've already hacked from two New York landmarks; why not a third? At 7:00, the building is pretty empty. Tourists are either taking the escalator down to the Guinness World of Records Exhibition or the elevator up to the Observation Deck. We're roaming the halls, scoping out pay-phone banks, and feeling rather conspicuous—six young men with a big black suitcase. A security guard, trying to be helpful, spooks us, and all six of us bolt simultaneously for six pay phones, pretending to be in midconversation. A ludicrous paranoia is setting in.

Eventually we find a velvet rope draped across a corridor, guarded only by a man polishing the floor. A few furtive glances down the hall, and we're over and in, ensconced in a secluded phone bank. We unpack our laptop, our modem, and our acoustic coupler; happily, the entire contraption fits on the phone's shelf.

Ikon starts pounding digits on the pay phone, trying to get that one dialup to work. But there is only continuous ringing. Suddenly he gets an idea. It's a long shot—a solution hopelessly simple. He calls the actual office whose computer he's trying to break into and politely asks the woman to (please) turn on the computer's modem.

Ecstasy.

"We're back on!"

"Yo! We're worth something!"

"It's MIZAR! It's everything!" "We have a reason to live!"

With access to NPSN, we now set out to "liberate" one of these pay phones, that is, to free it from its addiction to quarters. We get into the switching computer for this neighborhood and disconnect the pay phone. "The beast," Ikon declares, "is dead. We have killed it." Picking up the beast's receiver proves that he's right; no dial tone. "Now we bring the beast back to life," Ikon announces, and resurrects it as a regular phone, able to make local and long-dstance calls for free.

Kool takes out his black marker and writes on the pay phone in the wild style of graffiti artists: "The PLO Lives," and then adds, "Payphone Liberation Organization." We reconnect the computer to the liberated phone.

A second security guard happens along. He has a distinct interest in being told just what the—just what in *hell* is going on around here, anyway? Kool takes him aside for a bit of impromptu social engineering. "We're, uh, sending a story over the phones. We're with NBC." The guard notices the peacock logo on Ikon's white NBC baseball cap (NBC Studios gift shop, $10) and somehow makes sense of this—a bunch of teenagers, the middle of the night, Cheez Doodles, Jolt Cola; of *course* they're TV reporters. Now he wants to chat *us* up.

"What's the story on?" he asks eagerly.

"It's on the pay phones at the Empire State Building," replies Kool. "You know, uh, what kind of problems they have. . . ." Kool's improvisation is getting almost comically desperate, but the guard still buys it. After a moment, he moves on to complete his rounds.

From our current perch in NPSN, we want to hop onto the Brooklyn COSMOS maintenance system. The password we've been using no longer works; they've changed the locks. This is a serious problem. Social engineering at this level is extremely difficult, because the operators have been burned too many times to just hand over a password. What's more, there is no direct phone number to COSMOS, no dialup; COSMOS can only be reached from NPSN. But there is, as always, another way. This time it's called "pad-to-pad," probably the most advanced hacking procedure, because it calls for an artful use of both mechanical and social-engineering talents. Here's how it works:

Call an office in Brooklyn where you know they use COSMOS. Tell the person who answers that you're troubleshooting her COSMOS account, and you need her help. Ask her to type *stat* on her keyboard and read off the number that appears. With it, you can connect directly to her computer terminal; now *your* screen is *her* screen. Everything she types you can read, and vice versa. Begin the social engineering: Ask her to sign on to COSMOS and enter her password. She thinks everything is fine because she isn't telling you anything over the telephone, and she isn't, exactly; she's just typing on her terminal. And you type on yours, faking the computer's commands. When she types in her account number, you respond—as the computer would—by typing "Password?" Of course, her password won't get her onto COSMOS, since she's connected only to your computer; instead, it appears in glowing letters on your screen. You type "login incorrect." Before she tries again, detach your terminal from hers and keep talking, offering friendly advice.

At the Empire State Building, standing at a pay phone, our first shot at pad-to-pad works perfectly. Our victim puzzles over why the system won't grant her access and tries again. In a flash she hears the familiar clicks and squeaks that assure her she is safely on, and she and Ikon exchange cheerful banter as the COSMOS warning flashes on her screen:

ATTENTION ALL USERS

Under no circumstances should you disclose your logon password to anyone on the phone or in person.

Ikon strings her along for another few minutes, listening to her complaints, completing the lie: "Well, it seemed to be okay from this end. The first time it said 'login incorrect,' huh ? You think you might have typed it in wrong?"

But he's barely listening now, performing the coda by rote, because he's already connected to the Brooklyn COSMOS with her account, and he's exploring, looking for a backdoor program he installed here the last time he was on, before they moved the mainframe from Brooklyn to Massachusetts.

"It's here!" Ikon shouts.

"They're so stupid, man," says Kool.

"When they copied all the commands they copied our backdoor command over too," Ikon explains.

We execute this old command, disappear through the "back door," and surface on a higher, more powerful level of the machine. For the next few hours, we explore this strange new land, trying to figure out the look of the place. We are a dozen hands groping in darkness, feeling our way along the wall of a system somewhere in Massachusetts. While one hacker works the keyboard, the others throw out suggestions. Over time, ideas are winnowed, attempts are assayed. Failures are common, but they are relieved by moments of hope. A small obstacle is surmounted or a new passageway is discovered. The fun of gaining entry is over; now most of the hacking is trial and error, banging away at an obstacle until a path over, around, or through is revealed. At this remove—we are relayed off three computers and extended across four states—even the easiest hacking problems can suddenly become complex again.

We, the reporters, try to buoy our own interest by peppering the hackers with questions. But after a while, the answers are numbingly similar: "We're trying to get in." "We're just looking around." "We're trying to figure out what this does." After three hours, we are slumped against a wall, contemplating the significance of our boredom. At times, accompanying hackers is about as exciting as watching a graduate student flip through a card catalogue. During the fourth hour, several of the hackers grow restless. One leaves; another calls some friends. Kool slides down the wall to join us, and wistfully recalls the old days, when he could hack for twelve hours without a break.

Ikon outlasts everyone, which is not unusual. He's deep within the machine now, wired, intense, alert. He waves off the occasional call for food, ignoring his own hunger and fatigue. He's been standing before this unit for five hours without rest; he barely bothers to shift his weight from one leg to another. All we hear are the occasional staccato clicks as he attempts yet another entry. From time to time a security guard approaches and peers in. Our paranoia has yielded to exhaustion. We wave.

Ikon's reverie doesn't end until the battery pack on the laptop dies. Everyone else is relieved; we've been ready to go for hours.

As we pack up our equipment and head out into the night, Kool's attention is suddenly distracted by a low-slung, high-tech car. "Yo, check out that Porsche with the cellular phone. I'd give up hacking for that car."

"Who needs a Porsche?" asks Ikon. "We have MIZAR."

Kool looks at him with amazement, but Ikon goes on. "I'd rather have all of NYNEX than a Porsche. I mean, can you get passwords with a Porsche?"

Kool, still dumbfounded, states the obvious: "You can get *girls* with a Porsche! Can you get girls with a password?"

They're laughing, but we all know it's true: For Ikon, there is no higher purpose than hacking NYNEX. Kool, on the other hand, is willing to make a few exceptions. As they discuss the next day's hacking agenda, Kool admits that he's getting a little bored with the endless exploration, and suggests that they try some *cool* stuff. "Maybe we could forward calls to a radio station and be the only ones who can get through," he suggests. "We could win tickets to, like, a Depeche Mode concert."

Ikon is dismissive. "No. The Project."

"C'mon, let's think of something to do."

"No, wait. The Project, the Project." He is insistent: We will continue to chart the landscape of the telephone company. Nothing else matters.

We're with Kool, frankly: When do we get to start changing the orbit of satellites and listening in on Madonna's phone calls? For that matter, when do we conquer the entire NYNEX system? When does it end?

"The thing that keeps us so interested," Ikon tells us later, "is that with NYNEX, or any other system with good security, we'll *never* have permanent access. We'll always lose what we need, and we'll be forced to find another way to get back into it. It's almost like a game. It's like a never-ending role-playing adventure game, but it's real. The thing that makes it interesting is that you can never win."

"So why play?" we ask. "Why spend years at a keyboard, risking jail, to play a game you'll never win?"

"It's like having the edge. That's the whole thing," says Ikon. "The name of the game is having the edge."

"Over whom?" we ask.

"Over anyone else," he replies. "Some people spend their whole lifetime trying to find the one thing that they're really good at. We've found it already. We're hackers. You know, there are always these computer know-it-alls who say, 'Oh yeah, I used to be a hacker.' That's crap. If you're an ex-hacker, you were never a hacker to begin with. It's not something that dies. It's a way of life. It's a way of thinking."

What's the purpose of all this exploration? After a dozen nights, it hits us: Hacking *has* no practical purpose. Every hacker starts as a utilitarian, viewing phone systems as means to an end, such as free calls or high-tech pranking. But over time the means *become* the end. Advanced hackers are nothing more than aestheticians; they marvel not at the system's use but at the system itself. Suddenly a nagging contradiction makes sense. Throughout our apprenticeship, the hackers consistently scorned our "juvenile" requests to hack into TRW. Now we understand why. The best hackers are *bored* by TRW (and other record-keeping systems, like those at hospitals and schools) despite the juicy information they contain. These computers are simple data-retrieval units, not much more complicated than the word processor used to write this article. The TRW computer isn't worth hacking, because, as Kool so sweetly puts it, "it's a piece of [___]." The phone networks *are* worth hacking, not because of what a hacker can use them for, but because of their vast size. "It goes back to what Crunch said," Ikon explains. "The phone system is the largest network in the entire world." It's the hardest thing to hack, and therefore, it's the only thing *worth* hacking. It is from these hackers that the law and the corporations have the least to fear. Ironically, these are the ones getting busted.

It is true that everything Kool and Ikon do when hacking is illegal. All their calls are paid for fraudulently; all the systems they enter are proprietary. This fact occasionally provides a frisson of excitement (probably more so for us, the amateurs, than for serious hackers); more frequently, it is just ignored. What these hackers are doing makes absolute sense to them: They are gaining knowledge. If there are laws against that, they reason, they're not worth taking seriously. They've probably never heard Bob Dylan's code for the outlaw—"to live outside the law, you must be honest" but they instinctively follow it.

If pressed, they will describe the havoc they could unleash on the phone system; they could easily write a simple virus that would disable switch after switch, shutting down phone service for all of New York and New England in a few hours. The damage, they estimate, could take NYNEX engineers months to repair. "We could handle it," says Ikon flatly. But asking them what sort of harm they could do to the phone system is like asking a surgeon what sort of harm he could do to a patient he's operating on. They could destroy it . . . but what kind of question is that?

A couple of weeks after the night at the Empire State Building, we're sitting with four hackers in the appropriately named Cosmos Diner, watching four rail-thin adolescents attack four huge plates of meat. We ask them what had become an obvious question: What if the phone company actually offered them jobs?

"If NYNEX offered me a good job in an intelligent position, I'd take it in a second. I wouldn't even think about it," replies Ikon.

"Have you ever applied?"

"I called," Kool says. "They said all they had was repair, installation, and outside plant."

"Doofus stuff," explains Ikon. "All they have is [__] jobs."

We ask how many people in the phone company know as much about the systems as they do.

"To tell you the truth," says Ikon, "I don't think there are *any*. I'll tell you why. Each person in NYNEX specializes in a single network, or just a part of a network. We, on the other hand, could easily assume the position of any person in any department for any reason."

"What would happen if they did hire you, and they said, 'Okay, you're in charge of stopping hackers'?"

"There's a problem with that," Ikon explains. "There's this Legion of Doom member from Michigan who was busted last year for something minor. They gave him a job in some bogus department within Michigan Bell security. They'd get him to try to engineer departments, or try to guess passwords and get into systems. And then they canceled the project."

"Would you do a project like that if they asked you?"

"Yeah!" replies Kool. "That would be my perfect position."

"And could you make NYNEX secure?"

"Sure," says Ikon. "I could do it in a minute. We know every single aspect of how to get into these systems. I could tell them in a minute how to—" He stops himself. "But the thing is, it wouldn't be worth it. They would hire us, they'd get a few secrets and tips from us, and then they'd fire us. That's what they did to the guy in Michigan. They found out exactly what he could do, and then they fired him.

"If we were offered a real opportunity to help," Ikon continues, "then we would help. But they'll never do that. They would never admit that they could possibly be helped by people half their age. They just have too much pride."

"When I called up NYNEX to ask for a job," says Kool, "I talked to this guy in Corporate Security. This guy didn't know [__] about his network. I told him all these secrets, ways to break in; all they did was block all those entry points. I have yet to hear from anybody offering me a job."

"And later the same day, at home, we got back into the network through another entrance," says Ikon. "There's always another way."

"So [___] them," concludes Kool.

Over the last ten years, this country's relationship with technology has changed profoundly, in ways that we are only beginning to understand. Ten years ago, when we wanted to send a letter across town, we'd need a stamp and a few days to spare. Now we fax it in seconds. When we wanted money, we'd have to go cash a check with a real live bank teller. Now we don't even know when our banks are open. Personal computers, long-distance calling cards—we who have them can't imagine life without them.

During the same period, the many systems that we depend on—phone networks, banking transfers, even our national-security apparatus—have become increasingly dependent on computers. We trust these machines, sometimes unwittingly, with enormous amounts of personal information. This rarely concerns us; we have developed an almost religious faith in computers and in the people who run them. When we think of these systems at all, we trust that they are safe.

We are wrong.

Every one of these technological advances has made us less secure. Now our phones can be disabled; our credit histories can be changed, our medical profiles can be stolen; our social security information can be accessed. And it can all be done by an untraceable teenager at a pay phone, thousands of miles away.

There are no alarms being sounded by the people who run these systems. NYNEX, in fact, refused to allow any of its security personnel to be interviewed for this article. If computer-security professionals were to admit that the systems they manage are vulnerable, they would be asked how they could be made invulnerable. And at that point, they would have to admit that the systems cannot be, can never be.

Much of the public debate over computer hackers involves a search for the right metaphor. Are hackers simple trespassers, gliding through our houses without harming the contents? Are they armed robbers, breaking and entering? Are our computer systems like our homes, locked and protected? Or are they just a huge open field with a tiny sign saying KEEP OFF THE GRASS?

From a distance, a computer network looks like a fortress—impregnable, heavily guarded. As you get closer, though, the walls of the fortress look a little flimsy. You notice that the fortress has a thousand doors; that some are unguarded, the rest watched by unwary civilians.

All the hacker has to do to get in is find an unguarded door, or borrow a key, or punch a hole in the wall. The question of whether he's allowed in is made moot by the fact that it's unbelievably simple to enter.

Breaking into computer systems will always remain easy because the systems have to accommodate dolts like you and me. If computers were used only by brilliant programmers, no doubt they could maintain a nearly impenetrable security system. But computers aren't built that way; they are "dumbed down" to allow those who must use them to do their jobs. So hackers will always be able to find a trusting soul to reveal a dialup, an account, and a password. And they will always get in.

It is gradually dawning on us, thanks mostly to the exploits of hackers, that we have much less control over the computers that run our information society than we did over, say, file cabinets. Our general reaction has been to blame the messengers. In fact, to try to imprison them. Although they have never harmed the systems they hack, Kool and Ikon will probably be indicted early next year for a variety of acts made illegal by the Computer Fraud and Abuse Act of 1986; the charges they will face carry maximum sentences of many decades in prison. But even if hackers are jailed, hacking won't be eliminated; it's just too human an instinct, and just too easy a practice.

Toward the end of the summer, we decide to attempt the kind of hack the government says is the main threat: We will try to hack the White House—specifically, the PROF system installed in 1982 by Admiral John Poindexter, then President Reagan's national security adviser. Poindexter chose PROF in an attempt to *eliminate* security breaches. If any system is unhackable, we reason, this is the one.

By the time we finally get together, however, a week after we first discuss PROF with the hackers, we learn that one of them has already called the White House computer center. He laid on the usual line about doing work on the system, and he got a dialup. The more difficult task, still ahead, is obtaining an account and a password.

We are sitting, as always, around a phone, safe in what one hacker describes as "a covert, undisclosed location somewhere in the tri-state area." He thumbs through a Federal Yellow Book, the publicly available directory for the executive branch of the U.S. government. "Why don't I call one of these people?" he suggests, pointing to the page headed, EXECUTIVE OFFICE OF THE PRESIDENT. He scans down the page—the staffs of Fitzwater, Sununu, Scowcroft—and decides randomly on a target a few doors down from the President.

"I'll just talk to him really basic," he explains, dialing the target's direct number.

"I need a name to use." As the phone rings in the White House, he glances around the room and his eyes settle on a T-shirt, signed just above the pocket by the French designer Francois Girbaud.

The White House answers. The hacker's voice drops an octave.

Hacker: Yeah, how're you doin'? This is Francois Girbaud with the computer operations division.

White House: Mmm-hmm.

H: Yeah, I was just wondering if you had any access to the PROF system.

WH: Yeah, I do. I don't use it very often, though.

H: Yeah, I know. Cause we're, like, troubleshooting your account.

WH: Oh.

H: It seems that something's wrong with it. And, you know, we're wondering if maybe it's, like, one of the dialups that you're using to get in or something.

WH: Well, let me see. Hold on, I'm just getting out of what I was doing.

H: You know, if you're too busy I could call back later.

WH: No, that's okay, this is fine. Hold on one minute, I'm just saving what I was working on. Okay. [He logs into PROF too fast for the hacker to get his account.

H: Wait, wait. Why don't you go back a little? We have to verify the account as you're typing it.

WH: Oh, I'm sorry.

H: Yeah, we want to make sure that it's your account and not somebody else's.

WH: How do I get out of this?

H: Ah, don't worry about it. Just repeat your account. Just tell me the account you're using currently.

WH: Oh, I'm sorry. [And he reads off seven characters.]

H: [trying to decide his next move] Umm, okay . . . [but his next move is made for him].

WH: And do you need my password too?

H: Uh, yeah, sure. That would be good.

With an account and a password secured, the hacker politely concludes the conversation, hangs up the telephone, and bursts into laughter: "Yo, man, *Francois Girbaud!* I just read the name off his shirt! It's like saying 'Levi's'—Hi, this is Joe Levi's!' I shoulda said 'Calvin Klein.'" . . . For the rest of the evening, Francois Girbaud is the punch line to every joke. No other hack could top this one, so we head out to McDonald's for burgers and Cokes—just a bunch of teenagers, hanging on a Friday night. Maybe tomorrow we will read George Bush's mail.

Jack Hill and Paul Tough are writers living in New York.

Management Policies and Procedures Needed for Effective Computer Security

Stuart E. Madnick

In general, much of the literature and research on computer security-related matters has focused either on privacy and its associated social and legislative implications[1] or on technical mechanisms to enforce a specific security objective.[2] In comparison, the managerial and organizational issues, lacking the emotional tone of the privacy issues and the precision of the technical implementations, have received limited attention. This situation is especially unfortunate since, even after generally accepted privacy legislation is enacted and the major technological security mechanisms refined, the managerial security issues, by their very nature, will persist.

Managerial security (sometimes called operational or administrative security) is concerned with the policies and procedures adopted by management to ensure the security of their data and computer installation. Although certain of these policies and procedures may be externally defined, such as those relating to privacy laws or government regulations (e.g., IRS rules), most are internally defined.

A typical definition of data security found in the literature might be: " . . . protection of data against accidental or intentional disclosure to unauthorized persons, or unauthorized modifications or destruction."[3] Key to such a definition is the notion of authorization. Major managerial control issues include the questions:

1. Who should be authorized?
2. How is this determined?
3. How is the authorization process operated?

In recent years various authors have attempted to address some of these policy and procedural issues.[4] With few exceptions these studies either have been imbedded within elaborate privacy or technical security reports or have been intended to serve as introductions to particular aspects of the problem area. As a result, the literature on managerial security is largely diffuse and unorganized. This article introduces a comprehensive framework for organizing and studying the diverse aspects of managerial security. This framework places issues of management policies and procedures into four categories:

I. Operational considerations
II. Organizational impact

III. Economics

IV. Objectives and accountability

Using this framework, the key issues regarding management policies and procedures for effective computer security are categorized and analyzed. Specific emphasis is placed on this author's proposals regarding surveillance and authorization.

I. Operational Considerations

Many managerial decisions must be made regarding the procedures to be used in the operation of an organization's computer facility. Although most of these decisions are intended primarily to increase the degree of data security, they must also be viewed in light of the organization's overall objectives.

Operating Environment

Physical and operational procedures can be used to limit significantly the number of people that have any access to the computer facility. The three major categories of access are:

1. *Closed.* Only a very small number of operators have direct access to the computer facility. All computation to be performed is submitted to one of the operators who will then oversee the actual run.

2. *Open.* In principle, any member of the organization may have access to the computer facility. The user must physically appear at the computer facility to perform computations and may be screened at that time.

3. *Unlimited.* Access to the computer facility is via communication lines, usually the public telephone network. The user need not ever physically appear at the computer facility nor have any personal contact with the operators of the facility.

There are, of course, variations on the operating environments listed above. Each environment has implications for the organization's data security as well as the utility of the computer facility. By severely limiting access, such as in a closed environment, controls similar to those used for a bank vault can be enforced. In fact, most high security military installations use this approach, and the "computer room" is often actually a vault. Although a closed environment can provide high physical security, it may not be consistent with the organization's needs. Many of the important modern applications of computers are dependent upon the concept of on-line access—leading essentially to an unlimited access environment.

The open and unlimited access environments introduce different types of risks. In an open environment it is possible to screen out external intruders, but the computer facility is still exposed to the actions of internal users who have legitimate physical access to it. An unlimited access environment cannot easily constrain access by external intruders, but direct physical contact with the computer can be prevented and the actions that can be performed via communication lines may be restricted in various ways.

Types of Authorization Control

As noted previously, operational security is, to a large extent, concerned with the authorization process. The most critical aspects of this process relate to:

1. Who wishes to access or alter information?
2. Which information will be accessed or altered?
3. What operation (e.g., read, modify) is to be performed on the information?

These aspects should be analyzed in terms of the controls appropriate to and/or necessary for the individual firm's security goals. (A complete security system would likely include controls on when, from where, and why information is accessed or altered.)

Identification and Verification

The verification process usually involves something that the user: (1) knows (e.g., a password), (2) carries (e.g., a badge), or (3) is (e.g., a physical characteristic, such as a fingerprint). In many organizations, it is common to use surrogates, such as using an administrative assistant to obtain reports on behalf of the president. Considerable attention is warranted for both the technical mechanism for assigning roles, such as giving someone the "president's badge," and the procedural mechanisms for ensuring the correct and legitimate behavior of an individual acting as a surrogate for someone with more security authorization. In many systems there is no way to distinguish among the multiple individuals that are allowed to take on a specific role (e.g., acting for the president). Without such a differentiation procedure it is difficult to audit effectively such a system or to trace responsibility.

Classification of Information

The classification procedure can be complicated by many factors, such as granularity and security level. Granularity denotes the level of detail of information to be classified, such as an entire document, a record, or a specific data item. A single document may contain a variety of information that may warrant separate classifications. Furthermore, in certain types of computerized data bases, the concepts of documents or even records may not explicitly exist. In such a situation it becomes necessary to authorize on the basis of specific data items or data types.

The use of security levels is largely motivated by the military concept of security classifications, such as confidential, secret, and top secret. Most nonmilitary organizations also use this concept to some extent (e.g., company confidential, company registered confidential). Various combinations of information classification schemes could be employed in organizations. Combining "horizontal" partitioning (i.e., functional) with a "vertical" partitioning (i.e., security level) is a common choice.

Operations upon Information

Once the "who" and the "which" have been established, it must be determined what actions are to be allowed. As a simple example, one can distinguish between the operations "read" and "write." In the first case, an individual may be authorized to obtain certain information, such as a customer's bank balance, but have no authority to change it. In the latter case, authorization to change the information, such as changing the customer's bank balance, may be given.

Variations of these two basic operations should be considered. For example, the actions of "creating" or "destroying" records are often treated differently from "reading" and "writing." An inventory control clerk may be authorized to update the inventory balances, but only the engineering department personnel may be authorized to create new part records. Other versions of "reading" can be used. For example, some systems allow access to statistical information (e.g., average salary) without providing access to the individual salary information. Also, especially for proprietary software, there is the notion of "execute-only" access, where someone may be authorized to use the program but not allowed to modify or read the program (reading the program would allow it to be copied and thereby stolen).

Operational Ease

Many people fail to recognize the fact that security mechanisms may cause additional hardship or inconvenience for their users. If such mechanisms are not easy to operate, it is likely that they will not be used effectively. This is important because, for most users, security is not their sole job function. For example, an inventory control clerk's primary responsibility is to maintain up-to-date information on the company's inventory. If the security mechanism requires extra time to update the inventory status, it will be at odds with the clerk's primary job function and, implicitly, encourage shortcuts that may compromise the security mechanism.

When one is devising an authorization and security mechanism, it is important to consider the operational environment and pick an approach that is likely to be easy and convenient to use. This decision may involve compromises between degree of security and ease of use.

Reliability and Recovery

As the capabilities and cost effectiveness of information systems have increased, the systems have become closely integrated into the operation of many organizations. This has, in turn, increased the concern for reliability and recovery.

In some cases, reliability and recovery procedures are concordant with security procedures. For example, reliability mechanisms often include additional tests for potential errors in either the hardware or software. Some of these tests may directly, or with minor extension, also be used to test for potential security violations. On the other hand, other reliability mechanisms produce redundancy and duplication. For example, one way to safeguard the company's key files and provide for effective recovery is to make one or more copies.[5] Thus, if the original is destroyed, a copy can be used. Unfortunately, these copies may increase the exposure to security violations. In fact, since under normal operation the duplicates are not used, stolen or replaced copies may never be missed. In order to address this specific problem, many companies are adopting new procedures whereby both the original and copy are used in normal operation, such as on alternate days. In this way it is more likely that missing information will be detected. In addition, the reliability of the copies can be confirmed. In one organization a spot check of their "backup copies" revealed that 25 percent were not usable due either to errors during the copying operation or to deterioration during storage.

Transition

At time of transition, the system is extremely vulnerable to security violations, especially if the transition is from a manual to a computerized system.

This vulnerability is caused by various factors, including: (1) most users are not used to the new system and are likely to be careless; (2) the system itself may not include all the "ultimately desired" security facilities, and the facilities provided may not be fully tested;

(3) the operational and technical problems that usually accompany a transition may act as significant diversions for concurrent security violations. Security considerations must be carefully factored into the transition plan to minimize these vulnerabilities.

II. Organizational Impact

Computer system security often requires or causes organizational changes. Some of these changes are desirable and are concordant with the security objectives. Other impacts may be detrimental to the security objectives and, possibly, to the organization as a whole. Several of these key issues are discussed in this section.

Awareness and Education

The degree of awareness of data security as an issue and the possibility of security threats vary widely. Although awareness is increasing, it is likely that the situation has not changed significantly from that reported in one study where it was concluded that only a small proportion of computer users use security features.[6] As one senior manager of a timesharing firm states, "Some customers are concerned about security, some are not; but they are all naive." Furthermore, it was found that although most systems provided various special security mechanisms, only a handful were actually used and those were used by the most sophisticated users. The majority of the users assumed that the computer system was secure and that they were adequately protected.

Surely the need for user education is an important aspect of improved and effective security procedures and enforcement. Part of this increased education and awareness will come about as a result of external factors, such as (1) press and media coverage, (2) increases in direct personal contact with computer systems as these systems become more pervasive in organizations, and (3) advances in security, in both technique and cost effectiveness, that would provide a more natural and easier use of modern systems. Organizations may also find it valuable to accelerate the awareness process by developing or sponsoring specific security education activities.

Attitude

When extensive computer security is introduced into an organization, some personnel may react negatively because of a difficulty in getting their work accomplished and/or a feeling of loss of power. The first problem was briefly discussed earlier.

In a secure system people no longer can have unlimited, unrestricted access to the entire system. Management must explicitly determine each individual's access rights. To the extent that possession of information is a form of power, individuals may resist and resent any decrease in information access rights, even if the information is not necessary for the normal operation of the individual's job. Furthermore, restrictions on or the elimination of "hands on" computer access by most applications and systems programmers is often a serious blow to the programmers' egos.

Personnel and Responsibility

To a large extent the security-related aspects of personnel selection and assignment are very similar in both the computer and noncomputer environments; thus, much of the existing literature on such subjects (e.g., embezzlement) is applicable.[7]

Computerized systems have introduced several new problems:

1. A computerized system often allows for much more streamlined and efficient operation by eliminating many of the traditional steps. The loss of an intermediate step may also negate an existing internal check.

2. The operation of computerized systems introduces many new roles and procedures for which the concepts of division of responsibility are not well established from experiences with prior manual systems. Since computer programs, to a large extent, act as surrogates for what were traditionally manual steps, one individual may inherit the conflicting responsibilities of writing both operational and auditing programs.

3. Finally, the separation of responsibilities between computer programmers and operators can easily lead to conflicting company objectives. For instance, whereas in some cases it would be advantageous to hire only operators with no programming ability, the company's advancement opportunities may contrarily encourage operators to aspire to positions as programmers. The correct balancing of these potentially conflicting objectives must be carefully studied. Various additional procedures and checks and balances can be developed to lessen the potential exposure due to security violations by computer operators.

III. Economics

Key issues that must be resolved in order to determine security economics include: (1) a determination of the value of information, (2) an assessment of likely threats to the information, and (3) a determination of the costs of available security mechanisms and their effectiveness. Aspects of these issues are discussed below.

Value of Information

It should seem obvious that the determination of the value of information is a crucial step in any security decision as well as in normal information management. Unfortunately, the evaluation process remains very subjective. The process not only requires placing a value on information, but also consideration of the fact that the same information may be perceived to have different values by different groups of individuals. At least three separate interest groups are involved:

1. *Keeper*—the organization that has and uses the information;
2. *Source*—the organization or individual that provided the information, or to whom the information pertains;
3. *Intruder*—an individual or organization that may wish the information.

The value of information depends, further, on its type. The following are general categories of information type:

1. *Critical* operating information, such as this week's sales orders and production schedule, may have a very high value to the keeper, but considerably less value to its sources (i.e., the customers) or potential intruders.
2. *Personal* information (e.g., an individual's census data or medical information in the employee personnel file) may have a much higher value to the source (i.e., the individual) than to either the keeper or intruder.
3. *Proprietary* information, including marketing forecast data gathered by a company, may be much more valuable to an intruder, such as a competing company, than to either the sources (i.e., sample customers) or the keeper, who may have already finished analyzing the data.

The categories listed above are aggregations. The value of a specific type of information may be perceived differently by different keepers (or different individuals or groups within the "keeper" organization), sources, and intruders.

Threats

In evaluating threats, one wants to know the economic impact (usually interpreted as a loss or expense to the keeper or source) should a particular operation be performed on certain information. Threat operations can be divided into major categories, such as:

1. *Interrupt*—disrupt the normal processing of the information. Note that an interruption may be an important concern even though the information itself may not be affected in any way.
2. *Steal or disclose*—read or copy information for use by either the intruder or a third party (e.g., publishing the psychiatric records of a competitor).
3. *Alter*—change information, such as the intruder's bank balance. This is probably the most obvious threat to most people.
4. *Destroy*—permanently destroy the information, by erasing a magnetic tape, for example.

There are, of course, alternative categorizations of threats as well as additional factors that may be considered, such as whether the action was intentional (e.g., an intruder breaking in) or unintentional (e.g., someone lost the data). Although the intentional threats are often of most concern, the unintentional may be more frequent and, possibly, have greater economic impact.

Risk

The threat assessment is intended to determine the value of a certain action upon information. In order to develop a rational security plan, it is necessary to assess the probability of each threat occurring. A common objective of most risk assessment strategies proposed is to arrive at a quantitative statement of risk, such as a decision analysis calculation of the expected value of the loss for each threat.[8] However, numerous problems are encountered in attempting to perform such a risk assessment. First, determining the precise monetary value of a threat may be very difficult. Second, there is usually a reluctance to assign a monetary value to threats that have social impact, such as disclosure of confidential medical information. Third, as noted earlier, different individuals and organizations may assign different values to a given threat.

There is also considerable difficulty in determining the probability of a threat occurring. Computer threats are too diverse and recent to have attained much statistical information. A threat assessment is, therefore, the most subjective aspect of the economics of computer security, and thus each assessment would have to be calculated in its particular context.

Countermeasures and Costs

For each risk usually one or more countermeasures are possible.[9] Countermeasures are intended to decrease the risk either by decreasing the probability of the threat occurring or by decreasing the impact of the threat should it occur. For example, the probability of losing information can be decreased by adding new procedures to monitor the use and location of the information. The impact of having lost information can be decreased either by having copies of the information available or by setting up procedures in advance that enable rapid and inexpensive reconstruction of the information.

The two major considerations for each countermeasure are its effectiveness and its cost. This information can provide the basis for a rational economic security plan.[10] In particular, a countermeasure is economically reasonable if its effectiveness, in terms of decreased risk, exceeds its cost. The organization can establish maximum risk levels and then select one or more economically justified countermeasures, as necessary, to reduce the total risk below the maximum risk levels. Of course, many of the same problems that prevent precise threat and risk assessment exist in determining countermeasure effectiveness and cost. On the other hand, several efforts have been made to enumerate countermeasures and, at least qualitatively, rate their effectiveness and cost.[11]

One final issue that is often studied in the context of threats by intruders is the cost of the threat. In theory an economically rational intruder will not expend more to initiate a threat than the expected gain from that threat (e.g., one would not reasonably spend $5,000 to break into a vault that one believed only contained $10). Thus, one of the significant objectives of a security countermeasure is to increase the costs to an intruder so as to raise the price above the value the intruder anticipates and thereby reduce the risk. The intruder's costs include resources necessary, such as technology, expertise, time and opportunity. In addition, penalty costs, such as the possibility of detection and the resulting economic, personal, and social penalties, represent a potential expense to the intruder. Therefore, countermeasures that are based on ex post facto detection rather than prevention of threats may be equally effective at reducing the risk of an intruder threat. This point will be discussed in more detail later.

IV. Security Objectives and Accountability

As part of a meaningful security plan it is necessary to consider the objectives to be accomplished and the specific organizational responsibilities necessary to carry out the plan. As one example, it has been noted that security violations by authorized insiders far outnumber those likely to occur by external intruders. Thus, a plan focusing only on the outside intruder may not provide much increase in security.

Unintentional mistakes by insiders may even be a comparatively important problem in many organizations.

Validation and Consistency

Techniques and procedures to validate the reasonableness and consistency of data are important in reducing the frequency of unintentional errors and in providing a means of detecting or preventing various forms of intentional security violations by either insiders or external intruders. Simple format and range checks are common to most, but not all, information systems. A typical format check would be the verification that the zip code of an address is five digits long. A range check would, for example, verify that an employee does not report working more than sixty hours per week.

More complex consistency checks can be very valuable, though they are less frequently used. For example, salary range checks may be conditioned upon organizational position. For the president of the company, a wage payment of $2,000 per week may not be unlikely, whereas it might be suspicious for a clerk to receive such a salary. In the same manner, shipments being sent to an address different from the customer's normal address may be suspicious. Such consistency checks are much more complex, and time-consuming, both to construct and to execute, than simple range checks, since the procedures require comparing several different sources of information to determine consistency within individual records. Although the specific mechanisms for actually performing validation and consistency checks are largely technical issues, a determination of the extent of validation and the specific rules and procedures to be followed requires careful managerial consideration.

Surveillance

As noted earlier, computerized systems have often provided ways to streamline operations and greatly reduce the number of steps and amount of paper work involved in various activities. These systems can also greatly increase the difficulty in detecting security violations. A simple example, based on an actual "computer crime," may help to illustrate this point:

> A company uses an on-line order entry system to allow salesmen in the branch offices to place an order directly to the warehouse by telephone. A salesman, former employee, or outsider who has learned how to remotely access and use the system may place a large order early in the month, then rent a truck and pick up the merchandise at the warehouse (since the order was in the system, the warehouse personnel would be expecting the pickup). Before the order

is transferred to the billing system at the end of the month, the thief can cancel the order and thus remove all traces of the order from the computer system, simply by accessing the system again. Over time the company may notice that its inventory records differ from the physical inventory. In a large warehouse with annual inventory turnover of $100,000,000 or more, a $500,000 discrepancy may be attributable to breakage or normal losses. If the discrepancy is large enough to be viewed as a problem, the most obvious assumption is that the warehouse workers are stealing the equipment or that an intruder is breaking into the warehouse. The remedy would then likely be to install closed circuit televisions and increase the number of security guards. The thief at a remote terminal would not be a likely suspect. (Donn Parker, Stanford Research Institute, has studied and documented several hundred actual computer crime cases.)[12]

Using the computer's capabilities, special surveillance procedures can be incorporated into the system.[13] There are at least two major forms: (1) audit log and (2) monitoring.

Audit log   Basic to the concept of an audit log or audit trail is a permanent record of every significant action executed by the system. Thus, as in the days of quill pen journals and ledgers, one log record is made of every order placed and another if the order is cancelled (rather than merely discarding or erasing the order record). In principle, log records are accumulated and never changed. Such an audit log can be used for several important purposes:[14]

1. *Security violation detection.* As illustrated by the example above, an audit log can be used to help determine and diagnose certain security violations (e.g., there would be a permanent record of the order entry, order pickup, and order cancellation).
2. *Traditional auditing.* An audit log, at least in part, is essential to tracing transactions through the system as required in normal financial auditing procedures.
3. *Minor and massive recovery.* In an on-line system, an audit log of some type is essential to allow effective recovery from malfunctions caused by software or hardware during normal operations. The periodic (typically nightly or weekly) backup tapes would not yet contain records of the transactions for the current day. With an audit log, it would be possible to reconstruct information that may have been destroyed or invalidated due to the malfunction. In cases of minor transient malfunctions, such a recovery may be automated and accomplished in a few minutes or even seconds.
4. *Correction of errors.* In many systems, especially on-line systems, an error may be detected by the user immediately, such as

accidently typing the wrong account number or incorrectly deleting a specific account. The audit log can be helpful in reconstructing data that may have been incorrectly altered.

5. *Deterrence*. The mere existence of an audit log may be a deterrent to many security violations, especially by insiders. Even if one knows how to circumvent a given system's security procedures and normal checks and balances, the fact that one's actions may be detected from the audit log can be a deterrent.

The concept of an ex post facto security mechanism as a deterrent is often neglected in the design of many security procedures. The important point to note is that the computer system is only one part of the security process. Just as in the case of a "successful" bank robbery, ex post facto pursuit and prosecution are important elements.

A careful managerial study is necessary to determine what information should be captured in the audit log and how it should be organized for most effective use. Furthermore, a definite plan of active examination is necessary if security violations are to be detected in a timely manner. In many installations, audit logs are generated and stored away, but never used. The audit logs should be used in both a systematic and nonsystematic manner. In the former case, standard reports should be devised that could be used to detect unusual situations, such as an unusually large number of invalid or incorrect log-in attempts, exceptionally large orders from certain customers, etc. An intruder who has sufficient knowledge of the standard report procedures may find a way to violate system security that does not appear on any of the standard security check reports. (The standard cliché in movie burglaries is for one of the robbers to say, "The guard makes his rounds every 30 minutes; that gives us 25 minutes to break into the safe.") Nonsystematic behavior can be accomplished by introducing an element of randomness into the examination either by having the checking programs randomly select transactions for examination or by providing on-line access to the audit log, enabling security officers or management personnel to browse arbitrarily through the information.

Monitoring Monitoring is a more active form of surveillance. While the system is in operation, various forms of information and statistics can be gathered and displayed on special monitoring terminals. This type of facility can be used for a variety of security and nonsecurity related purposes:

1. *Security violation detection*. Information system monitoring facilities can be used in a manner similar to closed circuit television and intruder detector systems. They may be used in

a summary mode to note any unusual situations, such as an incorrect log-in attempt, numerous data input errors, or an exceptionally large order or withdrawal, or in a viewing mode to monitor in detail the actions of one or more specific terminal users.

2. *Education*. Such monitoring facilities can be extremely instructive to both new and current managers. By actually seeing the system in operation, at both the summary and detail levels, one can gain considerable insight into the operation of the organization. Many incorrect preconceived notions can be corrected and new patterns of operation can be observed.

3. *System performance and utilization*. By being able to monitor the system, its designers can explore possible areas of improvement. In one case it was observed that the lengthy "English-like" interface to the information system, though very popular with the infrequent management users, required excessive typing for the full-time system users and was the cause of most data entry errors. This problem had not been brought to the attention of the designers during the previous six months of system operation, because the data entry activity was organizationally and physically quite removed from the system designers.

Many of the other points noted about the audit log apply to the use of a monitoring facility.

There are two additional points that must be made about surveillance facilities. First, the audit log and monitoring capability introduce additional possibilities for security violations (e.g., stealing the audit log may be easier than stealing the data base itself). Thus, the security of these facilities must be carefully studied. In some installations extensive precautions may be made to secure the computer facility and the operational data, while the backup and audit tapes are stored unguarded in the basement. Second, use of the audit and monitor facilities must itself be audit logged. Otherwise, a dishonest security officer or someone who finds out how to gain access to these facilities may be able to use them to violate security and operate undetected.

Needless to say, the various surveillance mechanisms and procedures described above have definite implications for the privacy of the system's users. The monitoring facility, for example, could essentially allow a manager to "look over the shoulder" of any terminal user indefinitely without the employee being aware of this monitoring activity. In this regard such facilities are similar to concealed closed circuit televisions. Thus, careful consideration should be given to their mode and purpose for use, as well as to the extent of knowledge about the existence of these systems that the company should allow.

Authorization

The authorization process is an extremely important issue with numerous facets. Two specific issues will be discussed in this section: (1) authorization control and (2) rigidity of authorization.

Authorization control   The access control rules to be enforced by the system can be viewed, essentially, as merely another type of information in the system, but this information and the ability to change it have sweeping implications. A possible analogy is the safe that contains the combinations to all the other safes.

Changing the access control rules (i.e., changes to authorizations) can be accomplished in various organizational ways. These methods can be divided into three major categories: centralized, hierarchical decentralized, and individual.

1. *Centralized.* A single individual or organizational unit, such as the security officer or data base administrator, handles all authorizations.
2. *Hierarchical decentralized.* The central authorization organization may delegate some or all of its authority to subordinate organizations. For example, accounting files may be placed under the control of the head of accounting. Authority may then be further delegated (e.g., authorization control for certain accounting files may be assigned to different managers within the accounting organization). In most implementations the higher authorities in the authorization hierarchy retain the ability to revoke or override authorization decisions made by their subordinates.
3. *Individual.* In this situation no static authorization hierarchy exists. An individual may be allowed to create information (authorization to "create" may be controlled by either of the earlier two approaches), and the system would then recognize that individual as the "owner" of the information. The owner may authorize others to access the information, pass ownership to someone else, or establish co-ownership arrangements.

Each of these authorization approaches has advantages and disadvantages, which has led some organizations to develop combinations or variations of these basic strategies to meet their organizations' needs.

The centralized approach, not surprisingly, is largely motivated by the military concept of "security officers." With the increasing concern over the corporate "information resource" and the establishment of a data base administration function in many organizations, this approach has been adopted by some companies and may be viable in small or highly structured organizations. However, in most large volatile or decentralized organizations, the rapidly evolving functions and information, especially for test cases and development activities, as well as personnel turnover and reassignment, can result in an extremely large number of security authorizations required every day. For example, in a study of a medium-sized but highly volatile organization (a university), it was found that authorization changes occurred at least once every three minutes.[15] Therefore, the centralized approach may not be desirable in organizations with a high volume of security authorization changes or where the organizational structure is too complex or decentralized to allow effective and intelligent centralized control over authorization changes.

The hierarchical decentralized approach has been widely recommended in the literature and is basic to the security implementation on certain systems, such as the Honeywell Multics system.[16] This approach allows the security authorization control to be delegated to the groups that can most effectively administer and monitor these controls. From an organizational point of view this may be very important. For example, if a division or function operates as a separate profit center with control over its own expenditures and plans, that division probably should have security authorization control over its internal data.

A major problem with most implementations of this approach lies in the authority of higher levels in the authorization hierarchy to revoke or override all authorization decisions. This ability is usually viewed as necessary for organizational (i.e., "the boss is the boss") and operational (i.e., to correct mistakes in authorization assignments) reasons. However, no "private" information can exist in this system. By analogy to the normal office environment, this would be equivalent to banning locked drawers in employees' desks (i.e., not accessible by superiors). This issue of "corporate privacy" (as opposed to the more commonly accepted concept of "personal privacy") has been a major factor in the reluctance of many groups within corporations to computerize their records. One salesman noted that he would rather destroy his personal notes on client companies, and the peculiarities of their purchasing agents, than risk having these notes computerized and thus allow the chance that this information could be seen by anyone else. Indeed, few individuals do not view as private at least some information, records, or notes pertinent to their organizations that are presently kept in the privacy of their offices. This problem is likely to increase significantly among white-collar workers and management as advances in office automation greatly increase the scope and diversity of information stored in computerized information systems.

The approach of individual authorization control is used in many simple systems. A convenient implementation is to allow the creator of a file to designate "owner" and "user" passwords for the file. The owner password allows one to change either of the passwords; the user password allows one to access the file. Various authorization objectives can be accomplished using such a system. Private information can be kept private simply by not divulging either of the passwords. (Note: it is assumed that no standard way is provided for anyone, whether president or systems programmer, to find the passwords for any file.) Access or ownership rights can be awarded by giving the passwords. One drawback to the password strategy is that it is impossible to identify all the people who know the password or to revoke access selectively. However, alternative strategies can be devised to accomplish the same results without using passwords in the manner noted above.

One problem with the individual authorization approach, though, regardless of the implementation, is the potential for situations where it becomes necessary to override the security mechanism (e.g., the individual dies, becomes ill, leaves the company). In general, any security mechanism can be overcome, though some mechanisms, such as cryptographic encoding, may be very difficult to break even by the system's designers. If the mechanism is easy to break, the "privacy" assumed above will not exist; if it is very difficult to break, the organization may suffer if adverse circumstances occur.

Rigidity of authorization Computer systems, lacking discretionary judgment, require a precise statement of access control rules to be enforced. This requires that very careful thought be given to the establishment of these rules and the specific authorizations assigned.

The rigidity of the authorizations has posed various problems in the past. While testing the experimental Resource Security System (RSS), IBM's Federal Systems Center noted that "A major concern in FSC was that the use of a secure system would hamper our ability to react quickly to priority situations. . . . What this means, for purposes of system design, is that effective security overrides must be available to the installation."[17]

Most existing security systems either do not provide any security override mechanism or the override is in the form of a "panic" button that can be invoked by the security officer or computer operator to suspend all security enforcement. This approach is very crude, awkward to use, and may expose the system to security violations while security enforcement is suspended.

As an example, consider the situation of a doctor who desperately needs information about a patient admitted in an emergency. If the patient's regular doctor is currently unavailable to give the attending physician access to the patient's files, it should be possible to use a formal procedure whereby the attending physician can request access to the patient's file. The system will record this fact and the action will be subject to later review by the patient's regular doctor. Certainly, less rigid access control rules are called for in such situations. For example, three levels of access control may be defined: The normal "access is allowed" or "access is prohibited" can be augmented by "access *may* be allowed." Thus, in environments where high ethical standards are the norm and/or ethical behavior is encouraged by particular constraints (e.g., ex post facto prosecution), certain users may be assigned "access may be allowed" permission to another user's private information. In these cases, any attempted access will trigger a special action which would inform the user that the requested access is to private information. The user would then be required to acknowledge that his access is deliberate and to provide a brief explanation of the reason. The final decision as to the appropriateness of the access is deferred to human review at a later time.

This type of flexible security enforcement is rare in current security systems. Further development of these concepts and capabilities is essential in order to avoid the extremes of impairing effective use of the system or reverting to ad hoc emergency procedures all the time.

Security Responsibility

As should be clear from the preceding discussions, effective security requires the cooperation and planning of many people in an organization. Although certain aspects, such as awareness, require the active participation of almost everyone in the organization, most of the planning and decision-making issues are best resolved by a small number of people. Who should be responsible for security planning?

The problem of responsibility is complicated by the fact that at least three types of issues can be identified, each implying a potentially different type of organizational responsibility. These three issue types are:

1. *Policy*. Policy issues regarding the use and types of security procedures require the active participation, formulation, and acceptance by top management personnel.
2. *Operational*. Mapping the policy decisions into practice requires a detailed knowledge of the organization's information processing activities and the available security enforcement technologies. This type of activity would require the skills normally found in the data base administration, systems programming, and computer operations functions.

3. *Economic*. It has been noted that many security issues are essentially economic decisions, involving uncertainty or incomplete information and risks. The decision to use a certain security procedure which costs X dollars and provides a specific but unquantified degree of protection against certain types of potential security violations is very similar to the decision to expend funds on a project to develop a new product. In this context the role of "risk managers" (i.e., individuals experienced in making such subjective decisions) has been suggested in the literature.[18]

The concept of risk managers has been used in a very broad context to accommodate the perception that important elements of risk exist at the policy and operational levels as well as for economic decisions. Therefore, some security experts have recommended to top management that ongoing risk analysis teams be formed that include: (1) EDP operations management, (2) department managers, (3) applications programmers, (4) systems programmers, (5) internal auditors, and (6) physical security personnel.[19]

The specific security roles and responsibilities may vary from organization to organization, but careful planning and defining of responsibilities are essential to effective and operationally viable information system security.

Summary

This article has identified and categorized the key management policy and procedure issues relevant to the attainment of effective computer security. Although social, legal, and technical factors may be relevant in certain cases, the primary factors in each issue identified center on management decisions. Management must carefully weigh the operational, organizational, economic, and accountability implications of each of these decisions.

As our reliance upon computer-based information systems continues to increase and to propel us onward towards an even more comprehensive "information society," these issues will become increasingly critical.

References

1. S. H. Nycum, "Legal Aspects of Computer Abuse," *Proceedings IEEE Computer Society International Conference*, February 1976, pp. 181–83.
2. K. S. Shankar, "The Total Computer Security Problem: An Overview," *Computer*, June 1977, pp. 50–73.

3. J. Martin, *Security, Accuracy, and Privacy in Computer Systems* (Englewood Cliffs, NJ: Prentice-Hall, 1973).

4. T. Alexander, "Waiting for the Great Computer Rip-off," Fortune, July 1974, pp. 143–50; C. F. Hemphill, Jr. and J. M. Hemphill, *Security Procedures for Computer Systems* (Homewood, IL: Dow Jones-Irwin, 1973); D. B. Hoyt, ed., Computer Security Handbook (New York: Macmillan Co., 1973); S. W. Leibholz and L. D. Wilson, *User's Guide to Computer Crime: Its Commission, Detection and Prevention* (Radnor, PA: Chilton Books Co., 1974); Martin (1973); D. Van Tassel, *Computer Security Management* (Englewood Cliffs, NJ: Prentice-Hall, 1972).

5. P. S. Browne and J. A. Cosenting, "I/O—A Logistics Challenge," *Proceedings 74 Eighth IEEE Computer Society International Conference*, February 1974, pp. 61–64.

6. IBM, *Data Security and Data Processing*, vol. 6, International Business Machines Corp., Data Processing Div., form no. G320-1376 (White Plains, NY, 1974).

7. B. R. Allen, "Embezzlement and Automation," *Proceedings IEEE Computer Society International Conference*, February 1976, pp. 187–88; J. Honig, "Company Security and Individual Freedom," *Datamation*, January 1974, p. 131.

8. R. H. Courtney, Jr., "Security Risk Assessment in Electronic Data Processing," *AFIPS Conference Proceedings* 46, National Computer Conference (1977): 97–104; S. Glaseman, R. Turn, and R. S. Gaines, "Problem Areas in Computer Security Assessment," *AFIPS Conference Proceedings* 46, National Computer Conference (1977): 105–12.

9. N. R. Nielsen, "Computers, Security, and the Audit Function," *AFIPS Conference Proceedings* 44, National Computer Conference (1975): 947–54.

10. D. Clements and L. J. Hoffman, "Computer Assisted Security System Design," Electronics Research Laboratory, ERL-M468 (University of California, Berkeley, 1974).

11. IBM (vol. 3, pt. 2, form no. G320-1373, 1974).

12. D. B. Parker, *Crime by Computer* (New York: Charles Scribner's Sons, 1976).

13. P. Hamilton, *Computer Security* (London: Associated Business Programmes, 1972).

14. E. Myers, "News in Perspective: Computer Criminal Beware," *Datamation*, December, 1975, p. 105; Nielsen (1975); J. Wasserman, "Selecting a Computer Audit Package," *The Journal of Accountancy*, April 1974, pp. 3–34.

15. IBM (vol. 4, form no. G320-1374).

16. B. J. Walker and I. F. Blake, *Computer Security and Protection Structures* (Stroudsburg, PA: Dowden, Hutchinson & Ross, 1977).

17. IBM (vol. 6, form no. G320-1376).

18. "News in Perspective: Risk Managers Urged for Curbing Fraud," *Datamation*, June 1976, pp. 155–57; D. Firnberg, "Your Computer in Jeopardy," *Computer Decisions*, July 1976, pp. 28–30.

19. A. Weissman, "Security—The Analyst's Concern," *Modern Data*, April 1974, p. 28; Nielsen (1975).

Stuart E. Madnick is Associate Professor of Management at the Massachusetts Institute of Technology.

CASE 7
The Mercy Hospital Pharmacy Department

THE LITANY of security problems seemed endless for Dennis Farmer, director of pharmacy at the 180-bed Mercy Hospital. His assistant had prepared a report listing the security breaches associated with the new computer system, and was about to read it to him. The phrase "data trespassing" had now been added to his already extensive medical vocabulary.

Dennis had worked in various hospital pharmacies for 15 years and had seen, almost universally, that the majority of the pharmacists' time was spent writing orders, pricing, or doing clerical work. In a move to increase productivity, Dennis had conducted a cost-justification study on a stand-alone, modular mini-computer system. Purchased almost a year ago, the system virtually eliminated most of the time consuming paperwork in the pharmacy. Dennis calculated that the new system would save the hospital approximately $50,000 annually through time savings and the savings gained from allowing reallocation of staff time for additional duties. These savings included monetary savings from more accurate Medicaid documentation and better inventory control; clerical labor savings, since a billing clerk was no longer needed to fill out forms to third-party payers and patients; and nursing time savings, since the system cut nurses' work loads by automatically writing stop-order reports and compiling medication administration records.

All these savings might now be offset by the computer security controls that would have to be considered.

Mary Sanders, assistant director of pharmacy, summarized the recent problems:

> I'll try to be brief and present you with these problems by listing the most recent incidents. First of all, one of the printers was stolen last week. Unfortunately, it was the new laser printer everyone loved. We've lost about 300 of our outpatient profiles, and I'm not sure whether we can get them back. The supervisor of nursing was here yesterday and said the automatic stop-order reports and medication records for twelve patients in ICU were not consistent with their manual back-up system. I think someone, and I'm not sure who, has tampered with the inventory records. The physical inventory amount of Valium is different than our inventory records on the computer. And last but not least, our young pharmacy intern is using the pharmacy's computers to write his research report. When I confronted him with this, he said he assumed it was all right, since everyone else uses the computers for personal business. He asked if could use the laser printer for his completed research report. I told him it went bye-bye last week.

Dennis resolved to address these problems immediately, but recognized that the particular nature of the issues were complex. Once an intruder enters into the picture, it's often too late; when information has been changed or removed, the damage is already done. Whether pilfering or tampering had been done maliciously or not, the issue remained that this was his responsibility, and he needed to act. A multitude of questions had to be addressed. How much security was actually needed? What kind of technical and administrative measures needed to be taken? What precisely were the security problems that led to the present situation? What were the economic risks associated with security procedures?

In preparing a strategy for implementing a security plan for the pharmacy, Dennis reflected on the problem. It was evident that the physical security of the hardware and software was lax. Furthermore, people were able to get into the system and change the data. And finally, people were using the computer for personal business. It was, therefore, apparent that controls needed to be initiated on when, where, how, and why information would be accessed or altered.

Questions for Discussion

1. Describe the major security problems in the pharmacy.
   a. Evaluate the security of each problem.
   b. Prioritize these problems in terms of action that must be taken.
2. What factors associated with a computerized MIS affect the security of data in the pharmacy? How do social, legal, and organizational issues complicate the matter?

3. Develop a set of operational considerations that would serve as bases for the management policies and procedures of the pharmacy's security system (i.e., who, when, where, how, and why).
4. List the technical and administrative measures that would accompany these operational considerations.
5. Develop a strategy for implementing a new security plan. From Dennis's perspective, consider the organizational, group, and individual implications.

MAINTAINING INFORMATION PRIVACY

J UST AS the computer security issue has inspired many books, so, too has information privacy. Jeffrey Rothfeder's *Privacy for Sale*, for example, is based on the notion that computerization has made everyone's private life an open secret. He describes the random carnage sometimes caused by the carelessness and false assumptions of powerful institutions, and portrays the computer sharks who have learned to invade theoretically secure computer systems for private gain. Suggesting that the misuse of personal information in the U.S. is on the increase because of the growing computerization of records, he warns that millions of Americans are violated or otherwise abused by privacy invaders.[1] This chapter focuses on what health care professionals can do to prevent the erosion of information privacy.

The privacy and security issues in computer management are closely related. However, security is a technical and administrative matter on which there is general agreement about the problem and its solution, while privacy is a social and political issue that involves considerably less certainty and consensus. The privacy issue concerns what *should* be done to control information, while the security issue deals more with what *can* be done to protect information.

That securing information privacy is a serious matter is suggested by a report of the United States Privacy Protection Commission.[2] This concern for privacy is discussed at length in health care conferences, the health care literature, and the general press. A number of examples illustrate an increasing consciousness of the importance of information privacy:[3]

- The Director of the government's Office of Information Systems and Development Agency for Health Care Policy and Research listed privacy as one of four primary issues being addressed in Federal health care reform.
- The American Civil Liberties Union is mounting a campaign to tighten the laws protecting the confidentiality of medical information.
- The Joint Commission for Accreditation of Healthcare Organizations revised the Manual for Accreditation to include an information management chapter addressing a number of security requirements that guard against abuses of privacy.
- Court decisions in lawsuits such as *Behringer vs. Princeton Medical Center* have confirmed the patient's right to privacy, and have held health care organizations and their managers liable for preserving that privacy.

The matter becomes complex in that the right to privacy is not explicitly defined. Most people would probably agree with Supreme Court Justice Louis Brandeis who once identified "the right to be left alone" as a prerequisite for a tolerable life. Nonetheless, as Lawrence H. Tribe, a professor of constitutional law at Harvard University notes: "The debate over the outer boundaries of a right to privacy will continue for some time."[4]

The Nature of the Information Privacy Problem

A major misconception, occasionally presented in the popular press,[5] holds that privacy is a small matter chiefly concerned with keeping information secret. A few representative anecdotes can illustrate that privacy is a multifaceted issue with serious implications for computer users:

> "Do you have any skeletons in your closet?" Millstone was asked by his insurance broker. "No," he answered with a surprised laugh. "Why do you want to know?" "Some problem with your car insurance. The company wants to cancel it." So began a four year, $4,000 ordeal for James Millstone, assistant managing editor of the St. Louis Post-Dispatch. He asked the company for specifics and they directed him to a consumer credit investigating firm. It said that Millstone had been much disliked by his neighbors when he was in Washington, DC, that he was a hippie with a beard and long hair, and was strongly suspected of being a drug user. He was accused of lacking judgment, failing to discipline his children, and driving peace demonstrators to and from demonstrations. Millstone was outraged. Not only did he dispute every piece of adverse material, he wanted to know where the damning allegations came from. He sued the investigating firm.[6]

On a blustery day in late November, a woman was filling out papers at an automobile dealership in suburban Vienna, Virginia, on a new car she and her husband were buying. She needed her husband's social security number but couldn't remember it, so she asked to use a phone to call him. "Oh, don't bother him," a clerk said. "I'll get the social security number for you." He turned to a computer console at his desk typed in a code number and her husband's name, and within 30 seconds the computer was printing out the couple's life history: where each worked and their salaries; where they lived, the cost of their home and size of their mortgage; the fact that the husband had been married before; the credit cards each held, and a credit rating for each card.[7]

Dateline Miami (AP)—A 35-year-old North Miami man, released after spending five months in jail for two robberies he didn't commit, was rearrested because someone failed to clear his name from a police computer. Charges from the first arrest were dropped, with apologies from the prosecutors, on January 6, about a week after Matthews had been released on bond. On Wednesday, Matthews was walking down a northwest Miami street when a police cruiser pulled up behind him. Two officers stopped him, got his name and ran a computer check. It showed two outstanding robbery warrants.[8]

There are six major aspects of the privacy issue: they involve information collection, use, updating, purging, accuracy, and secrecy.

The information collection issue concerns limitations on the kinds of information that organizations are allowed to collect and maintain. For example, should health organizations be restricted to collecting only what is demonstrably needed, and prohibited from collecting certain kinds of information? A recent *Time*/CNN poll confirms the public's concern about this issue. The poll found that 76 percent of the respondents are "very concerned" about the amount of computerized information collected about them.[9]

The trend in privacy legislation is to limit information use solely to the purpose for which it was collected and given. For example, information obtained by a health clinic to treat a drinking problem could not be provided to an insurance company or to an employer. In this regard, both the American Hospital Association and the congressional Office of Technology Assessment are proponents of legislation that would put more comprehensive and stringent laws on medical record confidentiality applicable to the collection, storage processing and transmission of individually identifiable health care information.[10]

Should there be requirements to update information collected and maintained, that is, to keep it current? In the vignette above, for example, the Miami man was subjected to a police investigation simply because computerized information had not been updated to show that the charges against him had been dropped. Many people have been denied credit because a computerized data bank said they had unpaid debts, even after the debts had been paid.

Should personal information be automatically purged after a reasonable period of time? For example, should a health record always include the fact that a person contracted venereal disease as a teenager, or should that item be dropped from the record after, say, ten years? Should teenagers convicted of burglary, who never again stray, have the conviction on their record into middle age, or should records be cleared after a reasonable time period without an offense?

Perhaps the most serious aspect of the privacy issue concerns information accuracy and verification.[11] Should organizations be required to ensure the accuracy and completeness of the data they maintain, and should there be penalties for using erroneous or incomplete information? Should individuals have the right to inspect and verify personal information? Should patients have a right to verify their medical file? As computer science professor Early puts the problem:

> Most errors in computer files remain undetected. They are the simple keypunch errors, simple in execution but devastating to the person whom they affect; programming errors which remain undetected long enough to cause untold anguish to many; errors of omission and commission which cannot be rectified except by the action of the party whose reputation is besmirched.[12]

Aggravating this situation is the victim's own ignorance of the cause of the problem, either because he or she has not seen the file or is unaware of its existence and use.

Finally, information secrecy is a significant part of the privacy issue.[13] Should organizations be prohibited from holding information on people without their knowledge? Should organizations be required to notify any person on whom it maintains a file? Should there be a ban on secret information files?

These questions are complicated by legal, political, fiscal, operational, and inferential factors.

The legal dimension of the privacy issue comprises laws, court decisions, and accreditation standards. The United States now has federal, state, and local laws that place legal requirements on the organizational use of information. At the federal level, for example, the Privacy Act of 1974 protects the confidentiality of health information in the patient records system maintained by federal agencies. While these laws currently apply only to governmental data banks, legislators and health care organizations continue to push for a federal law that specifically protects the privacy, confidentiality, and security of information for everyone. As efforts to get specific legislation continue, many health care organizations are taking a wait-and-see approach.[14]

One particular problem relevant to health care service organizations today is the disconcerting fact that providers and payers operating in more than one state must comply with a multitude of often "inconsistent" laws and regulations.[15] Organizations, information users, and managers who do not know the laws that apply are in considerable jeopardy. These privacy laws, however, are further complicated by freedom of information or "sunshine" laws that provide no clear legal solution to disclosing data or maintaining confidentiality.[16]

While there is still considerable ambiguity, courts are beginning to recognize personal information as private property, resulting in profound privacy implications. For example, personal harm from a violation of privacy is currently judged under the law of torts, which means that it is a civil matter involving financial penalties. If the law of property is applied, the violation of privacy becomes a criminal matter involving possible jail sentences. Recent litigation in the courts supports the contention that personal information is a serious privacy consideration.[17] For example:

- A physician who worked for a medical center was diagnosed as having AIDs, but the information was not kept confidential. He filed suit against the hospital and some of its employees, claiming breach of confidentiality and violation of the state's anti-discrimination law.

- A patient sued a hospital for unauthorized release of patient records. The patient, an employee of the U.S. Postal Service, was judged unfit for the job by a psychologist who reviewed the employee's inpatient records without the individual's permission.

- A patient sued a regional health center, charging that employees of the hospital shared test results with individuals who were not associated with the hospital.

There is also a pseudo-legal dimension of accreditation. For example, the accreditation standards of the Joint Commission on Accreditation of Healthcare Organizations' (JCAHO) require that medical records be "confidential, secure, current, authenticated, legible and complete."[18] A health care organization that fails to meet this requirement can lose its accreditation.

Politically, the atmosphere is charged as a result of recent studies and of policies in other countries. In Great Britain, for example, lawmakers are trying to protect information in computers with a statute that makes unauthorized prying into a computer a crime punishable by up to six months in jail.[19] Sweden has enacted strong privacy policies that are being used as a model by United States grass roots interest groups. Under several acts of parliament, Sweden (1) requires that all data banks be licensed before being implemented; (2) prohibits any information gathering unless authorized; (3) recognizes a new felony crime, "data trespass," for unauthorized collection or use of personal data or for maintaining inaccurate, incomplete, or outdated information; and (4) applies these policies to all data banks in the country, whether private or public.[20]

In the United States, in light of increased use of computerized patient records, Congress is currently examining proposals for new federal medical records confidentiality laws that would preempt state laws and require protection that goes beyond current responsibilities of individual institutions.[21] These laws include (1) requiring hospitals to permit patients to inspect and correct their records; (2) making it a crime to obtain medical records under false pretenses; and (3) authorizing suits for breaches of confidentiality or other mismanagement of personal data.

Some states have general statutes governing the confidentiality of patient records and patient information. For example both Montana and Washington have adopted the Uniform Health Care Information Act. California has also adopted a statute governing release of individually identifiable patient information by providers.[22]

The fiscal dimension of the privacy issue is simply that privacy protection can be expensive. After the first year of the federal Privacy Act, the Department of Defense complained that the new policy "put a heavy administrative burden on the Department and had proved very costly to implement."[23] It is expensive to double-check for accuracy, to provide for inspection, to periodically purge, and so forth. How much privacy protection can organizations afford?

Operationally, the key problem is the dilemma between the information needs of health care organizations and the harm that can result. Restrictions on data activities imposed for the sake of privacy can make it difficult for an organization to function efficiently. What are realistic limits? For example, in Texas an employee of a mental hospital who raped a patient was later found to have previously been convicted of rape. A state law had denied the hospital the right to screen his arrest record before employment. And what can be done when the medical record of an unconscious patient is needed for treatment but cannot be released because it was collected for other treatment? As a CBS reporter complains, privacy can be carried too far.[24]

The inferential aspect of the issues is a factor that concerns even those "with nothing to hide." Currently, credit card and phone call records are two easily accessed sources of information about the range of personal interests and activities: what people read, where they travel, who they call, what they wear, what organizations they support.

For example, consider the kinds of records that are kept on individuals. Could someone infer from your large credit card purchase at the ABC liquor store that you have a drinking problem, not knowing that your job entails heavy entertaining? Could someone infer from your record of frequent blood tests that you are concerned about venereal disease, not knowing that you are monitoring your cholesterol level? Could an employer who sees a psychiatrist's report of your treatment infer that your are unsuited for a high-pressure job? The power of information, even accurate and complete information, to generate unwarranted impressions is considerable, and is a legitimate concern in the matter of information privacy.[25]

How Computers Affect the Issue

Clearly, information privacy is a concern even without computerization. But why do many believe that, " . . . by far, the most important high-tech threat to privacy is not an exotic surveillance device but a familiar storage system: the computer."[26]

One aspect is that computers remove information from a guarded medical environment to a technical one in which patient contact may be lost and intuitive concern for privacy may be preempted by billing and data storage needs. The tendency of computerization to depersonalize can aggravate the problem.

The integration capability of computers poses an additional threat to privacy. With computers, scattered pieces of data can easily be compiled into a profile never before possible. With computers, an erroneous piece of data that previously would remain isolated in a manual file cabinet can now be integrated with other data and widely disseminated. The computer also facilitates wide access to data; it enables personal information to be "passed on and on at lightning speed from one user to another all over the world."[27] As two medical lawyers point out:

> In the past hospitals could restrict access to confidential information about patients simply by preventing unauthorized persons from entering the medical record area. However, with medical information potentially available to anyone with a connected terminal, there is a danger of multiple breaches of confidentiality without the knowledge of the hospital.[28]

Also, the storage capabilities of computers make it easy to keep personal information. In fact, computers often make it less expensive to store data than destroy it. This can in turn result in a failure to purge outdated or erroneous data. It has also encouraged more data collection. Thus, more personal data is now collected and maintained. The more complicated and sophisticated the technology becomes, the more prone it is to error. "There are two broad dangers," says Gary Marx, a sociologist at MIT. "One is that the technologies work and the other is that they don't work."[29]

In addition, technical and psychological factors of computers aggravate the privacy problem. Many people are inclined to regard a computer printout as infallible. In fact, a University of Missouri research team found that even the brightest people "tend to take the word of a machine over their own good sense."[30] Whereas a handwritten notation on a person might be questioned, a computer printout item might appear so "official" looking as to dispel any inclination to question.

Finally, did you ever try to correct an erroneous computerized bill? It takes a while. Correcting a computerized record is a technical task that involves more than erasing or lining out a sheet of paper. The use of computers does magnify the privacy problem.

Managerial Implications

Dealing with the privacy issue in computerization is a serious responsibility that requires wise use of the perception and sensitivity of the user-manager. What can a manager do? Blithely leaving the management of privacy to the technicians while using the technology is ill-advised, as well as irresponsible.

The first step is to reduce the amount of personal data collected and maintained to that which is actually needed. The storage capability of computers often prompts a tendency to collect and store whatever data might be useful. As long as the client is available and has to fill out a form, why not collect all the data possible? Clearly, the more personal data maintained, the greater the privacy problem.

Second, user-managers should know the privacy laws and regulations that apply to their work. Many unwittingly break privacy laws and rules simply because they have not kept abreast of legal and regulatory developments on privacy.

Third, managers attuned to the problem can establish in-house information handling policies that exceed legal requirements to clients who entrust the organization with personal data. These policies should outline what can be collected, how it can be used, who must verify its accuracy, when it will be updated, and so forth.

Fourth, managers and users can provide training on the nature of the problem and on policies in order to develop a "privacy consciousness." Most privacy breaches occur because information handlers are unaware of the power of the data they collect and hold. Training can develop this awareness.

Fifth, protecting privacy is largely a matter of properly managing information—of establishing verification procedures, of updating, purging, and protecting data that is collected and stored. To collect and use an inaccurate piece of personal data is mismanagement of the first order. Weak or nonexistent information management procedures breed the kind of carelessness that makes privacy breaches simple, likely, and serious.

Sixth, managers must institute technical and administrative security measures as were discussed in Chapter 7. Computerized personal data that is otherwise well-managed can be easily accessed and altered unless solid security measures are employed.

Seventh, managers should periodically audit privacy protection measures. It is the business of some firms to attempt to obtain sensitive data from an organization, test verification and updating procedures, and measure staff alertness to potential privacy problems. Employing a firm of this type to conduct periodic privacy audits can disclose weak areas and produce better privacy safeguards.

Finally, managers could opt to not computerize certain particularly sensitive personal data. Automation does aggravate the privacy problem—a deliberate decision not to computerize certain data can sometimes be a wise policy.

Notes

1. J. Rothfeder, *Privacy for Sale*, (New York: Simon & Shuster, 1992).
2. *Personal Privacy in an Information Society*, no. 052–003–003395–3. (Washington, DC: U.S. Government Printing Office), 1990.
3. D. Miller, "Preserving the Privacy of Computerized Patient Records," *Healthcare Informatics*, October 1993, 72–74.
4. *New York Times*, 5 June 1988, E-2.
5. For example, D. Singleton, Privacy Study: Another Peek," *New York Daily News*, 6 May 1979, and J. Caper, "The Privacy Scam," *Newsweek*, 18 June 1979, 3.
6. Related by D. F. Linowes, "The Privacy Crisis," *Newsweek*, 26 June 1978, 19.
7. Related in J. Heller, "Not-so-Private Lives at a Finger's Touch," *Newsday*, 29 May 1978, 4.
8. "Innocent Man Cleared Again," *Times Union* (Albany), 15 June 1980.
9. "Nowhere To Hide," *Time*, 11 November 1991, 36.
10. Quoted from *Hospitals & Health Networks*, 20 November 1993, 14.
11. D. Harris, "A Matter of Privacy: Managing Personal Data in Company Computers," *Personnel*, February 1987, 34.

12. E. Early, "Letter to the Editor," *New York Times*, 12 December 1978, 29.

13. P. Dewitt, "Can a System Keep a Secret?" *Time*, 6 April 1987, 68–70.

14. R. Bergman, "Laws Sought to Guard Health Data from Falling into the Wrong Hands," *Hospitals & Health Networks*, 20 January 1994, 62.

15. *Hospitals & Health Networks*, 20 November 1993, 14.

16. See D. O'Brien, "Freedom of Information, Privacy, and Information Control," *Public Administration Review*, July–August 1979, 323–28.

17. R. Hard, "Keeping Patient Data Secure within Hospitals," *Hospitals*, 20 October 1992, 50.

18. Joint Commission on the Accreditation of Healthcare Organizations, *Accreditation Manual*, MR.3 (Oakbrook Terrace, IL: JCAHO, 1994).

19. *The Economist*, 4 May 1991, 21.

20. For an overview of privacy policies in other countries, see Gabriel Rach, "Data Privacy," *Telecommunications*, May 1980, 43–48.

21. Bergman, 62.

22. A. Waller and D. Fulton, "The Electronic Chart: Keeping it Confidential," *Journal of Health and Hospital Law*, April 1993, 105.

23. A. Gerow, "DOD Officials Wage 'Hell' to Curtail Privacy Act," *Navy Times*, February 1976, 4.

24. F. Graham, "Carrying Privacy too Far," *The Washington Post*, 12 September 1978, 18.

25. G. J. Bologna, "The Ethics of Managing Information," *Journal of Systems Management*, August 1987, 28. J. Rothfeder, *Privacy for Sale* (New York: Simon & Shuster, 1992).

26. Quoted in *Time*, 11 November 1992, 34.

27. Linowes, *Newsweek*, 26 June 1978, 19.

28. A. D. Jergesen, and S. V. Schnier, "Medical Legal Forum," *Hospital Forum*, (September–October 1979): 24.

29. J. Markoff, "A New Breed of Snoopier Computers," *New York Times*, 5 June 1988, E-2.

30. L. Tomnick, "Electronic Bullies," *Psychology Today*, February 1982, 10.

Selected Readings

Betts, M. "Safeguarding Privacy: MIS Confronts a Sensitive Challenge." *Computerworld* (17 July 1986): 53–59.

Business Week. "Protection, Individual Privacy" (9 February 1987): 106.

Campbell, D., and S. Connor. "Records Protected—People Exposed." *New Statesman* (16 May 1986): 16.

Collins, J. "Computer Matching Draws Concerns." *Data Management* (December 1986): 6–8.

Creighton, H. "Right of Privacy: Limit?" *Nursing Management* (March 1985): 15–17.

Egan, J. N. "The Medical Confidentiality Sham." *Family Health* (September 1980): 16–20.

Field, A. R. "Big Brother Inc. May Be Closer than You Thought—Lists and Database Profiles of People Cause Invasion of Privacy." *Business Week* (9 February 1987): 84–87.

Fresse, J. "Computers, Medical Care, and Privacy." *Journal of Clinical Computers* (1985): 129–31.

Gilbert, F., and K. Frawley. "Do Computerized Patient Records Risk Invading Patient Privacy More than Paper Records?" *Hospitals & Health Networks* (5 November 1993): 8.

Haydock, B. "Your Medical Records: Not so Private Anymore." *Changing Times* (July 1981): 41–43.

Katz, J. "Telecommunications and Computers: Whither Privacy Policy?" *Society* (November–December 1987): 81–87.

Laycayo, R. "Nowhere to Hide." *Time* (11 November 1991): 34–40.

Linowes, D. F. "Computers and Privacy Problems: Their Impact on People and Programs." *Journal of Health and Human Resources Administration* (February 1980): 364–68.

Miller, R. A., K. F. Schaffner, and A. Meisel. "Ethical and Legal Issues Related to the Use of Computer Programs in Clinical Medicine." *Annals of International Medicine* 102 (1985): 529–36.

Newman, M., and D. G. Marks. "Employment and Privacy: A Problem for Our Time." *Journal of Business Ethics* (February 1987): 153–64.

Norden, G. "Do the Laws on Confidentiality Obstruct Hospital Efficiency when EDP Is Introduced?" *World Hospital* (February 1984): 26.

Regan, P. M. "Privacy, Government Information, and Technology." *Public Administration Review* (November–December 1986): 629–33.

Romano, C. A. "Privacy, Confidentiality, and Security of Computerized Systems." *Computers in Nursing* (May–June 1987): 99–104.

Rozovsky, L. E., and F. A. Rozovsky. "The Computer Challenge: More Data, Less Privacy." *Canadian Doctor* (March 1985): 46–48.

Scholes, M. "Computers in Nursing—Privacy and Confidentiality." *Nursing Times* (March–April 1986): 59–60.

Sieghart, P. "Medical Confidence, the Law, and Computers." *Journal of Social Medicine* (August 1984): 656–62.

Vidmar, N., and D. H. Flaherty. "Concern For Personal Privacy in an Electronic Age." *Journal of Communication* (Spring 1985): 91–103.

Vuori, H. "Privacy Confidentiality and Automated Health Information Systems." *Journal of Medical Ethics* (1977): 172–78.

Westin, A. F. "The Dimensions of Privacy." *Computers and People* (July–August 1979): 14–16.

———. "The Impact of Computers on Privacy." *Datamation* (December 1979): 190–94.

READINGS

T HE PRIVACY issue continues to be one of the most difficult managerial challenges facing health care professionals. The following readings provide some useful perspectives. The *Time* magazine cover story is helpful in developing sensitivity to the dimensions of the privacy challenge and in illuminating the need for a multi-faceted managerial response. Sheri Alpert offers some sound perspectives for responding to the threats to privacy in light of new information technologies.

Nowhere to Hide

Richard Lacayo

Using computers, high-tech gadgets and mountains of data, an army of snoops is assaulting our privacy.

Open up in there. The census taker wants to know what time you leave for work. Giant marketing firms want to know how often you use credit cards. Your boss would like your psychological profile, your bill-paying history and a urine sample. Is that enough to make you feel like hiding in a corner, muttering to yourself about invasions of privacy? Forget it—the neighbors might be videotaping.

Though the word privacy does not appear in the Constitution, most people would probably agree with the great Supreme Court Justice Louis Brandeis, who once identified "the right to be let alone" as the prerequisite of a tolerable life. But the fundamental instinct to shield one's personal affairs from the eyes of outsiders is always under pressure from the no less venerable human urge to pry—and the snoops just may be getting the upper hand these days. Items:

- In June executives of the Procter & Gamble Co. in Cincinnati complained to police that company information was being illegally leaked to a reporter. To identify the source of the leak, Cincinnati Bell, acting in response to a grand jury subpoena, searched the phone records of every one of its 655,000 customers in the 513 and 606 area codes. P&G executives later conceded that the investigation was an error in judgment.

- Public uproar forced Lotus Development, a software manufacturer, and Equifax, a company that compiles financial information about individuals, to shelve their scheme to market a data base that would have allowed anyone with a personal computer to purchase a list of names, buying habits and income levels of selected households. The system would have permitted small businesses such as dry cleaners, pharmacies and pizza take-out restaurants to get a bead on their local customers.

- The Employers' Information Service, a company based in Gretna, La., is creating a massive data bank on workers who have reported on-the-job injuries. For a fee, employers can request a report on prospective employees, including a history of prior job injuries and a record of worker's compensation claims and lawsuits. To keep from being added to other data banks, workers in Idaho are suing that state's industrial commission to prevent it from releasing such records.

It may be customary to think of threats to privacy in Orwellian terms, with an all-seeing Big Brother government as the culprit. But lately the threat comes no less from private companies, private citizens—and from our own imperfect notions of how to define which matters are properly kept confidential. The powers of government are fashioned under the pressure of society's own values and expectations. Lately those values have been in flux.

From the quiet frontiersman to the modern urban loner, the archetypal American is someone whose most sacred territory is the portable enclosure of the self. But if "Mind your own business" has long been a prime tenet of the national philosophy, "Let it all hang out" is now running a close second. It's hard to find a national consensus on confidentiality in a nation of tell-all memoirs, inquiring pollsters and talk shows—not to mention televised Senate hearings—whose participants air explicit sexual details that would have caused earlier generations to blush and turn away.

As the bounds of privacy dissolve under the demands for frankness, they also bend before the pressures for AIDS testing, drug testing and now even genetic testing, which promises to predict each person's inherited susceptibility to certain illnesses but could also create a pariah class of people that employers would regard as too prone to cancer, heart disease or other ailments. Into this volatile mix of half-formed attitudes and sharply felt anxieties, technology has arrived with a host of unprecedented temptations. Many new answering machines are equipped to surreptitiously tape whole conversations. Video-surveillance cameras quietly scan many workplaces. Neighborhood retailers now stock hardware that used to be the stuff of spy novels. But by far the most important high-tech threat to privacy is not an exotic surveillance device but a familiar storage system: the computer. Computers permit nimble feats of data manipulation, including high-speed retrieval and matching of records, that were impossible with paper stored in file cabinets. They have turned data collection into a $1 billion-a-year industry—one in which nearly every American supplies the data, often without knowing it.

To get a driver's license, a mortgage or a credit card, to be admitted to a hospital or to register the warranty on a new purchase, people routinely fill out forms providing a wealth of facts about themselves. Little of it remains confidential. Personal finances, medical history, purchasing habits and more are raked in by data companies. These firms combine the records with information drawn from other sources—for instance, from state governments that sell lists of driver's licenses, or the post office lists of addresses arranged according to ZIP code—to draw a clearer picture of an individual or a household.

The repackaged data—which often include hearsay and inaccuracies—are then sold to government agencies, mortgage lenders, retailers, small businesses, marketers and insurers. When making loan decisions, banks rely on credit-bureau reports about the applicant's bill-paying history. Employers often refer to them in making hiring decisions. Marketers use information about buying habits and income to target their mail-order and telephone pitches. Even government agencies are plugging in to commercial data bases to make decisions about eligibility for health-care benefits and Social Security.

"In the not too distant future, consumers face the prospect that a computer somewhere will compile records about every place they go and everything they purchase," says Democrat Bob Wise of West Virginia who heads the House subcommittee that oversees the

Figure 8.1 Time/CNN Poll on Privacy

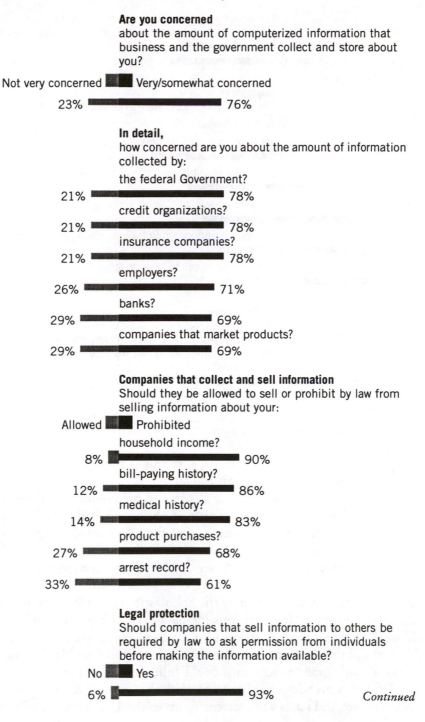

Are you concerned
about the amount of computerized information that
business and the government collect and store about
you?

Not very concerned ▮▮ Very/somewhat concerned

23% ━━━━━━━━ 76%

In detail,
how concerned are you about the amount of information
collected by:

the federal Government?

21% ━━━━━━━ 78%

credit organizations?

21% ━━━━━━━ 78%

insurance companies?

21% ━━━━━━━ 78%

employers?

26% ━━━━━━ 71%

banks?

29% ━━━━━ 69%

companies that market products?

29% ━━━━━ 69%

Companies that collect and sell information
Should they be allowed to sell or prohibit by law from
selling information about your:

Allowed ▮▮ Prohibited

household income?

8% ━━━━━━━━━ 90%

bill-paying history?

12% ━━━━━━━━ 86%

medical history?

14% ━━━━━━━ 83%

product purchases?

27% ━━━━━ 68%

arrest record?

33% ━━━━ 61%

Legal protection
Should companies that sell information to others be
required by law to ask permission from individuals
before making the information available?

No ▮▮ Yes

6% ━━━━━━━━ 93% *Continued*

Figure 8.1 Continued

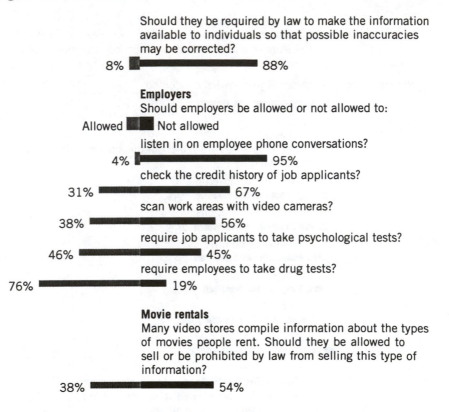

Should they be required by law to make the information available to individuals so that possible inaccuracies may be corrected?

8% ▬▬▬▬▬▬▬▬ 88%

Employers
Should employers be allowed or not allowed to:

Allowed ▬ Not allowed

listen in on employee phone conversations?
4% ▬▬▬▬▬▬ 95%

check the credit history of job applicants?
31% ▬▬▬▬▬ 67%

scan work areas with video cameras?
38% ▬▬▬▬ 56%

require job applicants to take psychological tests?
46% ▬▬▬▬ 45%

require employees to take drug tests?
76% ▬▬▬ 19%

Movie rentals
Many video stores compile information about the types of movies people rent. Should they be allowed to sell or be prohibited by law from selling this type of information?

38% ▬▬▬▬ 54%

From a telephone poll of 500 American adults taken on October 23 by Yankelovich Clancy Shulman. Sampling error is plus or minus 4.5%. "Not sures" omitted.

government's use of data. "I'm not sure this is the vision of the future that will make Americans comfortable."

Because computer information is stored on small disks, it tends to be more enduring than paper records of old, which had to be discarded from time to time to make room for new files. As a result, long-ago personal setbacks can now embed themselves in the permanent record. Two influential trade groups, the American Business Conference and the National Alliance of Business, have even joined with the Educational Testing Service, which conducts the Scholastic Aptitude Tests, in creating a pilot program for a nationwide data base of high school records. It would give employers access to a job applicant's grades, attendance history and the ancient evaluations of teachers. Just like Mother warned you—a ninth-grade report card could follow you for life.

Privacy watchdogs are warning that the combination of invasive technologies and lax laws threatens to make the U.S. a nation of people who live in glass houses, their every move open to scrutiny by outsiders. "I see no reason why McDonald's needs to know my Social Security number or my previous job title," complains New York Law School professor E. Donald Shapiro, a privacy specialist. "The danger is not that direct-marketing companies will clog your mailbox or call you during dinner to hawk commemorative coins," says David Linowes, former chairman of the U.S. Privacy Protection Commission. "The danger is that employers, banks and government agencies will use data bases to make decisions about our lives without our knowing about it."

At the same time, privacy is not an absolute value. With U.S. banks being used as a conduit for drug money, for example, law-enforcement officials have pressed them to report any suspicious movement of cash. Though that may involve a conflict with traditional notions of banker-client confidentiality, many banks have been willing to comply. "The social value of helping to fight drugs outweighs, at least to some extent, the privacy issue," says Jack Kilhefner, senior vice president at Wells Fargo Bank in San Francisco.

Business groups also argue that banning the sale of their customer data violates property rights. "The agenda of the privacy types is anti-technology, anti-free speech and anti-business," says Robert Posch Jr., vice president of legal affairs for Doubleday Book & Music Clubs and a leading defender of data collectors. "They're trying to play on the public's fear of computers and having their names on lists. But a computerized data base is only a file cabinet that's faster."

In the same sense, a car is just a buggy that goes faster—and yet the automobile revolutionized society. Data collection is doing the same. A number of catalog retailers and financial companies now make use of a business version of Caller I.D., a service offered by some phone companies, that lets them see the name, phone number and credit history of customers who call them. Once a company possesses a caller's name and address, it can dig up even more by linking with hundreds of data banks that also have the name on file. A phone number alone is so valuable to telemarketers that some companies advertise free phone-information lines as bait to gather numbers [Exhibit 8.1].

Three giant credit bureaus—TRW, Equifax and Trans Union—dominate the consumer-data industry, which also includes about 450 smaller outfits. Every month the Big Three purchase computer records, mostly from banks and retailers, that detail the financial activity of virtually every adult American. TRW and Equifax each have 150 million individual files. According to a report in the *Wall Street Journal*, anyone who applies for a credit card is listed on Equifax's "credit-seekers hot

Exhibit 8.1 Now We've Really Got Your Number

The new phone service known as Caller I.D. is a double-edged sword: it protects the privacy of some people, but at the expense of others. For about $6.50 a month, plus a one-time equipment charge of $45 to $80, customers get an electronic screen that displays the phone number of every incoming call. First offered four years ago in New Jersey by New Jersey Bell, Caller I.D. is now available in 20 states and under consideration in 13 others.

Caller I.D. is being touted as a way to combat obscene and annoying callers. It also gives florists, pizza shops and other delivery businesses a way to check that incoming orders are not pranks. Phone companies have been promoting the service as an electronic version of the peephole that lets apartment dwellers see who is knocking. "Caller I.D. protects subscriber privacy because it lets subscribers decide who to let into their house," says A. Gray Collins, a Bell Atlantic executive vice president.

But it also diminishes the privacy of callers. Some businesses use a commercial version of Caller I.D. that quietly displays the phone number of people who inquire about products, investments or insurance. The numbers can then be used to obtain other information about individual customers from consumer data bases. Privacy activists are also worried that the prospect of having phone numbers revealed will discourage anonymous police tipsters and callers to telephone hot lines that serve drug abusers, runaways and other people in trouble. Says Janlori Goldman of the A.C.L.U.: "The danger of Caller I.D. is that people lose control over when and to whom to give their telephone numbers."

Several states, including California, New York and Pennsylvania, have taken steps to prohibit Caller I.D. unless phone companies offer customers the ability to block their numbers from being displayed at any time. To pre-empt further moves by the states, the Federal Communications Commission has proposed that callers be allowed to block the display of their numbers on individual calls but not be able to demand that the phone company automatically block their numbers from being displayed at any time. The conflict may have to be resolved in the courts or Congress. The Senate has before it a bill that would permit the per-call restrictions proposed by the FCC. The House is considering a version that would allow the broader limits favored by some states. Telephone-company executives expect the two measures to be reconciled by the end of the year.

—*By Richard Lacayo. Reported by Jerome Cramer/Washington*

line," a popular buy for marketers, while the Bankcard hot line at Trans Union lists all credit card purchases.

The Big Three credit bureaus argue that their products do not disclose truly confidential details. But until recently, for instance, Equifax sold lists of consumers who used their credit cards more frequently than the average. Combining that with census data, the company then used a statistical model to estimate the general range of each card user's income, though not to specify the actual amount. "We would not disclose a person's total balances or how much credit they have available in absolute dollar terms," says John Baker, senior vice president of Equifax, which serves 60,000 business customers and whose profits for credit reporting and information packaging last year totaled $366 million.

That practice proved too controversial, and this summer Equifax got out of the business of selling direct-marketing lists based on its credit files. But smaller data banks have been breaking down figures to offer for sale such tidbits as the location of nearly every household in the U.S. that recently brought home a newborn child. For about $25 to $95 a month, plus search charges, customers of Information America, an Atlanta-based company, have access to profiles of 80 million households. By typing a name into a home computer, a subscriber can obtain that person's address, phone number, length of residence, records of property ownership, court appearances and business dealings. Some smaller outfits also have a reputation for selling personal data to people who may have no business seeing it—everyone from private investigators to bill collectors and spurned lovers.

Critics also charge that data collectors are deceptive. Few people realize, for instance, that when they fill out a product-warranty card, the information goes to a little-known data seller called National Demographics & Lifestyles. "People fill out product cards because they want the warranty," says Marc Rotenberg, Washington director of Computer Professionals for Social Responsibility. "But they end up on the mailing lists of stereo and record companies. Was that part of the stated bargain when they filled out the card?"

For marketers, detailed consumer profiles are an unmixed blessing, making it far easier to target thc households most likely to welcome their mail-order catalogs and other pitches. Direct marketers were once happy if just 1% of recipients responded to a mass mailing. A 5% response is now more common, which the marketers argue indicates that consumers are happier too. "We're matchmakers for parties with common interests," says John Cleary, president of Donnelly Marketing, one of the nation's largest list compilers. "We make sure companies don't try to sell lawn mowers to people in high-rises.

Each of the Big Three also operates a separate unit that compiles credit reports detailing the bill-paying history of nearly every American. The reports are sold to mortgage lenders, credit-card companies and anyone else who can show a legitimate business interest. The Big Three argue that their service is essential to the workings of credit-card and loan industries that most Americans could not do without. But their critics complain that the reports are frequently riddled with errors and that it is difficult and expensive to consumers to correct or even know about them. Earlier this year Consumers Union reported that nearly half the credit reports it studied from the nation's largest credit bureaus contained some inaccuracies.

Eugene N. Wolfe, a retired speech writer who lives in McLean, Va., knows all about that. In 1986 he was puzzled when a local bank turned down his loan request. To his horror, he discovered that for years an Equifax subsidiary called Credit Bureau, Inc., had merged his credit history with that of another Eugene N. Wolfe, who had a raft of debts. After weeks of conversation and paperwork, Wolfe thought he had cleared up the problem—until last year when he was turned down again for a new card and discovered that information pertaining to the other Eugene Wolfe had found its way back into his file.

"At one time I had to pay the highest interest rate on a car loan because the dealer was looking at bum debts that were erroneously listed in my name, but I didn't know it," Wolfe complains. "It makes you angry." Equifax contends that his case was unusual and that the company has recently adopted new software intended to reduce the likelihood of such confusion.

The issue of faulty reporting came to a head in July, when the attorneys general of six states—Alabama, California, Idaho, Michigan, New York and Texas—brought suits against TRW's credit agency operation, accusing it of violating consumer privacy and failing to correct serious reporting errors. The company filed countersuits in federal court arguing that the Federal Fair Credit Reporting Act Of 1970 supercedes state law. But recently TRW also announced that it would supply consumers on request with free copies of their own credit files, instead of charging up to $20 a copy. Trans Union and Equifax declined to follow suit, arguing that providing free reports would be too expensive. Equifax executives argued that there was no great consumer demand for cheaper reports.

The pressure on the companies seems likely to increase. On Capitol Hill, the House has before it legislation that would require written agreement from consumers before information about them is released by a bank, credit bureau or other institution. Credit agencies oppose the bill, along with another introduced by California Representative Esteban Torres that would update the Fair Credit Reporting Act, which gave consumers the right to see and, if necessary, correct their credit records. That bill would require all credit agencies to send consumers, upon request, one free copy of their report annually, as TRW has voluntarily agreed to do.

While data bases are an almost hidden threat to privacy, American workers are also finding themselves up against more visible measures to probe them and keep them under watch [Exhibit 8.2]. When Sibi Soroka interviewed for a job as a security guard in April 1989 at a Target store in Pleasanton, Calif., he was asked to take a three-hour written psychological test. The interviewer told him that he would assess Soroka's ideas about the world of work. Soroka was stunned to discover that many of the true-false questions on the test centered on sex, religion and political beliefs. "My sex life is satisfactory," read one. "I believe in the second coming of Christ," read another.

"I was astonished at how intrusive the questions were," he recalls. "But I needed a job." Though Soroka received a job offer after completing the test, he filed a class action against Target in September 1989. His suit is believed to be the first major court challenge to the increasingly common use of psychological testing as a condition of employment.

Defenders of the tests say they are needed for such workers as armed security guards, one of the few kinds of employees that Target subjects to the examination. "When we entrust individuals with weapons to protect the public, I think it's important to assess their emotional stability," says James Butcher, a psychology professor at the University of Minnesota, who helped revise the Minnesota Multiphasic Personality Inventory. An earlier version of that test provided many of the questions that were asked of Soroka. The revised version eliminates some of the inquiries about religion and sexuality.

Opponents of psychological screening say it is not only invasive, it's ineffective. "It just isn't the exact science people pretend that it is," says Lewis Maltby of the American Civil Liberties Union in New York City. "We have some ability to identify people who are potential thieves by a written psychological test. If you were to test 100 potential employees, you could probably catch 8 of the 10 thieves. But the only way you could do it is by rejecting 50 of the 100 people. So to catch 8 guilty people, you're denying a job to 42 innocent ones."

Surveillance at the workplace is also a concern for an increasing number of job holders. Drug testing is just the most publicized variety. One increasingly common tactic is to listen in on employees who deal with the public over the phone. Reservation clerks, phone-company operators and anyone who takes phone orders for catalog companies and telemarketers are all likely to be monitored. So are the customers they talk to. The Communications Workers of America, a union active in the fight against such surveillance, estimates that 6 million American workers are subject to monitoring. Surveillance at BellSouth, a group

Exhibit 8.2 Do-It-Yourself Espionage

Pssst. Want a briefcase that conceals a tiny video camera? How about a mini tape recorder that has a pinhead microphone disguised as a tie tack? You don't have to buy this stuff in a back alley. Just head over to your local CCS Counter Spy Shop, a chain with retail outlets in New York City, Houston, Miami and Washington that specializes in high-tech snooping gear. According to Tom Felice, sales manager for the New York City store, clandestine recording devices are the biggest sellers. "The more discreet they are, the more popular," he says. "There are a lot of paranoid people out there." Enough for the industry to claim total sales last year of $200 million.

Counter Spy is not alone. Other big electronics retail chains and smaller mail-order outfits are also bringing elite snooping into the mass market. New Jersey–based Edmund Scientific sells an electronic microphone for $625 that it claims can "pull in voices up to three-quarters of a mile away." Life Force Technologies in Colorado sells a briefcase with a hidden tape recorder for $1,195. "Invading someone's privacy has become as easy as walking into your local electronics store," complains Morton Bromfield, executive director of the American Privacy Foundation, based in Wellesley, Mass.

Many of these products can be used in ways that are not just obnoxious but illegal. For instance, federal law prohibits the taping of telephone conversations unless at least one of the parties on the line knows that the conversation is being recorded. But so long as retailers remain unaware of—and don't ask about—the potentially illegal purposes that a customer may have in mind, they cannot be held liable. Nine years ago, Radio Shack's parent company, Tandy Corp., was sued by Elizabeth Flowers, a South Carolina woman whose husband used a miniature recording device to secretly tape her phone calls after she filed for divorce. Lawyers for Radio Shack successfully argued that the company had no responsibility in the matter because it did not know what her husband planned to do with the device. "There would be nothing left to sell if we withdrew all the products that might be used illegally," says Robert Miller, a Radio Shack vice president. Besides, he adds, with unintended irony, it is not the company's business what customers do with the products "in the privacy of their own homes." But if the use of such devices becomes widespread, there may not be much privacy left at home—or anywhere else.

—*By Richard Lacayo. Reported by Thomas McCarroll/New York*

of phone companies in a nine-state Southern region, is typical—about two to five calls a month for each service representative and 30 a month for each operator, less than 1% of all the calls they handle.

Employers say monitoring is both legal and necessary to measure productivity and ensure that their telephone representatives are accurate and courteous in their exchanges with customers. Privacy and labor experts largely concede that employers have a right to monitor workers as part of training and supervisory functions. What they question is the value of employee surveillance—and the acceptable limits. "Supervisors have said to me, you're being too friendly, your voice sounds too sexy on the phone," claims Shirley Webb, a Southern Bell service consultant.

Barbara Otto, a director of 9 to 5, National Association of Working Women, a Cleveland-based women's advocacy group, says such monitoring can backfire. Telephone operators who are penalized for taking too much time with inquiries already tell of cutting short customer calls. At the same time, the personal calls of employees pass through the monitor's earphone. "Employers start catching non-work related information," Otto complains. "They discover that employees are spending weekends with a person of the same sex or talking about forming a union."

The House and Senate have before them bills that would require a visual signal or audible tone on the line when monitoring is going on. Among the leaders in the fight against them has been AT&T, which lobbied successfully to kill one such bill in Virginia. "Factory supervisors don't blow whistles to warn assembly-line workers they're coming," says an AT&T official.

Inevitably, Americans have been looking to Congress to resolve the questions concerning privacy. One irony is that the Federal Government is the nation's largest data compiler. At last count, in 1982, it possessed more than 3.5 billion files on individual Americans—an average of 15 per person, with more sure to come. Much of the data consists of uncorroborated information and hearsay, which could be potentially damaging to individual rights if it fell into the wrong hands. While the FBI has shelved plans to build a national computer bank that police could use to keep track of criminal suspects, it is still creating a data base on the 25 million Americans who have ever been arrested, even if they were not convicted. Meanwhile, the census is not just counting heads but peeking inside them. Instead of the usual short forms, 17% of all households last year received a longer questionnaire that asked such questions as How long is your workday commute? and How many people travel to work with you? Names of all individuals will be removed from the census files before the information is stored on personal-computer disks that marketers can buy.

Because the forms of privacy intrusion are so numerous and varied, no single remedy applies to them all. Congress is soon expected to tackle one of the most jolting new developments in telemarketing: the automated dialing machines that can call every number in a telephone exchange, one after another, to make prerecorded sales pitches. Over the objections of civil libertarians, who say the machines are protected by the constitutional right of free speech, both the House and Senate are considering measures that would ban or severely restrict the use of autodialers for most calls to private homes.

In response to a problem that lies closer to home, several law-makers have proposed legislation to beef up the 1974 Privacy Act, the federal law that defends citizens from government misuse of data. Enforcement is haphazard, and loopholes permit agencies to stretch the law. Though the act would appear to forbid it, agencies exchange information on individual citizens in the name of detecting waste, fraud and abuse of benefits. They claim that such exchanges seem justifiable in a time of tight budgets, but the precedent it sets for going around the law would encourage more ominous practices, such as using the records of people in drug-treatment programs to search for possible criminals.

West Virginia Democrat Bob Wise, chairman of the House sub-committee on government information, has gone further. In November 1989 he introduced a proposal to create a federal data-protection board to ensure that personal information in government computers is not abused. Demanding more sweeping action, privacy advocates want Congress to regulate private companies' use of data by requiring consent for the use of information and strict controls over its accuracy. They also call for the creation of a privacy ombudsman, like those in Canada and Australia, who can aggressively defend consumer interests.

Gary T. Marx, a professor at the Massachusetts Institute for Technology who specializes in privacy issues, even wants Congress to establish a royalty system to compensate individuals—or consumers en masse—whenever personal information about them is sold. "If we are to treat personal information as a commodity," he wrote recently, "it seems only fair that those to whom it pertains ought to control it and share in financial gain from its sale."

If nothing else, that scheme would have the virtue of framing what can be a metaphysical problem in simple market terms: Just what price do we put on privacy? No one can answer that question who has not sorted out the issues of how much privacy we need and how much we are willing to give up in exchange for things like convenience shopping, job opportunities, law enforcement and higher productivity. For unlike the nightmarish Big Brother world of Orwell, the question of how much privacy Americans preserve will depend more on the values of the people than the whims and dictates of government.

Reported by Tom Curry/Atlanta, Thomas McCarroll/New York and Dennis Wyss/ San Francisco.

Smart Cards, Smarter Policy: Medical Records, Privacy, and Health Care Reform

Sheri Alpert

> Current law does not adequately protect patients' privacy or their medical records. Proposals to computerize these records could further erode confidentiality unless new federal laws are enacted.

In the months ahead, policymakers in the United States will continue to debate how to control the ever-increasing cost of our nation's health care system. Several legislative proposals introduced in the 102nd Congress included provisions intended to reduce the cost of administering the system,[1] and similar proposals have already been introduced in the 103rd Congress.[2] Indeed, the President has recently unveiled his health care reform proposals.

A key feature of most of these reform proposals is the heavy reliance on computer technology to facilitate the flow of sensitive medical records (potentially on a national scale) to achieve administrative savings. A major impetus for relying on computerized medical records is the mobile nature of U.S. society. Census figures indicate that 44 percent of the American population changed their place of residence between 1985 and 1990. Approximately 25 percent of those people changed residences across state lines.[3]

Because the health care system is to be reformed on a national scale, conforming to a minimum set of standards, it is crucial that patients' right to privacy and the confidentiality of their medical records also be standard across the nation. Yet thus far, the fact that the law currently does not provide consistent protection for most medical records has been conspicuously absent from reform discussions. Only a handful of states have adopted any laws to protect these records, and those vary in scope and applicability. For instance, most states recognize a provider-patient privilege (discussed in more detail later). Some states also have specific laws to deal with highly sensitive medical information, such as mental health records and or/AIDS test results. A few states— for example, California, Washington, and Montana—have enacted laws defining access to health information generally, while statues dealing with licensing of medical providers and facilities, insurance transactions, or public health reporting. Moreover, state laws often contain provisions more favorable to information exchange than to patient privacy.[4] With the exception of records relating to substance abuse or records in the custody of the federal government, federal law does not protect the confidentiality of medical information. In fact, video rental records are afforded more federal protection than are medical records. As the law now stands, while the unauthorized disclosure of medical records may be ethically reprehensible, in the majority of states in this country, it is not illegal.

A patient's fundamental need to provide sensitive medical information to a practitioner without fear of the consequences should be fixed and not fluid—it must be consistent across every state. This will be especially critical with the advent of standardized and automated medical records and insurance claims. As a report to the secretary of health and human services noted,

> Historically, providers have stored medical information and filed health insurance claims on paper. The paper medium is cumbersome and expensive, two factors that led to the call for the use of EDI [electronic data interchange]. Ironically, it is this "negative" aspect of the paper medium (its cumbersome nature) that has minimized the risk of breaches of confidentiality. Although a breach could occur if someone gained access to health records or insurance claims forms, the magnitude of the breach was limited by the sheer difficulty of unobtrusively reviewing larger numbers of records or claim forms.
>
> From the provider perspective, EDI changes the environment dramatically. . . . Stringent security protocols may make it more difficult for intruders to access patient-identifiable data if the authorized review of unlimited health information. It will greatly increase the dimension of inadvertent and intentional breaches of confidentiality.[5]

If the disclosure of medical records is not legally bound and protected by enforceable standards, the security measures built into these systems will not prevent harm to the patient when records are released.[6]

This lack of protection for medical records has led to a situation in which people cannot be certain that the personal medical information they share with a care provider will remain confidential. This uncertainty on the part of the patient could undermine a physician's ability to provide treatment, because the patient may be reluctant to provide information crucial to his or her care. The introduction of vast computerized data bases (as are being proposed under several of the health care reform proposals) could further exacerbate this situation, because care providers may have even less ability to ensure the confidentiality of patient information.

The prospect of national health care reform, then, highlights the need to provide legal recognition of the value of privacy in the medical arena and legal protection for all medical records—paper and electronic. Federal laws to protect the confidentiality of medical records, regardless of the medium in which they occur, will become even more crucial to the integrity of our health care delivery system.

Reform Proposals in an Electronic Age

As stated earlier, most of the health care reform proposals currently circulating rely heavily on computer technology to facilitate the flow of medical records. Most envision a comprehensive electronic "cradle to grave" medical file on every individual in the United States covered by health insurance. These files would be contained in one or more data bases. Additionally, the proposals will introduce the use of "electronic" or "smart" cards to allow providers to gain access to a patient's medical information via telecommunications networks. While the magnitude of the proposed application of this technology is untried and unproven in this country, sufficient information is known about the capabilities of the technology to warrant careful examination of this use.

There are currently two types of card technologies available. One is similar to an automated teller (ATM) card or regular credit card. The other is known as the "smart" card. The proposals envision that individuals would carry their cards with them at all times to facilitate access to information in case of medical emergencies.

The ATM-type card is the size of a credit card, is often embossed on the front with the patient's name and health care identification number and has a magnetic stripe across the back. The stripe stores only a minimal amount of information, such as name, birth date, health insurance policy number, coverage codes, and deductibles. This kind of card could be used, in turn, to gain access to a patient's complete file of insurance and medical information from data base(s) maintained by someone other than the health care provider.

In contrast to the ATM-type cards, smart cards are essentially microcomputers. They are plastic cards that contain either one of more integrated circuit chips or employ laser technology. Smart cards are the only card technology that can process as well as store information (potentially the equivalent of several hundred pages). They are also typically the size of a credit card and function via a reader/writer device and a terminal that provides access to a host computer. The information stored on the smart card microchip must be customized for every individual and would contain comprehensive medical and insurance information.[7] The cost of using smart cards is a factor to be considered as well, of course. (The average cost of a smart card in 1988 was $10–$20.[8] In a recently initiated Houston health care application, the smart cards cost about $5 each.[9] The cost of the cards will not likely become any cheaper because of the probability that increased functionality will be incorporated into the cards.[10])

There is usually an enormous amount of personal information in a medical record, some of which can be quite sensitive. Aside from the patient's name, address, age, and next of kin, there also may be names of parents; date and place of birth; marital status; religion; history of military service; Social Security number; name of insurer; complaints and diagnoses; medical, social, and family history; previous and current treatments; an inventory of the condition of each body system; medications taken now and in the past; use of alcohol and tobacco; diagnostic tests administered; findings; reactions; and incidents.[11] Clearly, medical records contain extensive amounts of information that has nonmedical uses, and access to that information could be of interest to many parties. As the Workgroup for Electronic Data Interchange has noted, providers' obligation to maintain the confidentiality and integrity of that information "does not change with the medium of health information transmission or storage, whether paper or electronic. The providers' ability to carry out its obligation to ensure that confidentiality is maintained, however, can be greatly affected by the use of the electronic medium to store and transmit health information."[12]

We cannot fully appreciate the privacy implications of this technology, however, without discussing aggregation of data bases. The capability of disparate electronic data bases to be aggregated has been a major concern to many for several years. Stand-alone electronic files are today quite easy to link. This linkage is further facilitated if there is a unique identifying element common to each data base, such as a Social Security number (SSN). In fact, most federal and many state and local government agencies use the SSN as the means to identify recipients of services or benefits. For instance, roughly thirty-six states use the SSN as the driver's license identification number.[13] Additionally, some of the existing proposals would mandate the use of the SSN as the patient identifier.

The use of the SSN is not restricted to the public sector. Most credit-granting institutions (e.g., banks, credit card companies, department stores, etc.) require the SSN as their unique identifying number. Many physicians and insurance companies also use the SSN as their patient/customer identifier.

The implication of the proliferating use of the SSN or any universal identifier is simply this: once access to someone's SSN or identifier is gained, a floodgate of information about that individual is opened. The amassing of information from various data bases can result in very detailed dossiers on individuals. This can form the basis of adverse decisions about an individual, although the individual often knows nothing of this unless injury is done. Even then, the person may not become aware of the damage for years. Under current law, restrictions on the matching and aggregating of data bases apply mostly to records maintained by the federal government. Under the existing health care reform proposals, the custody of most of the electronic medical records would probably remain with the private sector.

Third Party Access to Medical Records

Much has been written in the last twenty years about third parties wanting and gaining access to medical records, without necessarily informing the patient of this access.[14] Private employers, for instance, have a strong incentive to see medical information, especially if they are paying for employees' health insurance.

There is a recent example of an employer beginning the process of computerizing its employees' medical records, ostensibly to improve the efficiency of its health insurance operation. A self-insuring company, it issued a release form to each of its approximately 9,000 employees:

> To all physicians, surgeons and other medical practitioners, all hospitals, clinics and other health care delivery facilities, all insurance carriers, insurance data service organizations, all pension and welfare fund administrators, my current employers and all other persons, agencies or entities who may have records or evidence relating to my physical or mental condition:
>
> I hereby authorize release and delivery of any and all information, records and documents (confidential or otherwise) with respect to my health and health history that you, or any of you, now have or hereafter obtain to the administrator of any employee benefit plan sponsored by Strawbridge & Clothier; any provider of health care benefits offered or financed through a benefit plan sponsored by Strawbridge & Clothier, and any insurance company providing coverage through any benefit plan sponsored by Strawbridge & Clothier.[15]

Not surprisingly, some of the employees were uncomfortable with the sweeping nature of the release authorization. Only about a dozen employees, however, challenged the form and succeeded in getting the company to add a clause (to their forms only) specifying that the medical records could only be used by the insurance companies to process medical claims. In subsequent years, the remainder of the 9,000 employees will also have their authorization forms amended in the same way. That change may have no impact on information the employer will already have collected under the current year's consent form.

It is quite likely all but these dozen employees either did not think to challenge the validity of their employer's claim for such a broad authorization for access to their medical records, or were afraid of the potential repercussions. This may be especially true because the company in question, a self-insurer exempt from many of the state regulations otherwise protecting patients' interests, has the power to threaten the employees' livelihood, if it so chooses. Those who did complain expressed concern over how their employer might use their medical information. Indeed, there have been cases of employers using medical information in making hiring and other employment decisions. The results of a comprehensive survey of employer practices regarding employee information conducted at the University of Illinois showed that 50 percent of the surveyed companies use medical records about personnel in making employment-related decisions. Of these, 19 percent do not inform employees of such use.[16] Similarly, a 1991 study by the Office of Technology Assessment found that many companies will not hire people with a pre-existing medical condition.[17]

Another little-known fact is that information on nearly half of the 1.6 billion prescriptions filled each year in the United States is passed along to data collectors who, in turn, sell the information to pharmaceutical companies.[18] Merck, the world's largest pharmaceutical manufacturer, recently announced plans to purchase the Medco chain of discount pharmacies. Merck plans to use Medco's pharmacy purchase data base information to promote Merck products.[19] Additionally, many physicians routinely allow information from their patients' records to be obtained by companies that provide computer hardware and software services. These companies provide the technology at a fraction of what it might otherwise cost in exchange for access to patient records. Typically, these exchanges of patient information take place without the knowledge or the consent of the patient. Most of the data is purchased to improve a company's direct marketing of its products and services. Indeed, one of the companies, while not including patients' names in the records it sells, does include the patients' "age, sex, Social Security Number, as well as their physicians' Federal ID numbers."[20] A goal of one company, which automates private physicians' insurance claims and files the forms for physicians (and keeps electronic copies of all claims filed), is to sell the records to drug marketers, insurance reviewers, and other companies. At the federal level and in most states, there is nothing to preclude these activities. In fact, in a few cases, state laws actually mandate some of them.

Concerned about the sale and exchange of prescription transaction information, Representative Pete Stark (D-Calif.) introduced H.R. 5615, "Prescription Drug Records Privacy Protection Act of 1992" on 9 July 1992. The bill would have restricted the disclosure of pharmacy records and allowed for civil remedy for unauthorized disclosure of such records. (No companion legislation was introduced in the Senate, nor was any action taken on H.R. 5615 during the 102nd Congress.)

Another type of access to medical records occurs through the Medical Information Bureau (MIB), a non-profit association based in Massachusetts formed to exchange underwriting information among its members as an alert against insurance fraud. MID is a significant source of medical information for almost all insurance granting companies. With a current membership of about 750 life insurance companies, its members "include virtually every major company issuing individual life, health and disability insurance in the United States and Canada."[21] According to its literature, "MIB's basic purpose was (and continues to be) to make it much more difficult to omit or conceal significant information."[22] It maintains computerized coded medical summaries on over 12 million American and Canadian policyholders, although its existence is not widely known. While Social Security numbers are not now included in MIB reports, "this may change."[23]

The information in MIB's data base is obtained when someone applies for life insurance. If the person has a "condition significant to health or longevity," then member companies are required to send a brief coded report to MIB. More than just medical information is reported, however. Information on adverse driving record, participation in hazardous sports, and aviation activities is also reported, presumably because these activities affect a person's insurance risk.

When an individual applies for insurance, he or she is given an MIB notice as part of the forms to be completed. This notice informs the individual that the insurance company may make a report to MIB, which will then exchange the information with all its member organizations to which the individual applies for insurance. The notice also informs the person that the insurance company may also release the information in its files directly to other life insurance companies to whom insurance applications have been made. Applicants must sign an authorization that reads:

> I hereby authorize any licensed physician, medical practitioner, hospital, clinic or other medical or medically related facility, insurance company, the Medical Information Bureau or other organization, institution or person, that has any record or knowledge of me or my health to give the _____ Life Insurance Company, or its reinsurer(s) any such information.[24]

Like the Strawbridge & Clothier authorization form, not many organizations or people would be excluded under this authorization from giving any medical or life-style information to an insurance company. This includes MIB, lab technicians, hospital workers, an employer, or a nosey neighbor. And because the underwriting process can sometimes result in erroneous information about an individual, information given to one MIB-member insurance company (which must be reported back to MIB) may well find its way to any of the 750 member companies. "The MIB does not investigate on its own, nor does it attempt to verify any information reported to it."[25] Information accuracy will only be investigated when a consumer requests a copy of his or her MIB file and formally challenges its contents.[26] It is the prerogative of the insurance company that filed the information with MIB to decide whether to change the file.

Information originating in medical or insurance files, then, may circulate widely through networks or data bases. Jeffrey Rothfeder has noted that:

> In fact, the medical records environment is so open-ended now that the American Medical [Records] Association has identified twelve categories of information seekers outside of the health care establishment who regularly peek at patient files for their own purposes, among them employers, government agencies, credit bureaus, insurers, education, institutions, and the media. Tack onto this list unauthorized data gatherers such as private investigators and people with a vested interest in uncovering all they can about someone they want to turn a dirty deal on, and it's clear the amount of medical information making the rounds these days is monumental.[27]

The Effects of Information Technology on Medical Records

Electronic filing of medical claim information will allow for greater mobility of patients in the health care system, which could foster competition for patients among health care providers. Additionally, the electronic cards would probably increase the speed with which patients' medical histories could be retrieved, thereby speeding treatment, particularly in the case of medical emergencies. Finally—and one of the major reasons electronic records and cards are being considered within comprehensive health care reform proposals—administrative costs should be reduced when claims are filed electronically. In Australia, for instance, where similar proposals have been suggested for using smart card technology, the estimated cost of processing claims with smart cards is about nine cents per claim, versus the current twenty-nine cents.[28]

But these electronic technologies can have negative effects as well:

> It is 1994. You are picking up an antibiotic at your local pharmacy. Your prescription and your insurance information are contained on a small plastic "smart" card that you give to the pharmacist. As she is filling your order, she calls out to you: "I see that your doctor says you have a mild case of eczema. Would you like to pick up a tube of 1 percent hydrocortisone cream on the way out?"[29]

In this illustration, the *Boston Globe* identified one of the more benign consequences of retrieving medical records by electronic cards. That pharmacist might just as easily have had access to information about a venereal disease or psychiatric treatment. The quote at least illustrates the fact that people other than the physician may be able to read medical records contained on or accessible through electronic cards, while the individual will probably have little control over what information is revealed. While new technology could hold the key to enhancing security procedures that restrict unauthorized access to and disclosure of medical and insurance records, the technology could also allow further erosion of patients' privacy, and on a much broader scale. New medical information systems should be designed to allow patients discretion in limiting access to portions of their most sensitive medical information, particularly where there is no compelling reason to allow access. This control could probably be exercised through the electronic cards, but realistically would probably only affect instances of information access to which the patient is present.

In and of themselves, smart cards could offer the technical capability to give the patient more control over medical information access than any other technology because the patient could most effectively control access to all or any part of his or her data—but only if the medical data is completely and solely resident on the smart card.[30] Yet none of the proposals suggests that medical data only reside on smart cards because of the possibility of loss or damage to the cards.

Depending on how the overall system is designed, the ATM-type card may or may not allow the patient to set any restrictions for access to his or her information. Absent any laws to the contrary, the patient could conceivably be totally dependent on the judgment of the designers and administrators of these various medical and insurance systems and data bases to determine what information should be accessible to which health care provider, insurer, or other third party.

Additionally, other uses will be made of the medical information, many of which will retain patient identifiers. Some of these uses are: administering the health care systems, performing audits of health care providers and insurers, and performing research on the adequacy and cost effectiveness of medical treatment and insurance. (Statistical and epidemiological studies of medical information can often be accomplished without the use of patient identifiers.) The individual patient may have little or no voice in how his or her information is used in these cases.

Each of the current proposals also calls for one or more massive data bases on the other end of medical and insurance transactions, keeping track of every claim filed and every medical procedure administered.

This prospect may be particularly pernicious given the tremendous demands by third parties for access to personal medical information. Indeed, electronic cards may do nothing to control access to data once the information resides in a data base. So, in reality, the cards could provide a false sense of security to a patient trying to control how much of his or her records someone else sees.

The electronic records environment may also expand a care provider's legal accountability to the patient because the provider would be directly responsible for ensuring the accuracy of the medical information placed in the system, as well as authenticating the identity of the patient presenting his or her electronic card. If either the medical information is entered incorrectly and a patient is harmed, or someone fraudulently uses an electronic card to receive medical care, the care provider may be held responsible in the eyes of the patient (and possibly the law).

Physicians have also expressed concern over the effect the electronic medical record will have on the physician-patient relationship and patient confidentiality. Some are concerned that the electronic record will interfere with physicians' ability to practice the "art" as well as the "science" of medicine. As one doctor wrote,

> Many physicians fear progressive emasculation of the special physician-patient relationship and greater erosion of confidentiality. Our medical record threatens to become less clinically useful as we are forced to include needless "necessary" details while we hesitate to include important information. Likewise, physicians fear patients will become less inclined to share needed facts. . . . We are entering a critical period as physicians. Our once sacred relationship with patients is engaged to marry the technology of the Information Age. We must serve as our patients' advocates and challenge this technology to evolve in a fashion which will promote their best interests. We must oppose any attempt by third parties to use this technology to further invade the privileged and confidential information trustingly given to us by our patients. . . . We must become literate with the emerging technologies of medical information management. We cannot allow information within the medical record to further threaten patient privacy or access to health care.[31]

Why Privacy Matters

Over the past century there has been much written about the nature and value of privacy—as a general concept, in relation to computerization of personal information, and in the health care context. For most of us, privacy is related to notions of solitude, autonomy, and individuality. Privacy is, thus, a very personal notion. Within some socially defined limits, privacy allows us the freedom to be who and what we are. The very fact that we are able to interact with others as we might like to is because our privacy allows us that choice. Legal philosopher Anita Allen writes that privacy "denotes a degree of inaccessibility of persons, of their mental states, and of information about them to the senses and surveillance devices of others."[32] Ruth Gavison speaks of privacy in terms of our limited accessibility to others, arguing that it is related to "the extent to which we are known to others [secrecy], the access to us [solitude], and the extent to which we are the subject of others' attention [anonymity]."[33]

Privacy has also been described as being fundamental to respect, love, friendship, and trust; indeed, some argue, without privacy these relationships are inconceivable.[34] Gavison explains that we enjoy our privacy "not because of new opportunities for seclusion or because of greater control over our interactions, but because of our anonymity, because no one is interested in us. The moment someone becomes sufficiently interested, he may find it quite easy to take all that privacy away."[35] When privacy is invaded, we are hurt because we are exposed, which may cause us to lose our self-respect and thus our capacity to have meaningful relations with others. In a similar vein, Edward Bloustein has argued that we should regard privacy as a "dignitary tort." He notes, "[T]he injury is to our individuality, to our dignity as individuals, and the legal remedy represents a social vindication of the human spirit thus threatened rather than a recompense for the loss suffered."[36]

Arnold Simmel likewise holds that privacy is related to solitude, secrecy, and autonomy, but argues that it also "implies a normative element: the right to exclusive control to access to private realms."[37] The difficulty with that argument, as Gavison sees it, is the way in which it suggests that the important aspect of privacy is "the ability to choose it and see that the choice is respected."[38] To her, this implies that once people have voluntarily disclosed something to one party, they can maintain control over subsequent dissemination by others—and that is generally not the case. Gavison argues therefore that the legal system should make a strong and explicit commitment to privacy as a value. She writes,

> Privacy has as much coherence and attractiveness as other values to which we have made a clear commitment, such as liberty. Arguments for liberty, when examined carefully, are vulnerable to objections similar to the arguments . . . for privacy, yet this vulnerability has never been considered a reason not to express this importance by an explicit commitment so that any loss will be more likely to be noticed and taken into consideration. Privacy deserves no less (p. 387).

In health care, the critical issue is the consequence to the patient when possibly very sensitive information is revealed. Vincent Brannigan and Bernd Beier contend that "[i]n the case of medical privacy, it is arguable that it is not the number of persons given the information, but their relationship to the patient that determines the scope of concern; there may only be a small number of persons interested in the particular patient, but disclosure to any one of them could be devastating."[39] They argue that the wide circle of persons many states consider to be "legitimately interested" in a person's health, such as a spouse or employer, can effectively destroy any right of privacy.

In the area of medical information, patients, for the most part, have the expectation that their communications with their health care provider are and will remain confidential. Because patients may presume that such communications have strong legal protection, they generally feel comfortable providing intimate details (if needed) in order to advance their medical treatment. As George Annas notes, "[p]atients are not likely to disclose these details freely unless they are certain that no one else, not directly involved in their care, will learn of them."[40]

Brannigan, however, stresses the fact that there are competing interests in privacy involved in the design and implementation of clinical information systems: the patient wants to ensure that no one has unnecessary access to his data; the hospital administrator sees privacy as an impediment to getting access to data needed for management; physicians view it as a time-consuming limitation on medical practice; and information system developers find it expensive, inelegant, and time consuming. He warns, however, that the balancing needed between privacy and the demand for information systems is not a medical or technical question—it is a political one. Because patients are not well represented in the design, development, and operation of information systems, the political process must ensure that their interests are protected in these activities.[41]

Even the doctor-patient privilege does not necessarily keep communications between doctors and patients confidential. The privilege, legally recognized by some forty states, is generally only applicable in a court of law. These laws do not apply to the many situations in which a doctor is allowed or compelled by law, regulation, or long-standing practice to reveal information about the patient to outside parties. Additionally, privilege statutes apply only in cases governed by state law. The Federal Rules of Evidence, which govern practice in federal courts, provide only a psychotherapist-patient privilege, not a general doctor-patient privilege. Therefore, the doctor-patient privilege is actually a narrowly drawn rule of evidence, not recognized as common law (as is, for example, the attorney-client privilege), and available only where it is specifically provided by statute.[42]

If privacy is the right individuals have to exercise their autonomy and to limit the extent of their personal domain to which others have access, in the "Information Age" this concept is largely defined by how much personal information is available from sources other than the individual to whom it pertains. The less ability individuals have to limit access to their own personal information, or to limit the amount of personal information they must give up to others (either voluntarily or by coercion), the less privacy they have.

Security, on the other hand, encompasses a set of technical and administrative procedures designed to protect or restrict access to information. The procedures are applied to the information and the technology handling, storing, and disseminating that information. Security measures are applied to information and the operation of information systems because of the need or desire to protect the privacy of individuals.

Security measures alone do not ensure privacy protection, however. As a result, legal recognition of the status of the information is needed, along with a delineation of an individual's rights vis-a-vis that information. To date there has not been a consistent public policy formulated, much less articulated, with equal applicability to all Americans, that protects the patient's and society's interest in privacy or in the confidentiality of an individual's medical information.

The major U.S. Supreme Court case addressing medical information privacy is *Whalen v. Roe*.[43] In *Whalen*, a unanimous Court determined that a New York state data base of lawful users of abusable drugs was allowable because the prohibitions on public disclosure of the information in the data base were adequate to prevent any constitutional harm to the persons listed in the registry. In reaching this decision, the Court looked at all the provisions in place to protect the data base. The stringent physical and administrative procedures protecting the patient's interest in privacy played an important role in the Court's finding. The Court did not address whether compilation of the information was itself a violation of privacy, however. They said, in part, that "New York's statutory scheme, and its implementing administrative procedures, evidence a proper concern with, and protection of, the individual's interest in privacy. We therefore need not, and do not, decide any question which might be presented by . . . a system that did not contain comparable security measures" (pp. 605–6).

Many interests compete in the collection, use, and dissemination of medical (or any personal) records. The Third Circuit Court of

Appeals, in its 1980 decision in United States of America vs. *Westinghouse Electric*,[44] tried to set out specific standards to be used by a court in weighing privacy rights in medical records against the need for information to be reported to public agencies. They held,

> The factors which should be considered in deciding whether an intrusion into an individual's privacy is justified are the type of record requested, the information it does or might contain, the potential for harm in any subsequent nonconsensual disclosure, the injury from disclosure to the relationship in which the record was generated, the adequacy of safeguards to prevent unauthorized disclosure, the degree of need for access, and whether there is an express statutory mandate, articulated public policy or other recognizable public interest militating toward access (p. 578).

A judicial commitment to privacy as a societal value is not enough; however. Indeed, to date, judicial decisions have been highly inconsistent and often hostile. Specific enforceable standards and procedures are needed to protect those privacy interests where the individual has no direct influence over the dissemination of information by and to others (generally secondary and tertiary dissemination). This notion plays an important role in the rationale for federal legislation to protect these interests, as well as in the recommendations laid out later in this paper.

Current Federal Law and the Confidentiality of Medical Records

In 1974 the Privacy Act became law in the United States. It provides a set of mandates for records in the custody of the federal government and delineates the rights individuals have with respect to those records. The act encompasses a code of five fair information practices originally set forth in the 1973 report by the Department of Health, Education, and Welfare Secretary's Advisory Committee on Automated Personal Data systems, *Records, Computers, and the Rights of Citizens*.[45] These principals are: (1) there must be no personal data record-keeping systems whose very existence is secret; (2) there must be a way for individuals to find out what information about them is in a record and how it is used; (3) there must be a way for individuals to prevent information about them that was obtained for one purpose from being used or made available for other purposes without their consent; (4) there must be a way for individuals to correct or amend a record of identifiable information; and (5) any organization creating, maintaining, using, or disseminating records of identifiable personal data must assure the reliability of the data for their intended use and must take reasonable precautions to prevent misuse of the data.[46]

The Privacy Act covers only the federal government, not other state or local governmental entities (with the exception of state and local government record systems using the Social Security number) or private sector entities.[47] In addition, it allows other uses of these records, if the purpose of the use is consistent with the reason the information was collected. This can (and does) lead to disclosures of personal information to other entities. As implemented, the Privacy Act has three major deficiencies: (1) it places the burden on individuals to protect their own interests; (2) its enforcement scheme provides remedies only after misuses have occurred; and (3) it is not sensitive to the existing power imbalance between individuals and federal agencies.[48]

One valuable outcome of the passage of the Privacy Act was the creation of the Privacy Protection Study Commission, which, in 1977, made several recommendations for federal legislation to protect public and private sector records, including medical records. The commission articulated three objectives for effective privacy protection, upon which all their recommendations were grounded:

> to create a proper balance between what an individual is expected to divulge to a record-keeping organization and what he seeks in return (to minimize intrusiveness) to open up record-keeping operations in ways that will minimize the extent to which recorded information about an individual is itself a source of unfairness in any decision about him made on the basis of it (to maximize fairness); and to create and define obligations with respect to the uses and disclosures that will be made of recorded information about an individual (to create legitimate, enforceable expectations of confidentiality).[49]

Many of the commission's fourteen recommendations on medical records were incorporated into federal legislation introduced in 1979 and 1980. Unfortunately, no legislation was passed, due to heavy lobbying by the intelligence community, which wanted to ensure easy access to medical records (particularly psychiatric records) in cases of national securities.[50] That was the last time Congress considered any measure to protect the confidentiality of medical records, although most of the commission's recommendations are relevant today.

The medical industry is, therefore, operating under the federal legal framework of the mid-1970s with technology anticipating the twenty-first century. The major practical differences between the industry then and now are extraordinary advances made in medical and information technologies, the medical industry's increased reliance on those technologies, and the increasing incentive for third parties to obtain access to medical records.[51]

According to a report issued by the Department of Health and Human Services, the regulatory framework governing providers' disclosure of patient-identifiable information is flawed. It dictates different disclosure rules for different types of providers . . . When protection is available, the remedy may be counter-productive. It usually cannot be obtained without litigation, an after-the-fact, costly process that might produce damages but typically will not prevent disclosure of the information. Also, patients have no workable way to "police" information practices to ensure that disclosure rules are being followed.[52]

Such flaws are troubling. As David Flaherty, who writes extensively in the area of information privacy, has noted, vital personal interests are at stake in the use of personal data by public and private sector organizations: "Such activities threaten personal integrity and autonomy of individuals, who traditionally have lacked control over how others use information about them in decision making. The storage of personal data can be used to limit opportunity and to encourage conformity."[53] He concludes that "the protection of privacy requires the balancing of competing values. Techniques available for legitimate purposes have the secondary effect of being invasive of individuals' perceived right to control their own lives" (p. 8).

Alan Westin gives more specific content to these concerns, noting that

the outward flow of medical data . . . has enormous impact on people's lives. It affects decisions on whether they are hired or fired; whether they can secure business licenses and life insurance; whether they are permitted to drive cars; whether they are placed under police surveillance or labelled a security risk; or even whether they can get nominated for and elected to public office.[54]

Given what's at stake, existing legal protection of patient privacy and medical records leaves much to be desired. The very fact that under virtually all of the health care reform proposals put forward so far enormous amounts of standardized medical data on millions of people will be compiled into centralized location(s) demands a centralized approach to the protection of these records. The current patchwork of state laws, court decisions, and limited federal regulation cannot assure a legally guaranteed set of rights that will place the individual patient on a more level playing field with those having access to his or her medical information. Federal protections should be placed on the collection, use, storage, disclosure, and access to all medical records prior to or as a concurrent effort with health care reform.[55]

It is urgent, then, that we reintroduce legislation at the federal level regarding patient privacy and medical information. In keeping with the fair information practices and objectives articulated by the Privacy Protection Study Commission in 1977, such legislation—which should apply to all care providers, researchers, insurers, and insurance support organizations like the Medical Information Bureau—should clearly define the rights patients have with respect to their own medical information; define what constitutes legitimate access to and use of personal health and medical information, as well as specifying prohibited uses; and provide oversight and enforcement mechanisms to ensure compliance. Enforcement strategies must include establishing civil and criminal penalties for prohibited activities to enable patients to collect damages. Moreover, legislation should set schedules for how long medical records may be maintained, and by whom (physicians, hospitals, insurers, etc).

Similarly, universally applicable, federal legislation should require that patients be notified of the use to which information in health and medical records is put and how patients may obtain their medical records. Mechanisms should also be put in place to audit use of patient records, to track requests for and disclosures of information, including reasons for which the information was requested. This information should be accessible to the patient to whom it relates.

To help assure that patients' privacy is respected, a unique identifier scheme should be put in place that prohibits all other uses of that identifier for purposes not directly related to providing medical care. To guard against the kinds of discriminatory use of medical information that is a central concern, employers' ability to review employee medical records and use medical or health information to make employment-related decisions should be strictly limited. So too, the marketing of personal health or medical data should be prohibited [Exhibit 8.3].

Dignity, Privacy, and Public Policy

Information technologies offer many benefits in a health care application, notably the prospect of lowering the administrative costs associated with health care delivery. However, because there will be one or more data bases capturing all medical and insurance transaction information, patients will probably never have substantial control over their own medical records or who sees them. This is why federal legal recognition of the patient's interest in privacy as well as protections for the confidentiality of medical records (consistent across states), while critical now, will become even more critical in a computerized setting.

Additionally, the lower cost of processing medical claims using an electronic card must be weighed against the cost of providing potentially tens of millions of the electronic cards to accommodate each insured person in the country. This includes the cost of initiating the

Exhibit 8.3 Federal Medical Privacy Legislation

To protect patient privacy effectively, federal legislation should:

1. Clearly define patients' rights with respect to their own medical information (i.e., their rights to gain access to, amend, and correct errors in their records, and have any control over others' access to their records);

2. Define what constitutes legitimate access to personal health/medical information; define the legal and ethical responsibilities of those with legitimate authorization to gain access to that information; and provide training for those persons;

3. Clearly define the types of both allowable and prohibited uses of personal medical information (e.g., in statistical research, for billing and insurance purposes, in employment situations, etc.) and provide an oversight and enforcement mechanism to ensure compliance;

4. Establish civil and criminal penalties for prohibited activities, allowing patients to collect damages;

5. Establish medical record retention schedules for each class of information recipient (i.e., physicians, hospitals, insurers, researchers, auditors, etc.), particularly where patient identifiers are attached to the information;

6. Require notice to patients of health/medical information record use, to include publishing information about the existence of health care data banks, and where and how patients can get access to their medical records;

7. Require extensive audit trails, accessible to patients upon request, to track all disclosures and requests for disclosure of personal medical information (i.e., whose records are released; a copy of the signed patient authorization for such release; names and addresses of the recipients of the records; the reason for the disclosure, such as billing, providing direct medical care, research, etc.);

8. Apply to all care providers (physicians, hospitals and their personnel, pharmacies, etc.), insurance companies, and insurance support organizations (e.g., the Medical Information Bureau);

9. Establish a totally unique patient identification scheme that prohibits all other uses not directly related to providing medical care;

10. Strictly limit employers' ability to see individual employees' medical/health records and use them to make employment-related decisions;

11. Prohibit "pretext interviews," where an insurer or employer conducts an investigation into a patient's medical history under false pretenses in order to gain access to health records;

12. Prohibit the marketing of personal health/medical data;

13. Give patients the prerogative to limit the authorization for the use and disclosure of their medical record information (to include specific references to the records subject to the authorization, the parties allowed access, an expiration date for the authorization, and a right to revoke that authorization).

program, as well as the cost of replacing lost or damaged cards. A further administrative challenge is loading patient information into the data bases and customizing each recipient's smart card with his or her unique medical records (if smart cards are the technology chosen). Mistakes are bound to be made in the process, which compounds the issue of who can have access to the data and the uses to which the data can be put (e.g., the harm that can befall the patient from the erroneous information). The potential for misuse of this data is also enormous, given third-party demands for personal medical information.

Privacy concerns dictate that any health care reform strategy relying on computer data bases and card technologies contain certain restrictions. These include setting limits to bound the types of situations beyond which electronic card access should not be allowed—for instance, whether a job applicant should be required to surrender access to his or her card, and its underlying data, to a potential employer. Enforcement standards should also be established to ensure compliance. This step could become increasingly critical as progress is made in genetic research. Efforts to map the human genome funded through the National Institutes of Health and Department of Energy have the potential outcome of providing everyone a "personalized map" of their genetic makeup. The temptation to include this information in a health care data base will be great, and without protections, this information will have an even greater potential for misuse.

With the sort of federal legal rights for individual privacy and "technology transparent" protections for medical records outlined in this paper, patients can be more confident that their medical information will be covered by stringent protections that respect their dignity and their privacy. Such legal protections will also enhance the effectiveness of the technical and administrative security measures built into the electronic records environment of the future, and guarantee that existing paper medical records are protected as well.

While the new information technologies carry potential threats to the privacy of our most intimate health and medical information, forward-looking public policy can assure that the enormous power of these technologies is made to serve patients' interests, not confound them.

References

1. These proposals include one by the Bush administration (orignally introduced as a nonlegislative proposal, and later, as an amended version introduced in both Houses as H.R. 5464 and § 2878, "The Medical and Insurance Information Reform Act of 1992") and four legislative proposals: § 1227, "HealthAmerica:

Affordable Health Care for All Americans Act," introduced by Senators Mitchell (D-Maine) and Kennedy (D-Mass); H.R. 1300, "The Universal Health Care Act of 1991," introduced by Representative Russo (D-Ill.); H.R. 3205, "The Health Insurance Coverage Act of 1991" introduced by Representative Rostenkowski (D-Ill.); and H.R. 5036, "Managed Competition Act of 1992," introduced by Representative Cooper (D-Tenn.).

2. The proposals introduced in the 103rd Congress include H.R. 191, "American Consumers Health Care Reform Act of 1993," introduced by Representative Gekas (R-Pa.); H.R. 200, "Health Care Cost Containment and Reform Act of 1993," introduced by Representative Stark (D-Calif.); and § 223, "Access to Affordable Health Care Act," introduced by Senator Cohen (R-Maine).

3. Printed report information from U.S. Bureau of Census Summary Tape 3A, U.S. Summary 1990, CPH-L-80, Table 1, "Selected Social Characteristics for the United States—1990."

4. For example, only in Colorado is it considered theft to obtain or use medical records, irrespective of the medium in which they occur, without authority to have them."

5. Workgroup for Electronic Data Interchange, *Report to Secretary of the U.S. Department of Health and Human Services* (Washington, D.C., July 1992), Appendix 4, pp. 3–4.

6. That security measures do not entirely project patient privacy was borne out during the 1992 election season. A congressional candidate to New York saw her privacy invaded when someone anonymously faxed her potentially damaging hospital records to various news organizations. Whatever the measures the hospital had in place to govern access to its records did not deter the person(s) bent on harming the candidate. At a press conference, the candidate said that she hoped the incident would be the subject of a criminal investigation. However, unless the hospitals records were obtained from a computerized system, it is probable that no crime related to the medical record themselves was committed—under either New York state or federal law. New York law makes intrusion into a computer system containing confidential personal or medical information a crime, but only under legislation dealing with computer crime, thus protecting only electronic, not paper records.

7. The cards are technically capable of storing information on an array of subjects such as finance, government benefits, credit transactions, etc. Most card schemes currently limit themselves to a single area of the card holder's life; however, in the context of health care reform, there have been discussions of including at least some financial record information on the cards as well.

8. *SmartCard Technology: New Methods for Computer Access Control*, National Institutes of Standards and Technology, September 1988, p. 34.

9. Joe Abernathy, "City Health Clinics Unveil Controversial 'Smart Card,'" *Houston Chronicle*, 11 October 1992.

10. Blue Cross-Blue Shield of Maryland recently lost about $14 million in its attempt to introduce "smart" cards on a mass scale. How much of this loss was due to company mismanagement has been under investigation. See Thomas Health, "The Card That Fizzled," *Washington Post*, 28 August 1992.

11. Robert M. Gellman, "Prescribing Privacy: The Uncertain Role of the Physician

in the Protection of Patient Privacy," 28 *North Carolina Law Review* 62, no. 2 (1984): 258.

12. Workgroup for Electronic Date Interchange, "Report," p. 3.

13. Testimony of Evan Hendricks, editor and publisher of Privacy Times, before the Senate Finance Committee, Subcommittee on Social Security and Family, 28 February 1992, p. 7. The Social Security Administration recently estimated that some 4 million people have more than one SSN. There is no estimate available of the number of single SSNs being used by more than one person. (Letter to Dr. Elmer Gabrieli from Andrew J. Young, Deputy Commissioner for Programs, Social Security Administration, 17 May 1993, p. 3)

14. What makes this situation particularly intriguing is the fact that in about eighteen states, patients do not have a statutory right to see what is in their own medical records.

15. Mubarak Dahir, "Your Health, Your Privacy, Your Boss," *Philadelphia City Paper*, 28 May–4 June 1993, p. 11.

16. David F. Linowes, *Privacy in America* (Urbana: University of Illinois Press, 1989), p. 50.

17. U.S. Congress, Office of Technology Assessment, *Medical Monitoring and Screening in the Workplace: Results of a Survey—Background Paper* (Washington D.C.: Government Printing Office, October 1991).

18. Michael W. Miller, "Patients' Records Are Treasure Trove for Budding Industry," *Wall Street Journal*, 27 February 1992.

19. Elyse Tanouye, "Merck to Exploit Medco's Database," *Wall Street Journal*, 4 August 1993.

20. Miller "Patients' Records Are Treasure Trove."

21. "MIB, Inc: A Consumer's Guide," distributed in March 1991, Westwood, Mass., p. 5.

22. "The Consumer's MIB Fact Sheet," MIB, Inc., distributed in March 1991, Westwood, Mass., pp. 2–3.

23. "MIB, Inc: A Consumer's Guide," p. 6.

24. "MIB, Inc. A Consumer's Guide," p. 7.

25. Privacy Protection Study Commission, *Personal Privacy in an Information Society* (Washington, D.C.: U.S. Government Printing Office 1977) p. 160

26. The nonmedical information (e.g., lifestyle information) in MIB files will be sent directly to the consumer. In some cases, decoded medical information will only be sent to a physician designated by the consumer.

27. Jeffrey Rothfeder, *"Privacy for Sale"* (New York: Simon & Schuster, 1992), p. 180.

28. Simon Davies, "The Technological Web: A Report to the Australian Doctors' Fund on the Proposed Introduction of Smart Card and Interactive Technology in the Australian Health System," 20 April 1992, p. 15. Because Australia has a universal health care system (that can be supplemented with private insurance), its overall administrative overhead costs start out lower than in the U.S. In comparison, therefore, the United States could see comparatively greater overall savings in administrative overhead.

29. Nathan Cobb, "The End of Privacy," *Boston Globe Magazine*, 26 April 1992.

30. This could occur through the segregation of information on the card and the setting of multiple Personal Identification Numbers for access to the different sections. This requires that the patient be technically sophisticated enough to understand how the smart card works, how then to segregate information within the card, and to set individual PINs to control access to the sensitive information on the card. It is possible that few patients would exercise these options, deferring instead to the care provider to decide what's best. Additionally, the issues of access, and to what information, in emergency situations need to be considered, because the patient may not be capable of controlling access to information.

31. Randall Oates, "Confidentiality and Privacy from the Physician Perspective," presented at the First Annual Confidentiality Symposium of the American Health Information Management Association, 15 July 1992, p. 4.

32. Anita Allen, *Uneasy Access* (Totowa, N.J.: Rowman and Littlefield Publishers, 1988), p. 3.

33. Ruth Gavison, "Privacy and the Limits of Law," in *Philisophical Dimensions of Privacy: An Anthology*, ed. Ferdinand D. Schoeman (Cambridge: Cambridge University Press, 1984), pp. 346–402, at p. 347.

34. Charles Fried, "Privacy (A Moral Analysis), *Yale Law Journal* 77 (1968): 475–93, at 477. See also James Rachels, "Why Privacy Is Important," in *Philosophical Dimensions of Privacy*, pp. 156–202, at 187–88.

35. Gavison, "Privacy and the Limits of the Law," p. 379.

36. Edward J. Bloustein, "Privacy as an Aspect of Human Dignity: An Answer to Dean Prosser," reprinted in Philosophical Dimensions of Privacy, pp. 156–202, at 187–88.

37. International Encyclopedia of the Social Sciences, s.v. "Privacy."

38. Gavison, "Privacy and the Limits of the Law," p. 349.

39. Vincent Brannigan and Bernd Beier, "Standards for Privacy in Medical Information Systems: A Technico-legal Revolution," *Datenschutz und Datensicherung*, September 1991, p. 470.

40. George Annas, *The Rights of Patients* (Carbondale: Southern Illinois University Press, 1989), p. 177.

41. Vincent M. Brannigan, "Protecting the Privacy of Patient Information in Clinical Networks," in Extended Clinical Consulting by Hospital Computer Networks, vol. 670 of the Annals of the New York Academy of Sciences, 1992, pp. 190–201.

42. Evan Hendricks, Trudy Hayden, and Jack D. Novik, *Your Right to Privacy: A Basic Guide to Legal Rights in an Information Society*, 2nd ed. (Carbondale: Southern Illinois University Press, 1990), pp. 155–56.

43. *Whalen v. Roe*, 429 U.S. 589 (1977).

44. *United States of America v. Westinghouse*, 638 F.2d 570 (1980).

45. Advisory Committee on Automated Personal Data Systems, *Records, Computers and the Rights of Citizens* (Washington D.C.: Department of Health Education and Welfare, 1973).

46. These principles have also formed the basis of European and Canadian privacy laws, although they have taken the principles much farther than the U.S., in that their laws apply to the private sector. Europeans see the protection of privacy as a fundamental human right.

47. It has been estimated that only about 5 percent of the medical data banks in the United States are covered by the Privacy Act. See Terra Ziporyn, "Hippocrates Meets the Data Banks: Patient Privacy in the Computer Age," *JAMA* 252 (20 July 1984): 317–19.

48. Priscilla Regan, "Privacy, Government Information, and Technology." *Public Administration Review* 46, no. 6 (November–December 1986): 629–34, at 633.

49. Privacy Protection Study Commission, *Personal Privacy in an Information Society*, pp. 14–15.

50. Rothfeder, *Privacy for Sale*, p. 179.

51. As a gauge of how the American public feels about personal and consumer privacy issues, Lou Harris and Associates and Dr. Alan Westin conducted a poll on the subject in 1990. Nearly four out of five Americans expressed general concern about threats to personal privacy in America today. ("The Equifax Report on Consumers in the Information Age," [Atlanta: Equifax, Inc. 1990] p. vii).

52. Workgroup for Electronic Data Interchange, *Report*, p. 17.

53. David H. Flaherty, *Protecting Privacy in Surveillance Societies* (Chapel Hill: University of North Carolina Press, 1989), p. 8.

54. Alan F. Westin, Computers, Health, Records, and Citizen's Rights (Washington, D.C.: United States Department of Commerce, 1976), p. 60.

55. The "Uniform Health-Care Information Act," written in 1985 by the National Conference of Commissioners on Uniform State Laws, provides a good foundation for medical record protection. To date, only Montana and Washington have enacted this legislation. This law protects the confidentiality of medical information between care provider and patient, and balances the need of the medical community for information with the patient's need to preserve his or her privacy. In fact, a 1991 report by the Institute of Medicine on computer-based patient records cited the Uniform Health-Care Information Act as a good example of the type of legislation needed before any consideration is given to nationwide scheme of computerized-patient records. The Computer-Based Patient Record (Washington, D.C.: National Academy Press, 1991), p. 166, fn. 43.

Sheri Alpert, a policy analyst working for the federal government, specializes in information technologies.

CASE 8
The Dilemma

HAVING JUST returned from a week-long conference on health care computing, Susan was not looking forward to her next task. Her administrative assistant normally placed high priority items in red manila folders. This morning she found two red folders on her desk. As executive vice president for hospital operations at St. Anne's Hospital for Women, she generally reserved the first morning back on the job from a trip for department head meetings. This morning, she felt, would have to be devoted to addressing the priority items on her desk.

Red Manila Folder #1

Memorandum
TO: Susan Wilbur
           Executive Vice President
           Hospital Operations
FROM: George Angell, M.D.

Apparently, in an effort to maintain the so-called privacy of some patients, this facility has put some patients in danger of not getting the proper care. Two nights ago a woman came into the emergency clinic with an acute infection and soon collapsed. Before she collapsed she mentioned she had been a patient here some time ago, and had been an intravenous drug-user. Requiring access to her past medical history would have been vital to assess her present condition. Not knowing her physician, I was unable to access her medical files from the computer immediately. "Access may be allowed" repeatedly appeared on the computer as a response to my inquiry, and I was informed this patient's medical file was "private information." I was required to acknowledge that the access desired was deliberate and then had to provide a lengthy explanation. After finally getting the information subsequent to an unreasonable waiting period, I was able to access the needed information. I was then informed that the appropriateness of access would have to be reviewed by another party. Had I had immediate access to this vital information, the patient would not have died. I later found out that some of the information on her record had not been updated, and that some of the information had been erroneous. Apparently at this hospital, computers, rather than individuals mediate care.

Susan winced at that last statement. The whole notion of protecting individual confidentiality has been a concern of both givers and receivers of health care since the formulation of the Hippocratic oath. It must have been frustrating, however, for Angell to have been prevented from getting the necessary information. But, didn't he realize that any effort in safeguarding privacy comes with a price? Although, in many respects, computers tend to depersonalize, they also help to prevent unauthorized intruders, compile and integrate patient data, and assist the hospital to store a great amount of information. The question, however, is whether the organization had taken the privacy issue too far.

Red Manila Folder #2

Ms. Susan Wilbur,
Executive Vice President
St. Anne's Hospital

Dear Ms. Wilbur:

As a former patient of your hospital and a resident of this town, I feel it's necessary to bring a matter to your attention that reflects upon the reputation of the hospital and the good of its patients. Are you aware that personal information concerning your patients is available to anyone?

I recently entered your hospital to deliver my first child. As an unmarried mother, for personal reasons, I chose to minimize the "publicity" associated with this event. The stay was uneventful, and I returned home with my child. Soon after I returned home, I encountered several disturbing incidents that led me to believe that the hospital was responsible for a violation of my rights. A representative from the Single Mothers of America called me, asking me to join their organization. Although they are a fine organization, it disturbed me that they knew my name and where I lived. Neither I nor anyone else I knew had contacted them. They informed me that my name was obtained from the hospital and I was now on their mailing list. Incidentally, they referred to me as Mrs. Smith, knew my religion, and listed me as the mother of five children. Is it possible you have too much information about me, or that some of the information is wrong?

In an attempt to find out how this information was obtained I discovered a disturbing fact. Apparently my medical record and patient chart, as every patients', is accessible to most people in the hospital. In talking with some of your personnel, they informed me that approximately two-thirds of the medical record is a collaboration of a variety of care-givers who preside in the overall care of the patient. The fact that such a large number of people have potential access to information that is sensitive is shocking, and now there is an electronic trace over which I have no control. How many patients have been compromised by this failure to maintain accurate, appropriate, and confidential information? How can I trust this hospital to maintain my privacy?

Sincerely,

Miss T.M. Smith

Obviously, the hospital had not taken the privacy issue too far in Miss Smith's case. Reading between the lines in both Dr. Angell's memo and Miss Smith's letter, Susan saw that the subject of privacy was complicated at best, and not just an issue of accessibility. Is sensitive information the property of the patient or of the hospital? What obligation does the hospital have to the patient? What can be done to ensure that the hospital can protect a patient's life, as well as a patient's confidentiality?

If a review of information-handling policies were to occur, there were a number of issues that had to be addressed, in light of the two red manila folders. Susan also had to consider the fiscal and operational nightmares that would accompany such an undertaking.

Questions for Discussion

1. Assess the privacy dilemma that confronts Susan.
2. What major aspects of privacy management must be considered in this hospital?
3. Discuss the legal and political ambiguities associated with privacy.
4. How does the use of computers complicate the issues and present special considerations in managing privacy?
5. Develop a set of principles that could guide Susan in a plan of action.

B. Essays for Discussion

MANAGING THE ECONOMICS OF HEALTH CARE COMPUTING

R ECENTLY, A 550-bed teaching hospital "switched-on" its state-of-the-art computerized information system during the month of January; by April of that same year, the hospital had nearly gone bankrupt.[1] Observers attributed this precipitous fall from financial grace to a lack of systematic consideration of the economic issues.

Similar stories about computer investments that turned sour are rampant. Whether it is the individual who purchases a computer that goes unused or the health care organization whose million-dollar investment falls short of the predicted financial benefits, the results often have serious economic consequences. When managers fail to consider systematically the financial costs and benefits of computerized information technology investments, they run the risk of cost overruns, misleading assumptions, and inevitable questions concerning managerial competence.

Numerous incidents have been publicized that reflect this failure. One of the more publicized cases is the California Department of Motor Vehicles (DMV), whose lack of systematic economic analyses led to a cost overrun of $35 million on a five-year automation project.[2] Designed to automate the registration and driving license processes and the collection of DMV-related fees, the DMV officials appeared to have failed in estimating economic impact and consequently, the project will eventually cost the state approximately $58 million in increased expenditures and unrealized savings.

Without a systematic economic analysis of the investment, ill-conceived predictions about the economic benefits of computerization also occur. Assumptions that are made concerning computer-induced financial return can easily mislead the manager. A *Wall Street Journal* article suggests the frequency of these kinds of mistakes. Studies reveal that computers in service industries often fail to produce the kind of financial benefits and levels of productivity that are predicted.[3] Richard Katzman, a data processing consultant, contends that, although the overall utilization of computer technology is high, it does not necessarily imply cost-containment. In fact, he notes that many organizations are misguided by promised benefits.[4] According to Ball and Boyle, while interest and investment in information technology have grown at an accelerated pace in recent years, this rapid growth has "left a gap between the decision to invest in information technology and the realization of benefits."[5] It is no surprise then, that many health care institutions are less than pleased with their information systems investment.[6]

How does a health care manager systematically consider the economic issues associated with computerization? Given today's emphasis on costs, market share and competition, an understanding of cost justification and "information economic analysis" is crucial. This chapter provides a basic understanding of these issues, and current thinking about the economic benefits that accrue with computerization.

Cost Justification

Cost justification is the process which clarifies the economic equation. One side of the equation is the cost associated with the activity, and the other side of the equation is the resulting benefit. Cost and benefit can be described in both qualitative and quantitative terms. Recent data help to shed light on health care executive thinking regarding both sides of the equation.[7] In a survey designed to examine the importance of qualitative and quantitative benefits in cost justification, 3,000 health executives were queried concerning their institutions' rationale for investing in computerized information systems. Although most stated that they hoped in part to achieve qualitative benefits (e.g., improved access to information), managers gave slightly more emphasis to quantitative benefits (e.g., improved cash flow) when making a decision to invest in computerization.[8] Table 9.1 lists the qualitative and quantitative benefits the respondents thought would accrue with computer implementation.

Current data concerning the other side of the economic equation, the consideration of cost, reveal that costs generally tend to be less a factor in decisions relating to computerization.[9] Michael A. Schmidt, Vice President of Finance for St. Joseph's Hospital, a staunch advocate of health care information systems, noted that decisions associated with the tradeoff of cost to benefits are far from easy, but "the increased need to install sophisticated information systems make the question not so much a matter of *how much* it will cost but what important benefits will be derived from the system."[10]

In the rush to implement information systems, this situation can be problematic. As Peter Van Etten, deputy Chancellor of the University of Massachusetts Medical Center observes, "All too often, investments are made without adequate cost justification. Top management or the data processing department decides to build or acquire a new system and then tries to justify their decision with cost-benefit analyses that are often grudgingly accepted by operating departments."[11]

Cost-Benefit and Cost-Effectiveness Analysis

Cost justification, the process of unbundling the two sides of the equation, is generally approached by using the techniques of "cost-benefit analysis" and perhaps "cost-effectiveness analysis."[12] These techniques are systematic approaches to examining the benefits and costs associated with a proposed program.

In health care computing, the term "cost-benefit" refers to the total expense associated with the acquisition or upgrading of a computer system or use of computer resources (i.e., cost) and the *dollar* value of all resources created by the project (i.e., benefits). As in the case

Table 9.1 Benefits Associated with Computer Implementation

Qualitative	Quantitative
Improved access to information	Decreased lost charges
Timely capture of information	Improved cash flows
Improved staff productivity	Reduced labor cost
Improved organizational communication	Increased revenue
Standardization of procedures	Reduced bad debt
Improved quality of care	Reduced length of stay
Better staff/patient relations	Improved market share

of acquiring a computer system, the benefit can be described as the economic *results* of the acquisition expressed in dollars. Expressed as quantitative benefits in the previously mentioned health care executive survey,[13] economic results include:

- Decreased lost charges
- Improved cash flow
- Reduced labor costs
- Increased revenue
- Reduced bad debt
- Reduced length of stay
- Improved market share.

The technique of cost-benefit analysis (i.e., comparing dollars spent with dollars created) can be illustrated with a simple example in Table 9.2. Assume that Hospital X presently uses a manual information system that employs ten people. A proposed computer system is being considered as an alternative to the manual information system. The following chart summarizes the costs associated with the present manual system and proposed computerized system. It also lists the benefits relating to the computerized system.

Note that the costs associated with the proposed system are less than the manual system. The financial or economic benefits of the computer system are illustrated by the reduction of staff and the gain by a more efficient accounts receivable system. The total costs of $110,000 incurred in acquiring the system are compared with the total derived benefits of $160,000. The total benefit is $50,000 per year and can be expressed as a benefit/cost ratio of 1.45 (i.e., for every $1.00 in costs, there is a return of $1.45) A ratio of less than 1.00 would mean the costs outweigh the benefits.

For the sake of simplicity, other potential costs relating to the computer system are not assumed. In general, relevant costs that should be measured include: direct capital outlays for project equipment or construction, salaries, supplies, labor, and overhead. There are also intangible or social costs associated with the project that are difficult to quantify. These costs have been alluded to in previous chapters. Absenteeism and turnover, are among the more elusive social costs that sometimes accompany computerization. Another point that must be considered is the fact that the benefits and costs of a proposed project extend over a number of years. The "present value" is therefore required in the calculations to account for the fact that a dollar of cost (or benefit) today, is more valuable than a dollar of cost (or benefit) tomorrow.

Table 9.2 Costs and Benefits of Proposed Computer System (1 year)

Manual System Costs

10 people @ $20,000 each	$200,000

Proposed Computer System Costs

Programmer @ $30,000	$30,000
2 clerks @ $15,000 each	30,000
Hardware and software	50,000
Total costs	$110,000

Proposed Computer System Benefits

Reduction of labor costs	$140,000
(7 people @ $20,000 each)	
Reduced bad debt	20,000
Total benefits	$160,000

Cost-Benefit Analysis

Benefits = $160,000
Costs   = $110,000
B/C ratio = 160,000/110,000
          = 1.45

Net Benefit

Benefits – Costs = $50,000 (economic results of proposed computer system)

A material consideration concerning this technique is its limiting characteristics in cost justification. One observer notes that when economic benefits only equals costs, there may be little justification for the impact of change[14] unless a demonstrable improvement in effectiveness is experienced. While cost-benefit analysis considers only the cost of acquisition and the economic results, (i.e., quantitative benefits), cost-effectiveness refers to the cost of acquisition and the effects for the organization (qualitative benefits). The survey of health executives listed the following qualitative benefits that are expected to be realized with computerization:[15]

- Improved access to information
- Timely capture of information
- Improved staff productivity
- Improved organizational communication
- Standardization of procedures
- Improved quality of care
- Better staff-patient relations.

Despite these expectations, several drawbacks exist in using cost-effectiveness as a systematic tool in examining the benefits of computerization. A major problem is the difficulty of putting a dollar value on such qualitative benefits as "improved access to information" or "improved organizational communication." These benefits are almost impossible to measure, and managers are often susceptible to "expert opinion" in the valuation of such benefits. Furthermore, there is very little hard data to suggest that realization of qualitative benefits necessarily occurs or occurs in a form that is expected. The anticipated "improved access to information," as well as most other anticipated benefits, may rest on a specious assumption. The notion that computerization "improves access to information" assumes that mountains of data will be turned into molehills. But as previously noted, without enlightened management, mountains of data often turn into mountain ranges. The problems with cost-effectiveness analysis, then, are its intrinsic inability to value benefits and its hidden assumptions, along with various unanticipated effects. Table 9.3 summarizes these issues.

Information Economic Analysis

Although some say they are impossible to quantify in dollar amounts, qualitative benefits nevertheless are a factor in many health care information technology economic decisions.[16] And, if intangible costs and benefits are not considered in measuring overall value, investment decisions will continue to be perceived as subjective.[17] In fact, a rising field of study in business management sciences—"information economic analysis"—deals with this issue.[18] Information economics gives decision makers a way to quantify and compare the importance of the intangible benefits (i.e., those not easily measurable in dollars) of the investment choice, while still showing the direct economic costs and benefits of the choice.

It is no surprise that, as Peter Van Etten puts it, a "grudging acceptance" exists regarding the value of many information technology investments. Many questions surround the value of information technology investments because the standard technique of measuring the return on investment—cost benefit analysis—generally fails to tell the whole story when applied to these kinds of technology investments.

Datamation and the Oracle Corporation have applied the technique of information economic analysis to information technology investment decisions by breaking the analysis into three basic decision factors:[19]

Table 9.3 Costs, Benefits, and Effects of Health Care
Computerization

Overt Costs	Anticipated Benefits
Hardware/software	Reduction of staff needs
Capital outlay for construction and/or equipment for space and storage	Increased accuracy of records
Design of system	Standardization of procedures
Salaries	Better staff/patient relations
System maintenance	Improved organizational communication
Supplies	Timely capture of information
Utilities	Increased staff productivity

Hidden Costs	Unanticipated Effects
Staff displacement	Morale problems
Staff disruption	Decrease in productivity
Absenteeism	Decrease in patient/staff contact
Turnover effort	Violations of privacy
Organizational disruption due to system failure	Misuse and abuse of computer resources
Time and effort needed to overcome conflict	Constraints in individual creativity
Loss of work effort and quality due to frustration and change	Creation of more work, rather than less
Personnel training and education	Duplication of work
Running new and old system simultaneously to insure accuracy	

- Tangible cost-benefit analysis
- Intangible benefits analysis
- Intangible risk analysis.

While the traditional cost-benefit analysis addresses the tangible costs and benefits (dollar costs of the system and direct dollar savings), information economics measures the importance of intangible technical benefits and technical risks-uncertainties.

Information economics measures the importance of these two factors as weights in the analysis, rather than as direct dollar measurements of costs and benefits. Weights are assigned by managers to measure the importance of the intangible factors to the organization's overall strategy. The investment option with the highest weighted scores end up as the investment choice. The technique of information economic analysis can be illustrated in Table 9.4 with a simple example that compares two technology investment options.

Table 9.4 Information Economic Analysis

	Weight (%)	Mainframe Option		Build Option	
		Rate	Score	Rate	Score
Tangible Benefits					
Labor savings	25	3	75	4	100
Other savings	15	2	30	3	45
Intangible Benefits					
Reduction in staff	7	2	14	1	7
Increased accuracy	8	2	16	3	24
Improved communication	4	1	4	2	8
Timely capture of information	3	3	9	4	12
Increased staff productivity	9	2	18	4	36
Intangible Risks					
Staff displacement	7	−2	−14	−1	−7
Staff disruption	3	−3	−9	−1	−3
Absenteeism	1	−1	−1	−1	−1
Turnover effort	1	−1	−1	−1	−1
Organizational disruption	5	−2	−10	−2	−10
Time and effort to overcome conflict	2	−1	−2	−2	−2
Loss of work quality	6	−2	−12	−1	−6
Staff resistance	4	−3	−12	−2	−8
Total	100		105		194

Degree of likelihood/Support for each option		
	Benefits	Risks
None	0	0
Minimal	1	−1
Moderate	2	−2
Strong	3	−3
Very Strong	4	−4
Maximum	5	−5

The method suggested by Datamation and the Oracle Corporation is as follows:

1. Form a committee of those who will be affected one way or another by a decision to invest in a new technology.
2. Come to consensus on the intangible benefits and risks.
3. Weight the importance of tangible benefits, intangible benefits, and intangible risks in the investment decision. (As in the illustration, for example, tangible benefits might be 40 percent, intangible benefits a combined weight of 31 percent, and intangible risks 29 percent.)

4. Estimate on a scale of zero to five the likelihood of each benefit and risk coming to fruition.

5. Multiply each estimate of likelihood by the weight for that factor and sum all the resulting numbers for the given options. The option with the highest total is the best bet.

Managerial Implications

Considering economic and cost justification issues is a significant part of coping with the managerial challenge of computers. Understanding the complexities of economic analysis can help the manager plan for computer use and will help to determine the extent of productive use of the technology. The real value of economic analysis may be the consensus-building process. It forces the manager to ascertain what he or she hopes to achieve with the investment, and puts a value on the importance of these goals. Taking one step beyond simple cost-benefit analysis, by deciding what the impact of the investment will be, forces participants to build consensus on benefits and risks and the relative importance of each.

As of yet, however, no single applied economic analytic methodology is regarded as absolute. It can be assumed that as technology costs stabilize and experience improves system design, computerization will provide a favorable return on investment.[20] What remains as a major stumbling block in considering the economic issues is the fact that benefits are often overpromised and some effects are typically unanticipated. This results in unfulfilled expectations, dissatisfaction, and disappointment.

Despite the apparent rationality that underlies such techniques as cost-benefit, cost-effectiveness, and information economic analysis, managers must resist the temptation to automatically assume that quantitative and qualitative benefits will accrue. Rather, effective, rational decisions concerning computerization hinge primarily on the fact that we manage people, not machines. Consequently, the economics of computing in health care is both subtle and complex.

Notes

1. *Computers in Healthcare*, March 1987, 41.

2. M. McEneney, "Cost Overruns Plague California DMV Automation Project," *Computerworld*, 20 January 1986, 15.

3. *Wall Street Journal*, 19 April 1988, 31(W).

4. See "The Expert's Opinion," *Journal of End User Computing*, Spring 1993, 31–33.

5. J. C. Henderson and J. B. Thomas, "Aligning Business and Information Technology Domains: Strategic Planning in Hospitals," *Hospital & Health Services Administration*, Spring 1992, 71.

6. D. A. Ryckman, "Information Technology Is Not Enough," *Healthcare Executive*, May–June 1991, 39.

7. C. W. Axelrod, "The New Economics of Computers," *Infosystems*, June 1985, 66–69.

8. T. K. Zinn and L. W. DiGiulio, "Actualizing System Benefits," *Computers in Healthcare*, May 1988, 38–40.

9. F. Cerne, "Prices Stabilize," *Hospitals*, 5 June 1988, 70.

10. *Computers in Healthcare*, April 1988, 20.

11. Quoted in *Computers in Healthcare*, November 1990, 51.

12. H. B. Wolfe, "Cost-Benefit of Laboratory Computer Systems," *Journal of Medical Systems*, February 1986, 1–9.

13. Zinn and DiGiulio, 38.

14. Editorial, "Making Effective Information Technology Investments," *Research and Development*, October 1986, 27.

15. Zinn and DiGiulio, 38.

16. R. Parker, "Realizing Benefits: The Role of Management and the Computer," *Computers in Healthcare*, March 1988, 57–60.

17. R. Lane and R. Hall, "Yes There Is a Way to Measure MIS Investments," *Business Month*, August 1989, 73–74.

18. J. W. Semich, "Here's How to Quantify IT (Information Technology) Investment Benefits," *Datamation*, 7 January 1994, 45–48.

19. Semich, 45.

20. R. E. Carlyle, "ROI in Real Time," *Datamation*, 15 February 1987, 73–74.

Selected Readings

Cox, G. H. "Technology's Rewards without the Risks." *Datamation* (1 February 1990): 69–75.

Faye, D. "Computers, Input-Output, and the Future." *Journal of Economic Issues* (June 1986): 499–507.

Kriebel, C. H., and A. Raviv. "An Economics Approach to Modeling the Productivity of Computer Systems." *Management Science* (April 1982): 446–47.

Maslia, D., and R. Boggs. "Using Automation to Control Receivables: How Computers Can Improve the Revenue Cycle." *Topics in Health Care Financing* (Fall 1993): 32–40.

Peterson, R. C., and K. M. Hanneman. "Gaining a Competitive Edge Through HIS Technology." *Healthcare Financial Management* (June 1991): 26–38.

Sparish, B. J. "Computer Expansion: An Issue to Be Reckoned With." *Journal of Systems Management* (December 1986): 16–22.

Zmud, R. W. *Information Systems in Organizations*. New York: Scott Foresman and Company, 1983.

READING

Harry Wolfe's article illustrates the kind of economic analysis discussed in this chapter. He uses "before-and-after" cost-benefit analysis in formally evaluating the system. The article provides a useful perspective associated with the economics of computerization in a health care setting.

Cost-Benefit of Laboratory Computer Systems

Harry B. Wolfe

The Tri-Service Medical Information (TRIMIS) Program Office (TPO) has installed computerized medical laboratory systems (TRILAB) in a number of military hospitals.

The TRILAB system is designed to support the following laboratory activities: patient files, test order entry, specimen accessioning and control, work document preparation, quality control, test result entry, inquiry and test retrieval, test result reporting at wards and clinics, and management reporting. The system is designed to have automated, high-volume test instruments on line, with the goal of reducing clerical work of laboratory technicians and transcription errors, and of monitoring quality control samples in order to check for correct calibration of instruments and proper handling of specimens within the laboratory. The system produces interim test result reports, daily cumulative reports, and cumulative summary discharge reports. In addition, the system produces management information, such as laboratory work load summary reports.

Reprinted with permission from Harry B. Wolfe, "Cost-Benefit of Laboratory Computer Systems," vol. 10, no. 1 of *Journal of Medical Systems*, 1986.

The system supports terminals outside the laboratory, such as in wards, clinics, and satellite facilities, for transmission of results and for inquiries as to test status.

Arthur D. Little, under contract to the TPO, conducted an evaluation of the TRILAB system. The evaluation was based primarily on a comparison of information and data on operations collected at a medium-sized hospital with an average daily inpatient census of 244 patients and a service volume of 376,000 outpatient visits per year. The clinical laboratory performs approximately 2.6 million tests (including quality controls) per year.

In addition to the comprehensive evaluation for this hospital, supporting "mini-evaluations" were carried out for two other hospitals.

Evaluation Approach

The basic evaluation design was a "before-and-after" comparison of manual (preimplementation) laboratory operations with operations of the laboratory using the TRILAB computer system (postimplementation).

Four types of data were collected during both pre-and postimplementation studies: (1) time spent by personnel within the laboratory in information-handling activities (using work sampling and time observations); (2) performance of services (turnaround time for test results in the laboratory, process time, transcription discrepancies, number of telephone inquires about test results, and patient waiting time); (3) staff perceptions of performance of services (staff questionnaire survey); and (4) staff and patient satisfaction (staff and patient questionnaire survey).

In addition, postimplementation interviews with providers and laboratory staff were carried out to obtain further data and information related to the impact of the laboratory computer system on hospital operations.

Evaluation Results

This section summarizes the evaluation data collected during the baseline and postimplementation evaluations, organized according to the system goals and evaluation measures: (1) personnel time devoted to information handling, (2) performance of service measures, (3) attitudes and perceptions about services (collected via survey questionnaires), and (4) interview information.

Personnel Time Devoted to Information Handling

One goal of the TRILAB system was to reduce time spent by laboratory staff in clinical or information-handling activities. In both the baseline and postimplementation studies, time spent by laboratory personnel in information-handling activities was measured by an extensive work-sampling program conducted in the three major laboratory sections: Chemistry, Hematology, and Bacteriology.

Table [9.5] compares the time devoted to information-handling activities in the pre- and postimplementation periods, in terms of both percent of time and estimated hours per week. The comparisons of percentage of time are considered more accurate than the comparisons of estimated hours per week, due to minor difficulties in interpretation of the estimates of weekly hours and staffing levels in the three sections during the baseline sampling period.

Overall, the percentage of time devoted to information-handling activities was 2.6% lower in the postimplementation than in the preimplementation period; this difference was statistically significant.

Statistically significant (at a 95% confidence level) reductions in the percentage of time devoted to information-handling activities were observed in Hematology and Microbiology sections (2.7% and 1.6%, respectively). An increase of 1.2% of time devoted to information-handling activities was observed for Chemistry. This increase, however, was not statistically significant. The overall reduction in time devoted to information handling between two study periods was about 60 hours per week. Part of this reduction, however, was due to the difference in staffing. At the staffing level during the postimplementation study, a reduction of 2.6% was equivalent to a reduction of 35.8 hours per week devoted to information-handling activities, or slightly less than 1 FTE.

As might be expected, time devoted to transcription and recording of test results was reduced by about .9%, equivalent to about 16 hours per week. Time devoted to compilation of work load statistics, which accounted for 21 hours per week of time in the baseline period, was eliminated in the postimplementation period because the computer system assumed this function. Time devoted to quality control logging, calculation, and updating was reduced by 31 hours per week.

It was concluded that time devoted to information-handling activities in the postimplementation period was approximately 2.6% lower than in the baseline. Based on current staffing, this was equivalent to a net reduction of 34 hours per week (day shift, Monday to Friday) devoted to information-handling activities in the Chemistry, Hematology, and Microbiology sections. As expected, there were reductions in time devoted to transcription and recording of test results, compilation of work load statistics, and quality control reporting.

Table 9.5 Comparison of Baseline and Postimplementation Information-Handling Times

| | Percent of Time | | | Hours per Week | | |
	Baseline	Postimplementation	Difference	Baseline	Postimplementation	Difference
Chemistry	37.3%	38.5%	1.2%	208.6	161.7	−46.9
Hematology	18.1	15.4	−2.7[a]	68.0	73.9	5.9
Microbiology	22.6	21.0	−1.6[a]	103.5	84.0	−19.5
All	27.2	24.6	−2.6[a]	380.1	319.6	−60.5

[a] Difference is statistically significant.

Performance of Services

Another goal of the TRILAB system was to make information available to providers with increased efficiency. Data on two types of performance measures were collected during the pre- and postimplementation periods: turnaround time for laboratory requisitions, and volume of telephone calls inquiring about test results.

Turnaround times   Table [9.6] compares process or "turnaround" times observed in the two study periods. In the case of the STAT/urgent tests, the postimplementation averages presented are for the "CRT process time" (time results available via the CRT) as being most comparable to the process time measured in the baseline period (time when results were telephoned back to the requesting units). In the case of routine tests, the final results available via CRT are presented as being most comparable to process times measured in the baseline period (completed results slips available for pickup).

The results suggest that process times were reduced in the postimplementation period compared to the baseline period for Hematology STAT/urgent tests (by .4 hours) and for Hematology routine tests (by 2.6 hours); these differences were statistically significant at the 95% confidence level. The process times for STAT/urgent and routine Chemistry tests increased (by .23 hours and 8.3 hours, respectively); these differences, however, were not statistically significant. Average

Table 9.6   Comparison of Baseline and Postimplementation Average Process Times

	Mean Turnaround Time (Hours)			
	Baseline	Postimplementation	Difference	F test
STAT/Urgent				
Chemistry	1.27[a]	1.50[b]	.23	2.6[e]
Hematology	1.25[a]	.85[b]	−.40[e]	1.07
Routine				
Chemistry	16.1[c]	24.4[d]	8.3	2.8[e]
Hematology	4.7[c]	2.1[d]	−2.6[e]	12.3[e]
Microbiology	39.1[c]	59.6[d]	20.5[e]	3.5[e]

[a] Time from receipt of specimen by laboratory to telephoning results.
[b] Time from accessioning to availability of first results via terminal.
[c] Time from receipt of specimen to availability of results at distribution box.
[d] Time from accessioning to availability of final results via terminal.
[e] Statistically significant difference.

process times for Microbiology tests increased by about 20 hours; this difference was statistically significant.

The differences observed must be interpreted with caution for the following reason. In the case of routine tests, the process times are not entirely comparable because in the preimplementation period the process time represents the time when the requisition slip was *available for pickup*, whereas the postimplementation process time represents the time that the result was in fact *available to the requester* (via terminal look-up). Thus, routine results were available to the provider (via terminal inquiry) considerably sooner in the postimplementation period for routine Chemistry and Hematology tests, and probably in about the same time for Microbiology tests.

We conclude that, for routine tests, results were *available* to provider locations (via terminal) sooner in the postimplementation period than in the baseline period for Chemistry and Hematology, and in about the same time period or sooner for Microbiology. Hard-copy daily reports were generally available to providers later than the completed results requisition slips were in the baseline period. Interim hard-copy reports (for the surgical floors) were available sooner in the postimplementation period for Hematology tests, and in approximately the same time for Chemistry and Microbiology tests.

Number of telephone calls Table [9.7] provides a comparison of the number of calls per day received by the laboratory during the two study periods. In the postimplementation period, the laboratory received an

Table 9.7 Comparison of Pre- and Postimplementation Period Telephone Calls in the Clinical Laboratory

	Number per 8-hour Day		Ratio of Baseline to Postimplementation	
	Pre-implementation	Post-implementation	Unnormalized	Normalized for Work Load
For filed results	12.5	2.9	.23	.20
Information from laboratory	62.4	34.4	.55	.48
Supervisor	12.9	8.8	.68	.59
Technician	9.0	17.8	1.98	1.72
General information	5.6	3.5	.63	.55
Total	102.4	67.4	.66	.57

average of 67.4 calls per day, two-thirds that received during the baseline period (102.4 calls per day). The distribution of calls by type was similar to that received during the baseline period, with the majority of calls (51%) requesting information from the laboratory with regard to test results.

It should be noted that not all nursing stations or clinics had terminals and not all areas of the laboratory (e.g., Nuclear Medicine, Pathology, and Blood Bank) were on the system. If additional terminals are obtained, the volume of telephone calls could be expected to be further reduced.

The volume of telephone calls to the laboratory was thus considerably reduced by implementation of the TRILAB system. Normalized to study period work loads, the volume of telephone calls in the postimplementation period was almost half (57%) that in the baseline study period.

Staff Perceptions of Laboratory Services

Survey questionnaires were distributed to medical staff, nurses, administrative corpsmen and clerical staff, and laboratory staff during the baseline and postimplementation studies. The purpose of the questionnaires was to determine the degree of satisfaction of various providers and staff with laboratory operations.

Questions were included with regard to perceptions about such factors as relations with laboratory personnel; legibility, quality, accuracy, and format of laboratory reports; amount of time required to obtain test results; promptness and completeness of laboratory reports in patient records; and ease of and amount of time required to obtain information by telephone. Respondents were asked to rate satisfaction with each factor, using scale values of 5, 4, 3, 2, 1 (the conventional Likert scale).

Satisfaction levels of physicians, nurses and physicians' assistants, and other users increased in virtually all categories. Physicians showed the greatest increase in satisfaction levels with regard to turnaround times of both routine and STAT tests. Nurses and physicians' assistants showed the greatest increase in satisfaction with regard to accuracy of results, completeness of laboratory reports, and test turnaround times.

Users were asked to compare relative frequency of problem events under TRILAB operations with previous laboratory (manual) operations. The TRILAB system received relatively "high marks" for most problem categories. The median response was that the following occurred "less frequently" with the TRILAB system: tests repeated due to delays (43.4% felt they occurred less frequently); tests repeated due to lost results (46.7%); and telephone calls to the laboratory (64.6%).

Results of Interviews

During the study periods and implementation monitoring visits, interviews were held with a number of laboratory supervisors and with providers, with regard to benefits achieved with the TRILAB system, and any problems encountered. The following summarizes the results of these interviews.

Telephone calls Laboratory staff at all three sites felt that a very significant decrease had occurred in telephone calls to the laboratory, which had interrupted work flow and taken up staff time.

Work load reporting Supervisors at the three sites felt that TRILAB accomplished management and work load reporting tasks more efficiently than in the baseline. Supervisors estimated that in the three major sections (Chemistry, Hematology, and Microbiology), approximately 8.5 to 10 hours per week in total were saved by having the TRILAB system produce the monthly work load reports: these reports were previously prepared manually.

Quality control reports Supervisors indicated that the quality control reports of the system (Levey-Jennings charts) were a significant benefit. Supervisors estimated that 11 hours per week were saved in preparing the quality control reports, which were produced by the TRILAB computer system.

Patient exception reports It was estimated that approximately 10 hours per week were saved in review of patient exception reports, due to the highlighting of abnormal results by the computer system.

Logging of specimens and preparation of work sheets Staff estimated that reduction of time spent in these activities averaged 14 staff hours per day.

Duplicate tests It was anticipated that the number of duplicate or repeated tests may be reduced with the TRILAB systems. Laboratory staff suggested that this could occur for two reasons: (1) Providers could easily check on the status of tests and would be less inclined to repeat an order if they saw a test was pending or in process. (2) Abnormal results and unusual "delta checks" (abrupt changes from the previous day's results) showed up on the screen as they were entered, so that extra attention was given to such results. This may have resulted in fewer result report errors.

Supervisors at all three sites felt that duplication of tests was reduced, but that the effect was likely small, approximately 1% of total tests.

In addition to the above (quantifiable) estimates of benefits, laboratory staff cited the following benefits:

Reduction in transcription errors   Because abnormal results were highlighted on the CRT screens and received extra scrutiny by technicians and reviewers, there was potential for reduction of transcription errors. It was felt, however, that such reduction in errors was likely small.

Normal ranges data   The system provided the capability to provide normal ranges data with each test (which is a CAP accreditation requirement). This may not have been universally provided previously, at least for the majority of tests for which the users were expected to know what the normal ranges were.

The following is based on interviews with providers (nursing staff and physicians):

Reduced staff time   Nursing staff estimated that there was considerable reduction in staff time associated with telephoning the laboratory to receive test results and to inquire about late or missing results, in filing time due to having cumulative reports available, and in chart review. Staff at all three sites estimated that savings amounted to about 4 hours per inpatient unit or clinic (which had terminals). Thus, time savings were thereby made available for other nursing activities.

Duplicate tests   Nursing staff estimated that there was less duplication of tests, perhaps resulting from the fact that results appeared on the terminal as they became available, and there was less chance they would be lost.

Decreased turnaround time   Turnaround time for test results, especially for routine tests, had been reduced, contributing to the reduction in telephone calls. Providers indicated that this may have resulted in improved patient care.

Improved morale   As a result of being able to look up test status on the terminal, and the reduction in telephone calls to the laboratory, nurses felt that relationships between nursing and laboratory staff had improved considerably.

Retrieval of information   Users interviewed relied heavily on TRILAB's information storage and retrieval capabilities. All comments in this regard were highly positive. This capability was reported to provide a great deal of information to users, possibly improving patient care.

Identification of abnormals Because abnormal results were identified, leading to faster and easier identification of patient problems, providers felt that patient care has been improved.

To summarize, both the questionnaire survey and the interviews indicated that health care providers were generally pleased with the TRILAB system, citing as advantages reduced telephone calls, decreased test turnaround times, improvements in relationships with laboratory personnel, an improvement in quality of care due to easier and faster access to test results, identification of abnormal values, and cumulative report formats.

A further indirect measure of approval of the system was the expressed desire of staff in those inpatient units and outpatient clinics that did not have terminals (and had to share a terminal in another location) for a terminal in their own location.

Cost-Benefit Analysis

The approach to the cost-benefit analysis was that of estimating total incremental life-cycle net costs and benefits over the period of the TRILAB contract, 8 years. The one-time and recurring costs associated with the acquisition and implementation of the TRILAB system were identified and estimated, using contract documents. Estimates provided by the facility were used for different components of implementation costs. Benefits were estimated by comparison of activities in the laboratory and in provider locations affected by implementation of the system, from the work-sampling and observation studies and interviews. The majority of quantifiable benefits resulting from the system were in the form of personnel time savings (Table [9.8]). These personnel resources saved through implementation of the TRILAB system have not necessarily resulted in fewer FTEs employed in the hospital, but in most instances have resulted in increased time made available to meet increased demand for services or to provide more directly related patient care activities. Thus, the value of the time freed up (measured by the associated hourly salaries and fringe benefits) was considered a benefit of the system.

The base-case life-cycle analysis showed that the TRILAB system is very cost-effective. Life-cycle benefits of $2.6 million exceeded life-cycle costs of $1.9 million by $750,000.

In addition, there were a number of benefits that could not be quantified, including improved turnaround time for test results, which

Table 9.8 Estimated Annual Savings Due to TRILAB System

Within Laboratory	
Information handling	$29,584
Reception desk	9,298
Reduction in duplicate tests	3,744
Outside Laboratory	
Nursing units	222,154
Outpatient services	127,738
Total benefits	$392,518

had the potential for improving patient care and reducing length of stay; improved and easier availability of test results to providers, which improved relationships between providers and laboratory staff; improved and more useful report formats, such as cumulative reports and highlighting abnormal results, which could improve patient care; and increased laboratory management reporting capability, which could improve overall effectiveness of laboratory operations.

CASE 9
Economic Analysis at Smiling Acres

P RIOR TO investing in the new computer system at Smiling Acres Nursing Center, Bob Sherman attempted to conduct an extensive economic analysis. Approaching the problem analytically, he realized that costs and benefits of the new system needed to be considered. Furthermore, the benefits had to outweigh the costs.

The health care management literature was replete with the virtues of computing and the benefits derived from switching to a computerized system. It was apparent that the potential existed for increased productivity and streamlined operations. Despite these exhortations, Bob proceeded to dig deeper into this analysis, and found the terrain a bit more complicated than expected.

Cost Displacement

Bob found that, generally, computer technologies have been sold to organizations from the perspective of "cost-displacement." This is a formula that calculates existing manual costs and compares the result with costs of performing the same work with a computer system. The calculation is:

Manual Costs − Electronic Data Processing Costs = Dollar Savings

or

$MC − $EDP = $Savings

To illustrate the calculation, assume that labor costs will be eliminated by computerization. This means that the costs of the computer displace the labor costs. For example, if the manual system requires ten individuals and the computerized system requires only five individuals to do the same work, and the salaries are constant, then dollar savings occur. Thus, the costs of the computer displace the costs of the manual system.

Bob noted in a glossy marketing brochure an impressive graph that helped to explain the economic relationships between computerization and costs (Figure 9.1). The graph suggests that with manual processing, as transaction volume increases, direct costs tend to increase. Indirect costs (occurrence of errors) also increase. With automation, costs tend to decrease with the volume of work.

Investment-Benefit Return

Another perspective that seems to serve as a basis for selling the idea of computerization is a formula widely used in business. The investment-benefit return formula focuses on the return on investment (ROI). This formula calculates the organizational investment and compares it with the return on that investment. The calculation is:

$$\$Investment - \$Benefit\ Return = \$Return\ on\ Investment$$

or

$$\$I - \$BR = \$ROI$$

To illustrate this calculation, assume that more dollars are returned than invested. For example, if the initial dollar investment for a computer

Figure 9.1   Economic Considerations in Data Entry

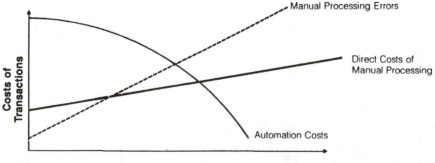

Information Systems in Organizations, by Robert W. Zmud (Glenview, IL: Scott, Foresman & Co., 1983).

system is $100,000, and the benefit returned from that investment is $200,000, then the net return on the investment is $100,000.

The economic relationships between costs of the investment and the return on the investment were illustrated in the marketing brochure Bob had. Assuming steady increases in workload, Figure 9.2 suggests that by introducing computers a company can avoid future costs. The difference between the costs avoided, and the initial investment is the ROI. The dollars that without computerization would have been spent can now be used to generate financial benefits (e.g., expanded services, increased market share, etc.).

Hidden Costs and Unanticipated Effects

While the cost-displacement and ROI formulas appeared to be partially helpful in the appraisal of the economic issues associated with computerization, Bob had a number of unsettling thoughts related to the uncertainty of the actual costs and effects related to any set of options. He was able to ascertain the tangible costs associated with the investment, but had little certainty concerning the associated hidden costs and unanticipated consequences of any option. What are the risks involved with each of the options? Will everyone see these hidden costs and risks the same way Bob sees them? Don't the cost-displacement and ROI formulas fail to tell the whole story when applied to the investment?

Figure 9.2   Return on Investment in Computers

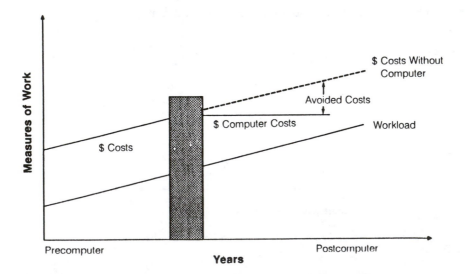

The Decision

Bob knew that considering the cost displacement and ROI issues associated with the investment would not be enough. In light of the inevitable staff resistance regarding any computerization effort, he needed both a consensus-building process and a way to put a value on the more uncertain costs and effects that would accompany computerization.

Questions for Discussion

1. How do economic analyses assist the decision maker?
2. Evaluate the "cost-displacement" and "ROI" perspectives as bases for a computerization decision.
3. Develop a strategy for Bob in implementing an information economic analysis. Use the prescribed method in applying an economic analysis as suggested in the text.
4. What major issues must Bob still confront in managing the economics of health care computing?

chapter 10

UNDERSTANDING SOCIAL IMPACTS

I N HIS engaging book, *The Social Impact of Computers*, Richard Rosenberg asks the kind of questions that raises the subject of computers in health care beyond the merely practical level: "Will technology bring about Utopia, or 1984? Are we entering an age of unprecedented access to knowledge and power, or are we becoming a fragmented society of technology haves and have-nots?"[1] While not proffering answers, he prods reflection on important questions for health care professionals. For example, is our use of computers in health related organizations moving our care-giving more in the direction of "Utopia," or of "Planet of the Apes"?!

Futurist Burt Nanus,[2] a quarter of a century ago, suggested an answer. He predicted that negative social impacts would inevitably appear if the implementation of computer systems were guided mostly by economic and technological considerations, with little managerial attention. According to some, his prediction has proven to be prescient.[3]

A case in point is the "progressive" long-term care facility that decided to automate its financial systems. During one weekend, manual systems were removed and a minicomputer with terminals and a printer were installed. After the financial files (including the personal accounts of the residents) were restored on the automated system, the old hand-copied files were destroyed. On Monday something happened that no one had anticipated: the elderly residents, to whom the computer age was a stranger, and whose last vestige of independence was their small personal account in the facility's office, were bewildered and shaken when an imposing printout was given to them in place of the familiar hand-written ledger. As a result, the happiness of these people was disrupted. The managers and users of the computer had not thought of the "social" impact in planning and designing the system.

Weighed against Rob Kling's disturbing contention that "the social problems of computer use and strategies for alleviating them are relatively neglected and poorly understood,"[4] the seriousness of the social impact of computer use becomes apparent. What is the nature of the problem, and how can managers deal effectively with the responsibilities it entails?

The Social Impact of Computers

The influence of computerization is apparent in nearly every aspect of life today. Students are educated on terminals and computers now even link parents to their children's schools so they can check attendance records, homework assignments, and lunch menus and have e-mail conversations with teachers. Clinicians use computers to diagnose and monitor patients. Pharmacy automation provides computerized dispensing units for medications. The technology of telemedicine enables care-givers to conduct two-way interactive video consultations. Elected officials use computerized mailing lists in campaigns and computerized opinion surveys in policymaking. Police use computerized fingerprints. The subway systems of San Francisco and Washington, DC are computer operated. On-line services like those from the Prodigy Services Company or America Online use the power of the personal computer to provide opportunities for social interaction as never before. New virtual communities are forming as a result of the Internet and other webs of computer networks.[5] As Terrell Ward Bynum, founder of the Computing and Society Research Center at Southern Connecticut State University puts it, "Computer technology and the information superhighway will change the world more than the inception of canals and roads . . . and by studying the effects of the computer revolution we can protect human values instead of damaging them."[6]

Few deny the social impact of computers, but many question and debate its results. Is the impact positive or negative? The dialogue basically splits between those who focus on the objective, tangible impacts and those who see subjective, invisible, subtle effects.[7]

On the surface, the social impact of computer applications in health care results in better service delivery, faster response, greater efficiency, and more sophistication.[8] Bringing telemedicine technology to rural communities, for example, could have considerable beneficial results. But, there may also be significant impacts below the surface.

The nursing home mentioned above did indeed improve its financial management and increase revenues through automation; it also, in the process, produced anxiety in the very people for whose welfare it presumably exists.

Similarly, *Time* reports the dawning of a new age using computer technology.[9] The "electronic superhighway," a new world of video entertainment and interactive services combining the switching and routing capabilities of phones with the video and information offerings of the most advanced cable systems and data banks will be in most of our homes in the near future. Instead of settling for whatever happens to be on at a particular time, subscribers will be able to select any item from an encyclopedic menu of offerings and have it routed directly to a television set or computer screen. Using relatively simple technological advances, such as translating audio and video communications into digital information, new methods of storing digitized information, and fiber optic wiring providing a virtually limitless transmission pipeline, users will have access to vast new video services.

"In the end," says *Time*, "how the highway develops and what sort of traffic it bears will depend to a large extent on consumers. As the system unfolds, the companies supplying hardware and programming will be watching to see which services early users favor. If they watch a lot of news, documentaries and special interest programming, those offerings will expand."[10] With economics driving the availability of services, a concern that this technology might endanger cultural diversity and pluralism may well be justified.

Most troubling to many skeptics is another kind of social impact. Neil Postman, a New York University professor and author of *Technopoly: The Surrender of Culture to Technology*, comments: "You already don't have to go out to the movies because you have your videos, T.V. and CDs. . . . With new technologies, you'd never have to go out and meet anyone. Is that great? It's a catastrophe!"[11]

These kinds of subtle impacts can occur in several dimensions. Politically, there is concern that the efficient use of computers by elected officials could lead to manipulation of the electorate. In reporting on the wide use of computers by American congressmen, for example, the *Wall Street Journal* added: "This causes concern both inside and out of Congress about whether the computer-using lawmakers can manipulate the voters back home in new and more sophisticated ways, thus making themselves even more invulnerable at the polls to opponents who have none of the perequisites the public purse supplies to incumbents."[12] Could health care professionals similarly manipulate clients? A recent article in *Management Review* entitled "Big Brother and Healthcare," reports survey results that more than 70 percent of Americans are concerned with how medical information on national electronic databases will be used.[13]

Psychologically, there is a concern that computers can cause feelings of alienation, fear, and depersonalization.[14] A Los Angeles bank that uses computers to improve operating efficiency sends the following automated letter to customers who fall behind in loan payments: "This is a reminder from your friendly computer. You are $48.88 in arrears on your payments. Please remit. If you do not, next time you will have to deal with a human."[15]

We might well ask, as some researchers have, whether computer systems in health care could similarly depersonalize professional-client relationships and dehumanize medical care.[16]

Considering the intellectual dimension of social impact, many commentators have expressed a concern about the proliferation of small, cheap electronic calculators among children who use them to count. Some writers go as far as warning that "today the question is no longer whether mental calculation is going to become less important but when it is going to disappear."[17] Could any health care computer applications tend to program decision making and leave the thinking to the machines? Certainly, the recent technological advancements for medical applications of artificial intelligence and virtual reality tend to stimulate this kind of conjecture.[18]

A sociological dimension is raised by many who, like Postman cited above, view the encroachment of computers in the home and workplace as a return to isolation in which people are removed from all but basic human intercourse. They see a society in which people never have to leave their homes because they can obtain what they need by ordering it on their home computerized video screen;[19] they see workers isolated from other co-workers, becoming "high-tech hermits," linked to co-workers only electronically;[20] and they see a bipolarization of society into those who know the technology and those who do not.[21] For health care organizations, in which human service is the raison d'etre, such loss of personal interaction could be serious indeed.

The psychological and social commentator Bruno Bettelheim talks in *The Informed Heart* about "seduction" by technology:

> The advantages we could enjoy from any new machine were always quite obvious; the bondage we entered by using it was much harder to assess, and more elusive. Often we were unaware of its negative effects until after long use. By then we had come to rely on it so much that small disadvantages that come with the use of any one contrivance seemed too trivial to warrant giving it up, or to change the pattern we had fallen into by using it. Nevertheless,

when combined with the many other devices, it added up to a significant and undesirable change in the pattern of our life and work.[22]

Bettelheim's words epitomize the concern of social impact thinkers and the responsibility of professionals to address the social implications of using computer technology.

Managerial Action

Jerome Wiesner, the former president of Massachusetts Institute of Technology and an eminent scientist and administrator, provides wisdom that is as relevant now as it was when he wrote about the impact of information technology:

> The great danger which must be recognized and counteracted is that such a depersonalizing state of affairs could occur without specific overt decisions, without high-level encouragement or support and totally independent of malicious intent. The great danger is that we could become "information bound" because each step in the development of an "information tyranny" appeared to be constructive and useful.[23]

Wiesner, and most writers, address the macro level, that is, society as a whole. We, as health care professionals, need to be concerned with the micro level, that is, the hospitals, clinics, nursing homes, etc. that we manage and work in. Deliberate managerial action at our micro level organizations is required to prevent undesirable social impacts from occurring as a by-product of otherwise useful efforts at employing computer technology.[24] For example, in the case of the progressive nursing home described above, managers could have chosen to maintain handwritten personal accounts, or they could have devised rituals to ease the residents into being comfortable with the change. With a little thought they could have improved the human situation along with organizational efficiency. The point is that it takes skill and effort to maintain a managerial perspective; economics and technology can blind us to the obvious.

Dealing with such a responsibility may be the biggest challenge that health care professionals face, for it is as difficult to anticipate such social impacts as it is to know how to counter them, and it will inevitably take more time and money. Recognizing and managing social impact requires broad awareness and sensitivity and a conscious effort to adapt perceptions to a specific health care organization. Precise thought is essential. As Bettleheim observes: "The most careful thinking and planning is needed to enjoy the good use of any technical contrivance without paying a price for it in human freedom."

Promoting social benefits and minimizing undesirable impacts require the institution of procedures and guidelines to safeguard such human values as individual respect and dignity, as well as interpersonal interaction. A need to focus on patients, clients, and workers in the design and use of computer technology, instead of solely on organizational efficiency, must surely be a hallmark that makes using computers and information systems a special challenge for health care professionals. As Thomas Sheridan has put it eloquently: "We will have our computers, but our subjective sense of what is right, beautiful, and consistent with a just and sustainable society, and what contributes most to human fulfillment, ought to dictate our use of these exotic tools with their enormous potential. Productivity in human terms should prevail over productivity in machine terms."[25]

In the past 40 years computer scientists have tackled and overcome enormous scientific hurdles to produce today's powerful computer technology. Now the challenge is managerial.

Notes

1. R. S. Rosenberg, *The Social Impact of Computers*, (San Diego, CA: Academic Press, 1992).
2. B. Nanus, "Managing the Fifth Information Revolution," *Business Horizons*, April 1972, 7.
3. Symposium, "The Third Industrial Revolution," *Impact of Social Science on Society*, no. 146, 1987, 107–201.
4. R. Kling, "Computing People," *Society*, January–February 1980, 14.
5. *New York Times*, 27 March 1994, 10.
6. *New York Times*, 6 March 1994, 10.
7. J. Danzinger, "Social Science and the Social Impacts of Computer Technology," *Social Science Quarterly*, March 1985, 3–21.
8. P. Mandell, "Computers that Humanize Health Care," *Ms. Magazine*, May 1986, 103–5.
9. "Electronic Superhighway," *Time*, 12 April 1993, 50–56.
10. *Time*, 12 April 1993, 56.
11. "The Next Revolution," *Newsweek*, 6 April 1992, 42–48.
12. J. M. Perry, "Congressmen Discover Computer and Use It to Keep Voters in Tow," *Wall Street Journal*, 15 March 1978, 1.
13. J. Szwergold, "Big Brother and Healthcare," *Management Review*, February 1994, 5.
14. W. H. Dutton, E. M. Rogers, and S. H. Jun, "Diffusion and Social Impacts of Personal Computers," *Communication Research*, April 1987, 219–50.
15. Printed in *Christian Science Monitor*, 1 June 1978.
16. E. McConnell, S. Somers O'Shea, and K. T. Kirchoff, "R.N. Attitudes toward Computers," *Nursing Management*, July 1989, 39.

17. S. Nora and A. Minc, "Computerizing Society," *Transaction*, January–February 1980, 30.

18. *New York Times*, 31 October 1993, F-11.

19. See *New York Times*, 13 February 1994, Sec. 13LI 2.

20. See *New York Times*, 8 February 1994, B-1.

21. See *Time*, 12 April 1993, 50–56.

22. B. Bettelheim, *The Informed Heart* (Glencoe, IL: Free Press, 1960), 16.

23. J. B. Wiesner, "The Information Revolution—And the Bill of Rights," *Computers and Automation*, May 1971, 8.

24. H. Gelman, "Computers: The People Factor." *CMA: The Management Accounting Magazine*, March–April 1986, 60.

25. T. B. Sheridan, "Computer Control and Human Alienation," *Technology Review*, October 1980, 72.

Selected Readings

Attewell, P., and J. Rule. "Computing and Organizations: What We Know and What We Don't Know." *Communications of The ACM* (December 1984): 1184–92.

Calhoon, C. "Computer Technology, Large-Scale Social Integration, and the Local Community." *Urban Affairs Quarterly* (December 1986): 329–49.

Davenport, T. "Saving IT's Soul: Human-Centered Information Management." *Harvard Business Review* (March–April 1994): 119–33.

Haglund, R. F. "Sociology, Economics, and Super Computing." *Academic Computing* (May–June 1988): 22–51.

Johnson, D. G. "Mapping Ordinary Morals onto the Computer Society: A Philosophical Perspective." *Journal of Social Issues* (Fall 1984): 63–76.

Powell, W. W. "Explaining Technological Change." *American Journal of Sociology* (July 1987): 185–97.

Sardinas, J., M. Blank, and G. Spiro. "Data Processing: Toward a Social Responsibility." *Journal of Systems Management* (January 1986): 7–11.

Symposium. "The Third Industrial Revolution." *Impact of Science on Society* 146 (1987): 107–201.

Wessel, M. R. *Freedom's Edge: The Computer's Threat to Society*. Reading, MA: Addison-Wesley, 1979.

READING

JOHN SEABROOK'S *New Yorker* article muses on the social impact of a relatively new phenomenon associated with computerization. "Flaming," a form of on-line communication, illustrates how "uncivilized" computer use can easily affect the way we think about ourselves and relate to each other. His insights can help health care managers "civilize" the use of computers in their organizations.

My First Flame
John Seabrook

It was love at first E-mail for the author. Then came the bitter realization that on-liners can behave just as badly as people in the real world—and sometimes worse.

I got flamed for the first time a couple of months ago. To flame, according to "Que's Computer User's Dictionary," is "to lose one's self-control and write a message that uses derogatory, obscene, or inappropriate language." Flaming is a form of speech that is unique to on-line communication, and it is one of the aspects of life on the Internet that its promoters don't advertise, just as rail companies around the turn of the century didn't advertise the hardships of the Great Plains to the pioneers whom they were hoping to transport out there. My flame arrived on a windy Friday morning. I got to work at nine, removed my coat, plugged in my PowerBook, and, as usual, could not resist immediately checking my E-mail. I saw I had a message from a technology writer who does a column about personal computers for a major newspaper, and whom I knew by name only. I had recently published a piece about Bill Gates, the chairman of Microsoft, about whom this person has also written, and as I opened his E-mail to me it was with the pleasant expectation of getting feedback from a colleague. Instead, I got:

> Crave THIS, asshole:
> Listen, you toadying dipshit scumbag . . . remove your head from your rectum long enough to look around and notice that real reporters don't fawn over their subjects, pretend that their subjects are making some sort of special contact with them, or, worse, curry favor by TELLING their subjects how great the ass licking profile is going to turn out and then brag in print about doing it.
>
> Forward this to Mom. Copy Tina and tell her the mag is fast turning to compost. One good worm deserves another.

I rocked back in my chair and said out loud, "Whoa, I got flamed." I knew something bad had just happened to me, and I was waiting to find out what it would feel like. I felt cold. People whose bodies have been badly burned begin to shiver, and the flame seemed to put a chill in the center of my chest which I could feel spreading slowly outward. My shoulders began to shake. I got up and walked quickly to the soda machines for no good reason, then hurried back to my desk. There was the flame on my screen, the sound of it not dying away, it was flaming me all over again in the subjective eternity that is time in the on-line world. The insults, being premeditated, were more forceful than insults spoken in the heat of the moment, and the technology greased the words—the toads, scum, shit, rectums, assholes, compost, and worms—with a kind of immediacy that allowed them to slide easily into my brain.

Like many newcomers to the "net"—which is what people call the global web that connects more than thirty thousand on-line networks— I had assumed, without really articulating the thought, that while talking to other people through my computer I was going to be sheltered by the same customs and laws that shelter me when I'm talking on the telephone or listening to the radio or watching TV. Now, for the first time, I understood the novelty and power of the technology I was dealing with. No one had ever said something like this to me before, and no one *could* have said this to me before: in any other medium, these words would be, literally, unspeakable. The guy couldn't have said this to me on the phone, because I would have hung up and not answered if the phone rang again, and he couldn't have said it to my face, because I wouldn't have let him finish. If this had happened to me in the street, I could have used my status as a physically large male to threaten the person, but in the on-line world my size didn't matter. I suppose the guy could have written me a nasty letter: he probably wouldn't have used the word "rectum," though, and he probably wouldn't have mailed the letter; he would have thought twice while he was addressing the envelope. But the nature of E-mail is that you don't think twice. You write and send.

When I got on the net, it seemed to me like a place where all the good things about E-mail had been codified into an ideology. The first thing I fell for about the medium was the candor and the lack of cant it makes possible. Also, although the spoken word can be richer and warmer than the written word, the written word can carry precision and subtlety, and, especially on-line, has the power of anonymity. Crucial aspects of your identity—age, sex, race, education, all of which would be revealed involuntarily in a face-to-face meeting and in most telephone conversations—do not come through the computer unless you choose to reveal them. Many people use handles for themselves instead of their real names, and a lot of people develop personae that go along with those handles. (When they get tired of a particular persona, they invent a new handle and begin again.) On the net, a bright twelve-year-old in a blighted neighborhood can exchange ideas with an Ivy League professor, and a businesswoman who is too intimidated by her male colleagues to speak up in a face-to-face meeting can say what she thinks. On the net, people are judged primarily not by who they are but by what they write.

My flame marked the end of my honeymoon with on-line communication. It made me see clearly that the lack of social barriers is also what is appalling about the net. The same anonymity that allows the twelve-year-old access to the professor allows a pedophile access to the twelve-year-old. The same lack of inhibitions that allows a woman to speak up in on-line meetings allows a man to ask the woman whether she's wearing any underwear. The same safe distance that allows you to unburden yourself of your true feelings allowed this guy to call me a toadying dipshit scumbag. A toadying dipshit scumbag! I sent E-mail to the people at CompuServe, which was the network that carried my flame to me, to ask whether their subscribers were allowed to talk to each other this way.

> To: John Seabrook
> Fr: Dawn
> Customer Service Representative
>
> Since CompuServe Mail messages are private communications, CompuServe is unable to regulate their content. We are aware of an occasional problem with unwanted mail and are investigating ways to control such occurrences. If you receive unwanted mail again, please notify us of the details so that we can continue to track this problem.

If the net as a civilization does mature to the point where it produces a central book of wisdom, like the Bible or the Koran, the following true story might make a good parable. In 1982, a group of forty people associated with a research institute in La Jolla established a small, private on-line network for themselves. For about six months, the participants were caught up in the rapture of the new medium, until one day a member of the group began provoking the others with anonymous on-line taunts. Before long, the community was so absorbed in an attempt to identify the bad apple that constructive discourse ceased. The group posted many messages imploring whoever was doing this to stop, but the person didn't, and the community was destroyed. Stewart Brand, who is a founder of the WELL, an on-line service based in San Francisco, and who told me this story, said, "And not only did this break up the on-line community—it permanently affected the trust that those people had for each other in the face-to-face world, because they were never able to figure out who did it. To this day, they don't know which one of them it was."

What would Emily Post advise me to do? Flame the dipshit scumbag right back? I did spend most of that Friday in front of the screen composing the most vile insults I could dream up—words I have never spoken to another human being, and would never speak in any other medium, but which I found easy to type into the computer. But I didn't send these messages, partly because I had no way of knowing for sure whether the person whose name was on the flame had actually sent it, and since this person was a respected author, with a reputation to consider, I thought someone might be electronically impersonating him, a practice that is known on-line as "spoofing." I managed to restrain myself from sending my reply until I got home and asked my wife to look at it. She had the good sense to be horrified, and

Although some of the language contained in the following reading is not consistent with Health Administration Press editorial standards, it has been reprinted in its originally published form to retain its substance and purpose in this book.

suggested sending the message "Do you know where I could get a good bozo filter?" But I wasn't sure I had the stomach for a flame war, so I settled on a simple, somewhat lame acknowledgment of the flame:

> Thanks for your advice on writing and reporting. The great thing about the Internet is that a person like me can get useful knowledge from experts, and for free.

In a few days, I received a reply from the writer, asking when my new column, "Pudlicker to the Celebrated," was going to start.

I was in a quandary that many newcomers to the net face. Newbies sometimes get flamed just because they are new, or because they use a commercial on-line service provider, like America Online or CompuServe, which shows up in their electronic addresses, just as Italian immigrants were jeered at because they had vowels at the ends of their names. Some people are so horrified by their first flame that they turn into "lurkers": they read other people's messages in the public spaces but are too timid to post themselves. (You see lots of evidence of the fear of getting flamed; for example, long posts that end, "Sorry so lengthy, please don't flame," and messages studded with smiley faces-":)"—and grin signs—"<g>"—which remind you of the way that dogs have to go through elaborate displays of cringing around each other to avoid starting a fight.) For other newbies, getting flamed puts the taste of blood in their mouths, and they discover that they like it. They flame back, and then a flame war begins: people volley escalating rounds of insults across the wires. Now that there are an estimated twenty-three million users connected to the Internet—ten million of which have come on-line in the last nine months, in what amounts to a massive cultural upheaval, as though a whole generation of immigrants to the New World had come over all in one day—the "netiquette" that prevailed in its early days is breaking down. And many of the new users are not the government officials, researchers, and academics for whom the net was designed; they're lawyers, journalists, teenagers, scam artists, lonely hearts, people in the pornography business, and the faddists who were buying CB radios in 1975.

On Saturday evening, some friends came over for dinner, and I told them about my flame. They asked to see it, so I went down the hall to print out a copy. But when I opened the electronic file where I store my E-mail I noticed that the title of my reply had turned into gibberish—where there had been letters there were little boxes and strange symbols—and that the dates for when the message was created and modified said "8/4/72" and "1/9/4." It occurred to me then to wonder briefly whether the person who flamed me had also sent some sort of virus into my computer, but I was cooking and didn't really have time to think about it, and when our guests left it was late, and I turned the computer off and went to bed. Just before six the following morning, however, I awoke abruptly and sat up in bed with a sudden understanding of what the last line in the flame—"One good worm deserves another"—might mean. A worm, in computerese, is one of the many varieties of viruses that infect computers. "One good worm deserves another": this guy had sent me a worm!

I got out of bed and went down the hall, turned on my computer, opened my E-mail file, and saw with a shock that the corruption had spread to the title and dates of the message stored next to my reply. The reply itself was still corrupted, but the gibberish and weird dates had mutated slightly. I tried to delete the two corrupted messages, but the computer told me it couldn't read them. The icy feeling inside my chest was back. I copied the whole file onto a floppy disk, removed the disk from my computer, dragged the original file into the electronic trash can, emptied the trash, and then sat there regarding my computer with suspicion and fear. I had the odd sensation that my computer was my brain, and my brain was ruined, and I was standing over it looking down at the wreckage. In my excitement over the new medium, I had not considered that in going on-line I was placing my work and my most private musings only inches from a roaring highway of data (only the short distance, that is, between the hard disk and the internal modem of my computer), and, like most highways, it didn't care about me. After thinking about this for a while, I noticed I was sitting in the dark, so I got up and pulled the chain on the floor lamp, and the bulb blew out. I thought, Wait a second, if my computer is connected to the outlet, is it possible that the worm could have gone into the plug and through the wall circuit and come out in the light bulb? The worm had entered my mind.

I waited for my computer to die. Even though I had removed the two corrupted messages, I was worried that the worm might have infected my hard disk. At my most paranoid, I imagined that I had received a "logic bomb," which is a virus that hides in your computer until a timing mechanism triggers it. (A few years ago, a rumor went around the net that a lot of computers had been infected with a logic bomb that was set to go off on Bill Gates' birthday, October 28th, but the rumor turned out to be false.) I felt creepy sitting in front of my computer, as though I weren't sure whether it was my friend anymore. Every time my software did something peculiar that I couldn't remember its having done before, my heart turned over a little. I'd think, It's starting.

When I tried to explain this feeling to a non-computer-using friend of mine, she said, "Yeah, it's like when someone breaks into your car," but actually it was more like someone had broken into my head. I sent E-mail to my computer-literate friend Craig Canine, a writer and farmer who lives in Iowa, asking what he knew about worms, and he E-mailed me back.

> Coincidentally, I just gave our goats their worm medicine. It's called Val-bazen, and it seems to work pretty well for ruminants—I'm not sure about computers, though. What does this worm do? Should I be communicating with you—might your e-mail be a carrier? Jesus, I've got my book on my hard disk. If your worm zaps it, I'll kill you first, then go after the evil perp. (then plead insanity, with cause).

I was a pariah.

On the Wednesday following my flaming, I took my floppy disk to work to show it to Dan Henderson, who set up the network here at the magazine. Every office where computers are networked together has a guy like Dan around, who is usually the only person who really understands the system, and is terrifically overworked, because in addition to doing his job he has to deal with all the people like me, who are mystified by their computers. Shelley said that poets are the unacknowledged legislators of the world; system administrators are the unacknowledged legislators of the net. Sysadmins are really the only authority figures that exist on the net. In small electronic communities, the sysadmin often owns the equipment that the community runs on—a personal computer, a modem, and a telephone line are all you need to run your own bulletin board—and therefore he has absolute power over what goes on in the community. If a sysadmin wants to read someone's mail, he reads it. If he wants to execute someone, electronically speaking—by kicking that person off the network—he doesn't need to hold a trial. A benevolent sysadmin can make the network a utopia, and a malevolent sysadmin can quickly turn it into a police state.

I sent Dan a QuickMail, which is the brand of interoffice E-mail we use, and told him that I thought my computer might have been infected with some sort of worm. I asked if he had time to see me, expecting that maybe he'd get to me before the end of the week. I was surprised when Dan appeared in my doorway within ten minutes.

"You QuickMailed me," he said. I noticed he was looking at me strangely.

"Yes . . ."

"You sent me QuickMail."

"I was slow getting his drift. So?"

Then I got it. "Wait. You mean you think I infected *The New Yorker's* network?" Dan was just looking at me, his eyebrows up around his hairline. "But I took the worm off my hard disk and put it on here," I said defensively, holding up the floppy disk.

Dan has that intense energy you often see in guys who are really into computers; the speed at which he talks and moves always makes me think of the clatter of fingers over the keyboard. He sat down at my computer with a couple of different kinds of software that looks for worms and viruses. After about ten minutes of probing my hard disk, he announced that he couldn't find any evidence of infection. He checked the floppy and found nothing there, either. The gibberish and weird dates had gone away. Dan explained that he didn't understand how I could have received a worm via E-mail, because worms are programs; most E-mail carries only text. A file containing a program can be sent over E-mail, but in order for it to infect your computer you'd almost certainly have to open the file and run the program.

Was it possible that my worm was just some weird software glitch I had never seen before, and that it just happened to choose my reply to the flame to make its first appearance, and that the line "One good worm deserves another" was just a coincidence? After thinking about this for a couple of days, I came up with a little experiment. My hypothesis was that perhaps the worm could have burrowed into the program I was using to set up a reply to the original message, and my experiment was to perform the reply operation again, in order to see if the worm would come back.

The next morning, my new reply and the message stored next to it were corrupted again. I tried to print out the gibberish, but again the machine couldn't read the characters, so I copied them down. I also got my wife's camera and took a picture of my computer screen. Then I called Dan at home.

"Dan? This is John. Dan, my worm is back. I'm looking at it now."

Dan was polite about it, but he made a sound that suggested he did not consider himself my sysadmin right now, at ten o'clock on a Saturday morning, and said, "Could we talk about this on Monday?"

I wanted to talk about my flame with someone else who had been flamed, but I didn't know anyone in my real-world life who had been. Then it occurred to me that I could use the net. This is one of the great things about the net: the spaces are organized around topics, so it's easy to find people who think like you and who share your interests. People who gather on the net to discuss a specific topic are called newsgroups, and each newsgroup has its own "site." In a literal sense a site is just a small amount of storage space in a computer somewhere in the world, which you can reach by typing its address, but it feels like an actual room. So, for example, if you think you might be a pagan, but you're still in the closet, you can go to the newsgroup "alt.pagan" for enlightenment. When you arrive there, the best thing to do first is to read the FAQ, the list of Frequently Asked Questions. FAQ files are more than the prosaic things they sound like; they are the repositories of the useful knowledge that has been exchanged and meaningful events that have occurred in that particular site since it was established. The table of contents for the alt.pagan FAQ reads:

1) What is this group for?
2) What is paganism/a pagan?
2b) What is Paganism? How is it different from paganism?
3) What are different types of paganism?
4) What is Witchcraft/Wicca?
4b) Why do some of you use the word Witch? Wiccan?
5) What are some different traditions in the Craft?
6) Are pagans Witches?
7) Are you Satanists?
8) What kinds of people are Pagans?
9) What holidays do you celebrate?
9b) How do I pronounce . . . ? What does this name mean?
10) What god(s) do you believe in?
11) Can one be both Christian and pagan?
12) What were the Burning Times?
13) How many pagans/Witches are there today?
14) Why isn't it soc.religion.paganism instead of alt.pagan?
15) Is brutal honesty or polite conversation the preferred tone of conversation around here?
16) What are the related newsgroups?
17) Are there any electronic mailing lists on this subject?
18) I'm not a pagan, should I post here?
19) How does one/do I become a pagan?
20) What books/magazines should I read?
21) How do I find pagans/Witches/covens/teachers in my area?
22) What's a coven really like?
23) How do I form a coven?
24) What does Dianic mean?
25) Aren't women-only circles discriminatory?

26) Can/will you cast me a love spell/curse my enemies?

27) Is it okay if I . . . ? Will I still be a pagan if I . . . ?

28) I am a pagan and I think I am being discriminated against because of my religion. What should I do?

29) What one thing would most pagans probably want the world to know about them?

Then you can scroll though a list of hundreds of discussion topics and see what people are talking about. Some are:

14 European paganism (16 msgs)

15 Statement (6 msgs)

16 College Pagan Groups

17 PAGAN FEDERATION GIG: Thanks (3 msgs)

18 Broom Closet Pagans Hurt Us All (3 msgs)

19 Pagan funerals? (27 msgs)

20 NIGGER JOKES (18 msgs)

21 Necromancy (2 msgs)

22 Another campus Pagan group (4 msgs)

23 When the Revolution comes was Re: New Forest Service . . . (6 msgs)

24 Looking for invocations to the following . . . (4 msgs)

25 New Community Pagan Group? Need help.

I suppose you could choose not to double-click on NIGGER JOKES, but it's harder than you think. This is the biggest drawback of the way newsgroups are set up: a really interesting post that enriches your understanding of a subject is next to a post that is appropriate only for the space above the urinal. There's nothing to stop someone in alt.misanthropy or alt.tasteless from coming into rec.pets.cats and posting a graphic account of what it's like to behead a cat or drink its blood, and although you can bozo-filter that person after his first post, so that you never have to read a message from him again, the horrible words tend to stay in your memory for a long time.

NIGGER JOKES turns out to be a collection of racist jokes and limericks about killing African-Americans, which was posted on April 5th. The name and address on the jokes is that of a student at the University of Michigan. The post has been "spammed," as they say on the net, which means that the student has spread it around to many different newsgroups, thus insuring himself an audience of hundreds of thousands, and maybe millions, since the jokes are still making their way through the net. (Some employees of Fortune 500 companies have recently reported finding the jokes on their office networks.)

When someone posts a message that offends the other participants in a newsgroup, the group metes out the only punishment at its disposal, which is to flame the offender, and in this case the student who posted the jokes has been getting flames by the thousand. Also, in typical net fashion, there has been much soul-searching in the newsgroups about the character of the net itself:

> The Last Viking <paalde@stud.cs.uit.no>
> We don't have to go around being racists like those fascists in the real world! PEACE ON THE NET!!!!

> Michael Halleen <halleen@MCS.COM>

> As offensive as this is, I do not believe this should put this person "under investigation." . . . He should get hate mail, censure (not censors), and universal condemnation. There should be open debate and discussion, but leave his right to speak alone. He may use the net for other constructive purposes and taking it away may hurt him, and he needs help.

> Richard Darsie<darsie@eecs.ucdavis.edu>

> Get a grip, man. Free speech *is not* and never has been an *absolute* right. There's gotta be some limits. . . . This person abused his First Amendment rights and should face some consequences for it. Can't have rights without responsibilities.

An investigation at the University of Michigan recently concluded that the student whose name was on the posts hadn't made them; someone had spoofed him. The wrongly accused and now flame-broiled student had used a university-owned computer to log on to his account, and someone had tampered with the software in that computer so that it captured his password. This person had then logged on in the student's name and posted the jokes. The day after the jokes went up, another student, who had used the same computer to log on, discovered that his identity had been used to send a message to the Islamic Circle, a campus organization, calling its members "Godforsaken terrorists."

I went to alt.flame, thinking this might be the site where people talk about flaming, but it turned out to be a place where people go to flame each other. I saw that an intrepid writer from *Wired* magazine, Amy Bruckman, had posted that she was writing an article about flaming and was getting flamed for doing it.

> Insert finger in appropriate orafice and shove off.

> Sod off bitch, we don't need your glamour here. . . .

> WHAT?!? Do you think I wanted to be publicated in your low-life-scum magazine??? . . . BTW, what kind of name is Bruckman? Are you kind of a German refugees' daughter from the 2'nd world war? Kraut? a sauceage woman? Anyway go to hell.

I decided not to post in alt.flame myself.

I considered posting a query about my worm in the newsgroup comp.virus, and I lurked around there for a while, but didn't post, because I was worried that my assailant might hear that I was posting queries about him in public spaces—it's difficult to keep secrets on the net—and devise some even more elaborate torture to inflict on my computer, or begin spoofing me in some diabolical fashion. I had already seen how the net could be used to hurt someone's reputation. One day, as I was wandering around inside the Electronic Frontier Foundation discussion space, which is one of the most interesting newsgroups on the net, I came upon a subject line that said, "Ralph Berkeley made homosexual advances toward me." Ralph Berkeley (I'm not using his real name) is a regular participant in discussions of net policy, who appears, on the evidence of his posts, to be an articulate and thoughtful man, and often takes the position that completely unrestricted free speech on the net might not be such a good idea—a position that causes him to receive his share of flames. However, this post upped the ante a bit:

> Ralph Berkeley made homosexual advances toward me when I visited him at his office approximately two weeks ago. As I went there just to chat with him and he's not my employer or anything I don't think I have any grounds for any legal action or anything like that. But I must say that prior to that event I had a lot of respect for him (not necessarily his opinions, but the evenhanded way in which he stated them). I am really disappointed.

This brought forth even more furious bursts of thinking and feeling over the nature of the net:

> Dik T. Winter<dik@cwi.nl>
> I think Ralph Berkeley has enough grounds for a suit on defamation of character. Ralph, I urge you, *do* sue. I do not agree with you but please, *do* sue.

> Jim Thomas<tkOjutl@mp.cs.niu.edu>
> No. Although we all assume the original post was homophobic sleaze, a suit is even more offensive. Such a suit itself constitutes "fag bashing," because it continues the stigmatizing of gays by suggesting that homosexuality is abnormal or pathological.

Then, in the best spirit of the net, Dr. Berkeley posted this reply:

> Thanks to readers whose responses showed such good sense. Of course it's false.
> Ralph

Everywhere I went in the newsgroups, I found flames, and fear of flames. In the absence of rules, there is a natural tendency toward anarchy on the net anyway, and in some stretches I'd come upon sites that were in complete chaos, where people had been flaming each other non-stop, absolutely scorching everything around them, and driving all the civilized people away. Sometimes I'd arrive at a dead site long after a flame war broke out; it was like walking through what was once a forest after a wildfire. Sometimes I came upon voices that were just howling at the world; you could feel the rage and savagery pouring out through people's fingers and into the net. Of course, you can hear this sound on the streets of New York City, but less often than you hear it on the net, and in the city it lasts only as long as the person who is making it has breath for it and is heard only by the people within earshot. On the net, it can be heard by millions and reverberate for a long time.

Sometimes I returned from these trips on the net feeling lonely, cold, and depressed. I would see the net less from the point of view of the acrobat and more from the point of view of the fish. Ironically, the net seemed most alive to me when I was off it and found myself using a word I had picked up in my travels. The net is a hotbed of language, because on the net language has to accomplish everything; the whole world is made of words, and people are constantly forced to coin new ones. And, because typing takes more effort than speaking, people are always inventing acronyms or abbreviations—"lol" for "laughed out loud," "f2f" for "face to face," "BTW" for "by the way," "RTFM" for "Read the Fucking Manual," which is a message people often send back to you when you ask them for technical help. There's something wonderful about all this, but it's also sad to go to a chat group and see the "lol's" scrolling by on the screen, sometimes with no other words attached to them, just people typing "lol" to each other. How much of the pleasure of laughter can you get sitting alone with your computer, typing "lol"?

I sent a copy of my flame to someone I know only as Jennifer, a woman I met on the net and feel I know in a strange way, although in fact I know hardly anything about her. She replied:

> I must say that I was shocked to read about your experience. . . . The magnitude of your assailant's tirade rends my heart. I have been thinking about those graphic words, unbidden, for the last two days.

Here was another good thing about the net—that a woman I didn't even know would be so concerned for me. I wrote to Jennifer that the net seemed to me in some ways a cold place, and she replied:

> You are right about the coldness of the net. There is an air of pre-established hierarchy there—if you're new to the net, or even to a particular group on the net, you don't belong a priori. As a woman, I have encountered an additional

barrier; the net is heavily male and women who want to play with the big boys either have to be ultra tough-talking—one of the boys—or else play off as coy, charming, "little-ol-ME?" feminine. (Even geeks have fantasy lives, I suppose.) Or use a male/neutral alias with no one the wiser.

So part of the boys' club, I imagine, is the smallness, the selectivity—the geek elite, if you will. For more than a decade these guys had their own secret tin-can-on-a-string way to communicate and socialize as obscure as ham radio but no pesky FCC requirements and much, much cooler. . . . But then the Internet—their cool secret—started to get press. . . . Imagine these geeks, suddenly afraid that their magic treehouse was about to be boarded by American pop culture. It was worse than having your favorite obscure, underground album suddenly appear on the Billboard charts.

As my assailant had suggested, I also forwarded a copy of the flame to my mother, whom I had got wired for E-mail. She replied:

I deleted that thing you sent me immediately. What a terrible man. He must have been drunk.

When you link your computer, through a phone line, to the Internet, you turn your computer into a printing press and your phone line into a broadcast system. Anything you write on your computer screen has the potential to be read by millions of people. You don't have to formulate your message in language suitable for publication in the letters column of the *Times;* you don't have to go to the trouble and expense of buying time on a TV channel; you don't have to pass out paper copies of your message on a street corner. And you don't have to be responsible for what you say.

The great question for the future of the net is: To what extent will this extraordinary freedom be allowed to remain in the hands of the people, and to what extent will it be limited and regulated? The Internet is not the information highway, but it might become part of the information highway. In order for this to happen, though, the Internet will have to be "civilized"—a word that gives many net users the willies. The net is, fundamentally, about free speech, while the I-way is about commercial and CIVIC transactions: It's a route for delivering videos, newspapers, and catalogues into people's home computers, for filing taxes on-line, eventually for voting on-line. Completely unrestricted speech, which is desirable in a free exchange of ideas and data, is less vital when you're talking to a business competitor or to your congressman.

The net poses a fundamental threat not only to the authority of the government but to all authority, because it permits people to organize, think, and influence one another without any institutional supervision whatsoever. The government is responding to this threat with the Clipper Chip, a fingernail-size sliver of silicon that was designed by the National Security Agency and that the government hopes will eventually be installed in everyone's phone, fax, and modem. (A.T. & T. recently began manufacturing telephone-security devices with the chip in them.) With Clipper, the government is attempting to regulate the net not at the level of content, which would probably be impossible in a network so diffuse, but at the level of code.

When you write into a computer, your words are turned into a code called American Standard Code for Information Interchange, or ASCII, which is made out of a hundred and twenty-eight permutations of eight-digit strings of ones and zeros. Each zero or one is called a bit, and a bunch of eight bits is called a byte. The letter "A" is a byte made out of eight bits, and it looks like this: 01000001. The purpose of the Clipper Chip is to encrypt the ASCII text as it leaves your computer and turn it (by using an algorithm) into a code so complex that it would take a hundred supercomputers a thousand years to break it. At the receiving end, another Clipper Chip converts the code back into ASCII, which your computer in turn converts back into human language.

Encryption is like a slightly weird older brother of software who would have remained obscure if his younger brother hadn't become the leader of the digital age, but because of their common ancestry in code, we have to reckon with the older brother, too. Both the net people and the I-way people recognize the need for encryption in the on-line world. Computer networks are insecure, because they are packet-switched; that is, after your message leaves your machine it is broken into bits and sprayed into a wire that is full of bits of other messages. Sometimes bits from a single message get separated, sprayed into different wires, and squirted through different computers, and then the software in the computer at the other end reassembles the bits. This makes it relatively easy for someone to intercept your bits without your knowing about it, which is no big deal if there's not much in your bits that people want to read. But if people are really going to live on the information highway—if bits containing their medical records, their credit-card numbers, their bank balances, and their intimate secrets are going to flow through the wires—then the general insecurity of the bit stream is going to be a problem, and encryption is the best way to solve it.

The obvious danger in supplying people with encryption is that encryption makes it easier to keep secrets, which makes it easier for people to commit crimes. With powerful encryption, the net would become an ideal place for criminals to organize conspiracies. If John Gotti had planned his crimes on-line instead of in the Ravenite Social Club and he had been using good encryption, there would have been no bugs, and he wouldn't have been convicted. Dr. Clinton C. Brooks, the N.S.A.'s lead scientist on the Clipper Chip project, told me, "You won't have a Waco in Texas, you'll have a Waco in cyberspace. You could have a cult, speaking to each other through encryption, that suddenly erupts in society—well programmed, well organized—and then suddenly disappears again." Therefore, in an effort to balance the good and bad sides of encryption, the United States government has proposed that people use a brand of encryption that the government has designed, which is powerful enough to take care of everybody's legitimate encryption needs but has an electronic "back door" that law-enforcement agencies could use, with a court order, to listen to the conversations of people they suspect of being criminals. This brand of encryption is inside the Clipper Chip.

On the net, where the single most popular topic of conversation is the net itself, Clipper is extremely unpopular, and President Bill Clinton and Vice-President Al Gore, both of whom have addresses on the net, have been getting royally flamed about it. It is easy to see why Clipper makes people nervous. You're taking the N.S.A., an agency whose main activity for the past forty years has been electronic surveillance—an organization so secretive that for many years the government tried to deny its existence—and you're putting it in charge of protecting people's privacy. I've noticed that my level of paranoia is higher now than it was before I got on the net, but I'm not sure which I should be more afraid of—criminals or spies. My feeling about Clipper is that the government is swimming upstream, against history. You actually feel sorry for the government; in order to get people to use their brand of encryption, the government is reduced to invoking the spectre of on-line cults and conspiracies. Orwell's idea of a totalitarian government using technology to subjugate the people was based on the technology of television, and you could argue that television has allowed large, centralized organizations to control and manipulate people. But the personal computer has transferred enormous power away from institutions and into the hands of individuals, and that trend is only accelerating with the exponential growth in computing power and the spread of the net. In the future, somebody will develop encryption that the N.S.A. won't be able to crack, and smart criminals will be able to talk without being overheard. The Clipper Chip initiative seems like a vain attempt to reverse the way the technology is going. In the digital future, it isn't just Big Brother we're going to have to worry about.

One day at work, I asked Dan Henderson if he knew of someone I could go to for the final word on my worm—the top worm man in the country, as it were—and he gave me the E-mail address of John Norstad, at Northwestern University. Norstad is the author of Disinfectant, a popular brand of virus-protection software for the Macintosh, and probably knows as much as anyone in the world about the viruses and worms that affect Macs. I sent him E-mail saying I would be coming out to Chicago in a couple of weeks on business and wondered if I could have him examine my PowerBook. Norstad promptly E-mailed me back to say that he was in the midst of fighting a new virus that had just broken out in Italy, and didn't have time to think about my problem now, but would be happy to see me when I came to Chicago.

We arranged, through E-mail, to meet at the Palmer House, where I was staying. Because my only contact with Norstad had been on-line, I had no clue what sort of man to expect, and as I waited for him in my room I tried to imagine what he would be like. I realized that I was envisioning Norstad not as a Western doctor but as a kind of tribal medicine man. Whether the corrupted messages in my computer were the result of a real worm or were caused by a software glitch, all my troubles seemed to me to be related to the general wizardry of software—the mysterious incantations of ones and zeros being whispered inside my computer. I felt as if someone had put a spell on my computer, and I was bringing it to John Norstad to have him heal it.

Norstad turned out to be about forty-five, not tall, with a beard that had some gray in it, glasses, and a shy, polite manner. He wore a flannel jacket over a loose gray shirt, and gray pants. He was carrying a PowerBook loaded with the dominant strains of all the nastiest viruses known to the Macintosh world; the viruses were safely corralled on his hard disk with Disinfectant, which he distributes free on the net to anyone who wants it. Norstad set his PowerBook next to my Power-Book and showed me his collection of infected programs. He moved his cursor over and pointed it at an icon, double-clicked on it, and said, "Now, if I didn't have any protection this little guy would start erasing my hard drive right . . . now. But because we do—there, see . . . Disinfectant caught it." It was awesome.

I asked Norstad about the Italian virus he had been fighting when I first E-mailed him, and he said that it had appeared in an item of software posted on a bulletin board in late February. Because the software was copyrighted, and had been posted on the board illegally, there was some suspicion that the virus writer was trying to teach the pirates a lesson about copyright infringement. Norstad opened the E-mail log in his PowerBook and showed me the hundreds of messages he had sent and received between February 28th, when he received E-mail from three people in Italy which said that a new virus was erasing people's hard disks, and March 3rd, when he and his colleagues produced vaccines. Upon hearing about the Italian outbreak, Norstad had immediately sent E-mail to a group of colleagues called the Zoo Keepers, a sort of on-line volunteer fire squad, to alert them to the existence of the new virus. The Zoo Keepers are a virtual community that live all over the globe—Australia, Germany, the United States—and could exist only because of the net. Norstad received a copy of the virus from Italy, made copies, and sent the copies out over the net to the Zoo Keepers. Keeping in touch over the net, the scientists reverse-engineered the virus and a number of effective vaccines for it. Norstad then updated Disinfectant—version 3.3 became 3.4—and posted it around the net, where people could download it for free. All this took fifty-six hours.

I asked whether virus writers were often motivated by politics, and Norstad said no, they were mostly relatively harmless hackers, at least in the Mac world. In the world of I.B.M.-compatible machines, which is much larger than the Mac world, there are many more viruses, and they tend to be deadlier. They are the stuff of legend. Norstad told me of an account he had once heard from a Bulgarian virus expert, about software engineers commissioned by the Communist government to crack the security seals on Western software. When the regime fell, the story goes, the unemployed engineers were said to have whiled away their empty hours writing viruses for I.B.M. compatibles.

I asked, "Is it possible that a terrorist could take down a large part of a country's computer systems with a virus?"

"It's possible. Of course, the problem with a virus that virulent is, How do they keep it from infecting their own system?"

I told Norstad the story of my worm, and asked whether it was possible for a technically sophisticated person such as I believed my assailant to be to send a worm through E-mail. This seemed like an important point to establish, because if it was possible to send a person a worm or a virus via E-mail, it would be like giving someone a cold by talking to them on the phone. I was thinking, If bad people can infect decent people's brains just by communicating with them, this medium is not going to work.

Norstad said, "I will not say it is impossible. Anything is possible. I'm saying I don't understand it and I've never heard of it happening before. I will say that the kind of symptoms you describe could be a software problem."

"Like what?" I asked.

"Who knows?" Norstad said. "It's software. It's weird stuff. People are always writing and calling me because they think they have some kind of virus, and in almost every case it's a software problem, not a virus—but these people are fearful and need my help. For example, quite a few people have written me to say a shrieking death's head appears occasionally in the top of their screens. You know what it is? If you have Apple's Remote Access program, hold down the option key, and hit the shift key three times, your computer makes this funny trilling sound and an object appears in the corner of your screen that could, if you were sufficiently paranoid, look like a death's head. It's not a virus. It's just a weird software thing."

While Norstad was talking, I brought my flame up onto the screen and asked him to look at it. He leaned toward me and silently read through the litany of insults. When he had finished, he sat back and sighed and didn't speak for a couple of seconds. Then he said, "I'm just so sorry when something like this happens." He lowered his head and shook it sadly. "Gee, that's terrible."

I said, "I have to admit it was upsetting. I've been thinking about it a lot. I ask myself, Do I recognize the right of this person to flame me? Yes, I do. Do I celebrate his right to flame me? I'm not sure. Do I recognize the right of this person to send me a worm? Definitely not. But at what point does a flame become a worm? I mean, can a virus be a form of free speech? In other words, could a combination of words be so virulent and nasty that it could do a sort of property damage to your head?"

I was rambling, and I could actually feel tears coming into my eyes, so I stopped there. But Norstad seemed to understand what I was talking about, and I felt better after I had told him. I realized that I would probably never know for sure whether my worm was real or just a software glitch. We chatted for a while longer, and then he said, "Don't get discouraged. The net is a fundamentally wonderful place. Most of this work I do could be done only on the net. Look at the work we did on the Italian virus, working with colleagues all over the world to reverse-engineer it. Can you imagine trying to do this by fax? Phone? Fed Ex? It would not be possible." He unplugged his PowerBook and began packing it up. "Of course," he said, "the net allows people to spread viruses much more easily than before."

"But that's the thing about the net," I said. "Each of the good things about it seems to have an evil twin."

"Yes, but you could say that about all new technology," Norstad said. "There is always going to be a dark side to it. That is why it's so important to be decent on the net, because the dark side is always right there."

As Norstad was putting on his coat, he said, "My thirteen-year-old daughter is a Pearl Jam fan, and the other night she asked me if there might be some Pearl Jam stuff on the net. So we logged on and looked around, and we were able to download some Pearl Jam posters, some music, some song lyrics—really neat stuff. But then we came to the Pearl Jam newsgroup, and there was a really terrible flame war going on in there. People were saying really awful things to each other, things I was embarrassed to be sitting next to my daughter reading." Norstad shook his head. "Terrible things. After a while, my daughter looked over at me and asked, 'Daddy, do these people have a life?' And I said, 'No, darling, most of them don't have a life.'"

John Seabrook is a freelance writer.

CASE 10
Wedgwood Health Center

CAROLYN WRIGHT, Director of Social Services, hadn't quite put her finger on what was going on in the facility. She could sense a kind of malaise, and at first attributed it to the cyclical disquiet so common in nursing homes.

Yet Wedgwood's recent conversion from a manual system to a computerized system, resulting in improvements in its financial and patient information systems, had gone on without a hitch. Wedgwood had gone "live" over the weekend, and Carolyn was surprised the installation and on-line activation could be done so quickly. The technological changes were seen, for the most part, as an effort to facilitate record-keeping and improve the facility's efficiency and productivity. Most of Carolyn's co-workers had accepted the fact that change was inevitable, and saw Wedgwood's computerization as minimally affecting their day-to-day contact with patients. Rather, it had the potential of expediting much of the bothersome, time consuming, paperwork many staff members disliked. For example, Carolyn no longer had to keep reams of files stored in her desk or in a locked file cabinet. When she needed to refer to a patient's file, she would simply press a button on her computer console and the patient's entire social service file would pop up on the screen.

Soon after the new technology came on the scene, the general feeling she sensed manifested itself in a number of disparate incidents.

It began with Muriel, the bookkeeper, asking Carolyn to speak to a patient, Mrs. Pettibone. Apparently, in a fit of pique, Mrs. Pettibone had angrily wheeled herself out of the bookkeeping office after Muriel attempted to explain the new computerized personal patient fund account form to her. Carolyn went to her room to quiet her.

> I couldn't make heads or tails out of that damn thing. I could understand the old ledger card; it was clear to me. All these new lines and numbers don't make sense. And that woman tells me she threw the old forms away. Now I don't know how much money I have. If you people wanted to confuse me anymore than I already am, you're doing a good job.

Carolyn left Mrs. Pettibone, making a mental note to ask Muriel to try again and explain the new computerized form to her. As she walked through the patient lounge on the way to her office she spotted Sam Finkle dozing in the chair. This seemed unusual, especially at 10:00 a.m. Sam usually delivered the mail to his fellow patients at this time. Carolyn gently shook Sam and asked why he wasn't delivering mail that morning.

> The girl in the office told me the mail goes through the machine now. I'm not sure why. They take it to the patients piecemeal now. I don't care, it was a pain in the neck. Everyone used to complain to me about every little thing, anyway.

Carolyn wondered if she could find Sam something else to do in the mornings. When Carolyn returned to her office, Mrs. Todd and Mrs. Jennings were waiting for her. Each in their early 80s, they had finally begun to adjust to living in the nursing home after a rocky adjustment, and both seemed to have come to terms with the fact that this was their home. Admitted around the same time and with similar backgrounds, they had begun to pal around together. Sitting on the couch across from Carolyn, they seemed concerned.

> We want to complain about the nurses. They seem grouchy lately and don't have enough time for us. I asked one of the nurses for something today and all she seemed to have time for was that typewriter and T.V. on her station. All I asked for was my granddaughter's telephone number.

Carolyn chuckled to herself, noting Mrs. Todd's reference to the computer, and proceeded to access her file. Out of the corner of her eye she felt a sense of anxiety from the two women. Mrs. Todd suddenly said that she remembered the telephone number and asked if she could leave. What had just happened? Carolyn tried to reconstruct the scene. Both women were in full view of the screen and both seemed surprised Carolyn could call up the file so quickly. Did it bother them that it was so easily accessible? Or did it bother them that their files were now contained in a big "TV" instead of a locked file cabinet?

It was lunch time and Carolyn could see the ambulatory patients coming off the elevator, making their way to the dining room. Once a week, Carolyn made a point to join the residents for lunch. The patients seemed to enjoy the opportunity for interaction with a key staff member, and she found people less inhibited and more apt to tell her what was on their minds in this kind of setting. As the trays were being distributed to her table, Mr. DellaRusso began tapping his cane noisily.

"What's the matter, Mr. DellaRusso?" asked Carolyn.

"They've given me the wrong diet," said Mr. DellaRusso.

A diet aide came over to the table, examined the diet card and said: "Sorry, Mr. DellaRusso, computer error. I'll go down and get you another tray."

"I guess we're just numbers now," snorted Mr. DellaRusso.

Carolyn quickly changed the subject and asked the patients about the newly redecorated dining room. The new wallpaper, carpeting, and furniture brightened up the room considerably.

"I guess it's O.K.," said Mrs. O'Brien, "but the old dining room was just fine. Why do they have to keep changing things? I was just getting used to the old furniture."

Other patients chimed in and began passing sentence on the color of the wallpaper, the feel of the carpet, and the sturdiness of the new chairs.

After Carolyn finished her lunch, she walked to the business office, expecting it to be busy, occupied by residents depositing, checking, or withdrawing their personal patient accounts or social security checks. Remarking on how quiet the business office seemed to be, Muriel's assistant said,

> The patients don't have to bother with most of the financial stuff now. The nurses can relay any requests for transactions on the system, and the system takes it from there. I kind of miss talking to them, though. How's Hobbe's gall bladder? Could you give a piece of this fruitcake to Mr. DellaRusso? I would always give him some when he came into the office to check on his finances.

Questions for Discussion

1. Evaluate the degree of social change brought about by the technology described in the case.
2. How did the change to computer technology affect the lives of some of the residents?

3. Describe the "ripple effect," or how changes in roles and procedures in one area result in widespread changes in other areas.

4. Defend the following statement: How technological changes occur in a health care organization are as important as what technological changes occur.

5. Develop a managerial strategy for minimizing the negative social impact of computer technology at Wedgwood.

PREPARING FOR EMERGING TECHNOLOGIES

A RECENT CARTOON in the *New Yorker* magazine highlights the importance of preparing for emerging technologies, even in the afterlife. Two angels are conversing and one dejectedly says to the other, "I put in for reincarnation, but they said if you don't know computers forget it."[1] While humorous, the cartoon underscores an important point: Success in a world of fast paced technological change means adaptation and adjustment.

The technological development of information systems (IS) within the health care field has accelerated considerably in recent years. In fact, it is predicted that the growth potential of IS technology within the health care industry during the coming years will be greater than in any other industry.[2]

Among the reasons that may help to explain this surge is the remarkable paradigm shift in the financing and delivery of health care.[3] Few circumstances hold greater potential impact for health care managers today than the reshaping of the health care system. The recasting of incentives, strategies, and relationships will have significant implications on innovation and technological change in information systems.

Some informed observers note that the increased scrutiny of costs and competition accompanying reform will change the ground rules for technology management. Acquiring and managing the "latest and best" technology will no longer be a major concern. Instead, the issue will revolve around a number of questions, such as: Will the technology advance the mission of the organization? . . . Will the technology address client needs? . . . Will the technology be of use to the medical staff? . . . Will the technology reduce operating costs?[4]

With institutions more and more at risk for the costs and outcomes of care rendered, the health services executive will likely be under increased pressure to maintain an awareness and understanding of emerging information system technologies and the concomitant skills to manage new, fast-changing technologies.

In this regard, the competent health care manager will have to be at ease with rapid technological change and the continued growth of information system functions and capabilities.[5] Accordingly, managers will need agility in adaping to the ever-changing nature of technology and proficiency in the "hows" and "whys" of shifting information needs.

Adjusting to New Information Needs

The paradigm shift occurring in the health care delivery system is spawning a new and complex environment. This environment is forcing health care service organizations to adapt to new information needs and priorities.

Driving these new information needs and priorities, in part, is the increasing presence of managed care. In a managed care world, understanding the cost of providing service and managing those costs is a prerequisite to viability. Of primary importance is the organization's capacity to capture detailed cost information for cost management, the establishment and monitoring of standardized data definitions (e.g., costs, outcomes), and the inculcation of an organization-wide emphasis on quality control and cost containment.[6]

Accompanying these structural finance and delivery changes is an increased insistence on new regulatory information standards and requirements. Accordingly, more robust information system requirements are emerging. New data needs are already appearing, as well as the need for increased reporting frequency.

Changing medical staff relations will undoubtedly occur in a more intense competitive environment, as will pressure to acquire patients. This will mean a broadening of the focus of technology systems. Looking to technology in order to improve services, to capture a wider market, or to enhance customer satisfaction will be strategies increasingly used as health-related organizations struggle to survive.[7]

Health care reform and the managed care trend are also driving a demand for greater information sharing. Health care service organizations are recognizing the need for an easier flow of information among operating entities. This information flow, for example, may take place within a single institution or among a wider community health network.

At the same time, autonomous units within institutions will have to understand the financial and administrative consequences of everyday decisions. Data access and exchange may be the most viable methods for achieving this "interoperability" within health care institutions and, more broadly, among health care facilities forming the emerging health care networks.[8]

In short, this new and complex environment demands that managers be comfortable with the new technology and the continued growth of information system functions and capabilities.

While earlier technology helped fulfill relatively basic needs through the automation of well-defined work processes, we have entered into a new era where rapidly changing technology, driven by a new environment, is reengineering the entire work of health care organizations. Because of this, the manager must continually adjust to the new technologies in order to accommodate those new needs.

Emerging Information Technologies and Health Information Systems

Until recently, the emphasis in the hardware, software, and user-interface technologies has been on the improvement of data processing technology, i.e., automation of routine well-defined work processes.[9] More currently, advances in office automation and teleprocessing technology have moved to the forefront.[10] Office automation refers to the technology of automated office systems that ostensibly increase productivity and reduce worker effort. Teleprocessing technology refers to the electronic processing of transmitted text, voice, or data from one source to another.

These technologies have played a key role in the development and expansion of health information systems. Since the 1960s, information systems have been used in health care primarily for administrative and financial purposes, not for patient care insights.[11] While health information systems offer providers and payers an opportunity to increase efficiency of health care delivery by automating claims processing, analyzing volumes of data on performance and quality, and tracking supplies through the system, it is commonplace now for most large institutions to have computerized systems that also serve the clinical aspects of the work of the institution. In this area, computer technology typically serves to improve the scheduling of patients, automates patient records into computer files that are readily accessible to physicians, monitors patient status, and provides computerized medical care information to assist physicians in making a decision about the course of patient care.

A number of experts have sought to classify these technologies and health information systems applications.[12] Typically, these technologies and systems are ordered along a number of levels. Table 11.1 depicts one way in which these technologies and health information systems might be classified.

Merging Information Systems and Technologies: Integration and Networking

Information Systems

As health care service organizations attempt to deal with a new and complex environment, there has been a growing recognition that information sharing among physicians, nurses, and administrators and systems specialized in the needs of different departments within an institution will become increasingly necessary.[13] As the clinical, financial, and administrative issues associated with rendering care coalesce, so must the applications. Moving away from fragmented, monolithic, mainframe-oriented systems and merging financial, clinical, and administrative information appears to be the next comprehensive shift in information system technology.

A recent Hewlett Packard/Healthcare Information Management Systems Society Leadership survey bears this out. According to the survey, 46 percent of respondents said that the primary information systems challenge in the coming years will be to integrate existing systems.[14] Open systems architecture, allowing multiple systems to share data regardless of their particular hardware and software components will become more the norm in health care institutions.

According to Erica Drazen of the consulting firm Arthur D. Little, if employees are to make good decisions, they must have integrated

Table 11.1 Information Technologies and Health Information Systems

		Information Technologies		
		Data processing	Office automation	Tele-processing
Health Information System Applications	Financial			
	Clinical			
	Administrative			

information.[15] Ms. Drazen suggests that organizations place selected data from all systems in a central data repository so that information is stored in one place. An integrated system, as she suggests, might be used to check whether applicable tests have been conducted when a physician orders specific procedures.

The trend toward integration of health information system applications is in evidence in the three categories of applications. Clinical HIS applications, for example, are evolving toward totally on-line, integrated patient-centered systems, collecting patients' status and delivering information when and where it is needed. This includes "point-of-care" on-line systems that permit bedside, examining room, or physician's office monitoring; clinical laboratory systems that handle comprehensive information, from test order to final patient reporting and billing; and pharmacy systems that provide on-line access to vital information, such as diagnosis, dosage, and drug interactions. These clinical applications ensure that proper information is available for making both clinical and administrative determinations. These examples illustrate the marriage of applications through integration of the clinical, administrative, and financial areas.

Accompanying the commitment to integration and open systems architecture is a requirement to adhere to standards. Standards are agreements on formats, procedures, and interfaces that permit designers of hardware, software, databases, and telecommunications facilities to develop products and systems independent of one another with the assurance that they will be compatible with any other product or system that adheres to the same standards. Standards are the single most important element in achieving integration of the information and communications resource.

The standard setting process can be cumbersome and lengthy because it involves negotiations among information technology providers and users, formal agreements and definitions, certification and testing procedures, and documentation and publication. One example of a standard is "IEEE 802.2–802.5," a standard for local areas networks (LANs) defined by the Institute of Electrical and Electronic Engineers (IEEE).

Technologies

Separate islands of technologies to support information systems within institutions have typically been the norm. However, in light of the cost-efficiency emphasis, the huge capital layouts for separate technologies, and the limitations of products based on only a single technology, the separate approach will necessarily decline. More attention will be given to applying information technology to improve the effectiveness of the organization and the managerial decision-making regarding the costs and quality of health services delivery. The use of fragmented information technology will decrease.

This trend is in evidence in many future-oriented technologies and information system applications. For example, integrated office products, artificial intelligence, and telemedicine are all examples of the merging of several sets of functions that signify a move from fragmentation to integration. A 1992 study looking at telemedicine, the technology that enables providers to do two-way interactive video consultations and transmit digital messages such as x-rays and MRIs to other sites, found that the use of videoconferencing in medicine could reduce the annual costs of remote consultation by as much as $132 million. Some states are funding telemedicine projects, while others have received assistance from the Rural Health Policy Office and the Federal Rural Electrification Administration.[16]

Another example of a future-oriented technology is the use of virtual reality as a training tool for students and physicians. Virtual reality uses electronic and computer-generated images to give an individual the illusion of participating in fabricated events. Virtual reality environments have great promise as a way to provide a "dry run" through risky or costly procedures. As a method for surgical planning, a software model of a patient can be programmed by using data from various electronic and computer-assisted diagnostic tests. By importing this outside data, a physician could operate in virtual reality to determine the most efficient or effective procedure.

A good illustration of technology integration is Harvard Community Health Plan's use of interactive protocols to collect information directly from the patient. HCHP has patients in about 150 households using home computers to receive medical advice and general health information. Plans for this system include service to over 5,000 households. The goal of the system is to improve patient education, raise the quality of health care, and lower costs by reducing the number of unnecessary visits.[17]

In this era of technological change and increased user expectations, the trend can be seen in other areas as well, especially through the marriage of small desktop computers with larger computers. This integration and expansion will continue to be seen through such operations as tracking patients throughout an entire system, automated medical records that are accessible by all locations, and the networking of community groups and facilities.[18] By most estimates, computerized patient care records will be an important feature of the reformed health care delivery system, drawing patient data currently scattered among various providers into an integrated format containing the most useful information.

The development of health information networks (HIN), where a combination of computer software and communications facilities permit multiple users to transmit, receive, and store all forms of health care data, including image and voice, can easily be envisioned. Although no existing HIN has yet to fully develop the complete range of functions that the technology is capable of achieving, hundreds of companies are providing support for these kind of electronic data interchange activities (EDI). The Blue Cross organizations, the regional Bell operating companies, and the Hartford Foundation are active in this regard.[19] The regional health care system of the future will have its internal clinical and administrative systems connected to each other and to an external HIN. In such a setting, new approaches to patient care and efficient operation are plausible. Each patient encounter, for example, could be tracked from initial complaint through treatment to final outcome. Physicians could also admit patients remotely and check inpatient status from their offices.[20]

The success of the Wisconsin Health Information Network in Milwaukee, provides support for the notion that the merging of technologies will make organizations better positioned for health care reform. This HIN has combined computer software and communications facilities so client users can easily transmit, receive, and store all forms of health care data, including image and voice. Leveraging of existing technologies permits physicians to pick up a telephone and send clinical and administrative information to hospitals, as well as to retrieve data. Ameritech, the Chicago-based telecommunication parent company of the Wisconsin Health Information Network, believes merging telecommunication technology with health information technology will serve the needs of health care organizations and reduce administrative costs for organizations.[21] Of course, a major challenge to effective implementation of all of these technologies is managing the security and privacy realities cited in Chapters Seven and Eight, as well as the concerns elaborated below.

Managing Emerging Technologies

While health care executives generally perceive great benefits from new technology, it is axiomatic that they will have problems managing the new and emerging technologies. It is easy to concede that every good thing about new technology has an "evil twin." For example, many hail the benefits of Internet, the global web that connects more than thirty thousand on-line networks. Its usefulness as a disseminator of information and its potential in the information superhighway is unlimited. The possibility of list servers on the Internet specifically attuned to health care topics carries great promise. Nonetheless, the sheer accessibility of the "Net" allows people to spread viruses much more easily than was possible before.

Voice recognition, a technology that allows a computer to translate spoken words into digitized text without the intervention of a human transcriptionist, has enormous potential but limited usefulness unless the technology is fast and powerful enough to accommodate normal speech patterns and large vocabularies. The likelihood of unintended consequences caused by unseen flaws in the technology increases if the technological limitations of the hardware and software are disregarded.

The fundamental issue in managing new and emerging technology, however, may not necessarily be the hardware or software. As Boxerman and Gribbens see it, the underlying concern is the logic of the systems that the computer executes.[22] According to Boxerman and Gribbens, health care executives must focus on the appropriateness of the various models, the accuracy of the databases and the skill levels of the functional specialists working with the new technology. Boxerman and Gribbens offer four issues to consider in the management of new technology: (1) the time constraints in implementing the new technology; (2) the institutional capabilities; (3) the degree of employee acceptance regarding the need for technological improvement; and (4) the degree of work interdependence existing in the organization and how that intensity of collaboration in the organization affects the smooth implementation of new technology.

In addition to distinguishing the underlying logic of the new technology, another major problem health service organizations face in managing new technology is the issue of responsibility. The responsibility for managing technology in health service organizations is often diffused among upper management, line managers of technology, and technology users.[23] Some suggest that, in order to improve the effective management of technology and to maintain a competitive technological edge, health care service organizations in the 1990s may benefit from a corporate level technology management function such as a chief technology officer (CTO). The CTO would effectively supervise technology activities in the organization, focus on technology health, acquire external technologies, and coordinate technology effort in the organization.[24]

As information systems play an increasingly important role in the success of the health care organization of the future, others suggest that someone in the organization must be designated to link information systems capabilities with the strategic direction of the organization. Accordingly, a number of health service organizations and health care systems are bringing information management into the senior level executive domain in the form of the chief information officer (CIO) position. It is asserted that the "true" CIO of the future goes beyond simply controlling data. The CIO is an executive team member, sitting at the planning table recommending computer solutions to executive strategy problems.[25] In some organizations, the coordinating focus of managing emerging information technologies will conceivably be the CIO, a corporate senior manager, who sets priorities to achieve organization/system-wide objectives. The eminence attributed to information system management is supported by a number of experts who predict that among the more important trends shaping the future labor force in health care will be the increasing prevalence of health information specialists.[26]

Technological innovation, brought about by the paradigm shifts in health care will further affect how we make decisions. As health services executives struggle to deal with financing and delivery system changes, the relentless onslaught of new technology and information system needs confronts them. Managing these issues can easily overwhelm, but allowing new technology and information systems to haphazardly proliferate is both irresponsible and imprudent.

With this in mind, the Wharton School at the University of Pennsylvania has produced a number of action guidelines that help in managing innovative technology.[27] These are starting points for managers who are continually challenged with the accelerated pace of new needs and urgent priorities.

First, determine the "risk personality" of the organization. How averse to risk is the organization? Does the organization generally cope well with shifts in strategies and adjustments to external pressures?

Second, assess business plans with a view toward technology. How can information system technologies be linked with the strategic direction of the organization?

Third, evaluate what significant developments in health care might affect the use of technology. How does the trend toward managed care and competition create new information needs and technological capabilities?

Fourth, integrate technology plans and assessments into a business plan. How does the organization use current and future information technologies to attain long-term and short-term goals and objectives?

Fifth, be prepared to induce change with leadership and rewards. How does the organization communicate its comfort level with innovation through senior level management attitudes and action?

We would add a sixth guideline, namely, carefully evaluate the security, privacy, and social implications of adopting the new systems.

The managerial challenges associated with emerging technology requires an in-depth understanding of its ramifications to the organization as a whole, to its employees, its patients, and to the future direction of the institution itself. As the changes in health care delivery and financing move forward and the industry shakes out, successfully managing innovative technology will undoubtedly play a significant role in the viability of health-related organizations. The concepts probed in the previous chapters are offered as aids for meeting that managerial challenge.

Notes

1. *The New Yorker*, 20 June 1994, 84.
2. J. K. Kerr and R. Jelinek, "Impact of Technology in Health Care and Health Administration: Hospitals and Alternative Care Delivery Systems," *Journal of Health Administration Education*, 8, no. 1, 1990, 5–10.
3. D. Johnson, "Hospitals Must Prepare for the Paradigm Shifts to Managed Care," *Health Care Strategic Management*, December 1993, 10–13.
4. See C. Heinemann, in *Health Care Executive*, January–February 1992, 32.
5. C. J. Austin and B. T. Malec, "An Ideal Curriculum Model," *Journal of Healthcare Administration Education*, 8, no. 1, 1990, 53–61.
6. Johnson, 10.
7. W. Wachel, "CIO—Roles and Relationships," *Healthcare Executive*, January–February 1992, 14–16.
8. J. Ferguson, "I/S Interoperability a Must in Tomorrow's Complex Health Care Environment," *Computers in Healthcare*, November 1993, 22–28.
9. J. K. H. Tan, "Graduate Education in Health Information Systems," *Journal of Health Administration Education*, Winter 1993, 33–34.
10. Ibid, 33.
11. R. Dick and E. Steens, eds., "The Computer-Based Patient Record: An Essential Technology for Health Care," Committee on Improving the Patient Care Record, Division of Healthcare Services, *Institute of Medicine*, 1991, 35.
12. For example, see the *1994 Reference Guide for the Health Care Technology Industry*, Health Care Technology Institute, 41.
13. P. J. Haigh, "CIH Survey Confirms Communication Networks as Vital Health Care Technologies," *Computers in Healthcare*, December 1993, 24–28.
14. T. Binius, "Conference Report: Executive Forum on Information Management," *Healthcare Executive*, September–October 1992, 38–39.
15. R. Bergman, "Integrated Information Paves the Way to Better Decision Making on Patient Care," *Hospitals & Health Networks*, 5 January 1994, 56.

16. ———, "Letting Telemedicine Do the Walking," *Hospitals & Health Networks,* 20 October 1993, 46–48.

17. ———, "Computers Make 'House Calls' to Patients," *Hospitals,* 20 May 1993, 52.

18. Wachel, 15.

19. J. E. Kasputys and S. Lazarus, "Health Information Networks: Connecting Your Healthcare Organization to the Future," *Healthcare Executive,* November–December 1993, 21–23.

20. Ibid, 23.

21. R. Bergman, "Telecommunicators Making Their Way into the Health Care Market," *Hospitals & Health Networks,* 5 September 1993, 60.

22. S. Boxerman and R. Gribbens, "Technology Management in the '90s," *Healthcare Executive,* January 1991, 21–23.

23. O. Heller, "The New Role of Chief Technology Officer in U.S. Hospitals," *International Journal of Technology Management,* 7, nos. 6–8, 1992, 455–61.

24. Ibid, 455.

25. R. Hard, "The Real Thing: Future Information Needs Will Require 'True' Hospital CIO's," *Hospitals,* 20 February 1993, 30–31.

26. J. L. Sherer, "Five Trends Shaping the Future Labor Force," *Hospitals & Health Networks,* 5 October 1993, 30–31.

27. R. Simpson, "Managing Innovative Technology," *Nursing Management,* 10 October 1993, 18–19.

Selected Readings

Binnius, T. "Community Health Information Networks (CHIN) Are Underway," *Healthcare Financial Management* (January 1994): 61.

Holusha, J. "Carving Out Real Life Uses for Virtual Reality." *New York Times* (31 October 1993): F-11.

Lumsdon, K. "All Connected: Infrastructure Is the Path to IS Growth." *Hospitals* (20 February 1993): 31.

———. "Medical Informatics-Point-of-Care Clinical Systems Gain Ground." *MedPRO Month* (February 1993): 28.

Seabrook, J. "My First Flame." *New Yorker* (6 June 1994): 70–79.

Sherer, J. L. "Clinical Information Systems: Up to Par?" *Hospitals & Health Networks* (20 August 1994): 28.

Smith, L. "The Coming Health Care Shakeout." *Fortune* (17 May 1993): 76.

———. "Study Forsees 17 Trends Altering Healthcare." *Health Industry Today* (January 1994): 10–11.

READING

MICHAEL CARRIGAN attempts to gear our perspective on information management to his estimate of the nature of the future health care environment. Already, he argues, "Information managers are being asked to accomplish impossible tasks with their currently installed systems." He outlines how health care managers might position their information systems to respond to the health care realities of the year 2000 and beyond. The managerial concepts presented throughout the book are, of course, essential in wisely evaluating Carrigan's vision.

The Future of Health Care Information Systems

Michael Carrigan

Health Delivery System of the 1990s

The health care delivery system in the United States is undergoing dramatic and widespread changes that will continue to occur through the 1990s. Mounting pressure to lower cost and to increase quality of care will continue to challenge health care executives. Hospital census continues to decline as our primary care facilities experience the traditional life-cycle curve that is encountered by other industries. Legislative action by federal and state government could have a profound impact on the health care delivery system. Competition will most certainly become more intense as hospitals try to remain in the anchor of their community-based health care delivery system.

Reprinted by permission from "The Future of Health Care Information Systems, by M. Carrigan. *Hospital Materiel Management Quarterly*, vol. 15, no. 1, 1–13. © 1992 Aspen Publishers, Inc.

Hospital executives recognize the importance of patient-centered care and the impact that it will have on the future of their respective hospitals. As a result, executives in many hospitals are in the process of implementing total quality management (TQM)/continuous quality improvement (CQI) plans. Patients become customers, each process in the health care delivery system is evaluated to ensure customer satisfaction, and departments and staff, recognizing each other as customers of their respective services, consider how each one's successful delivery of these services affects the other and customer satisfaction. Service offerings are continually evaluated, modified, and implemented to provide the best quality of care for the customers. Most executives now understand that successful implementation of a TQM/CQI plan is necessary to provide a cohesive foundation for the health care delivery system of the 1990s and beyond.

Many questions arise as health care executives position their organizations for the future. What role will the traditional hospital play in an altered health care delivery system? How will hospitals differentiate from competitive facilities? What factors will physicians consider when choosing an acute care facility for their patients? How will the successful implementation of TQM/CQI plans in health care facilities define the requirements for information systems? What role will information systems play in the future health care delivery system? How will future technology advancements, from an information systems perspective, be utilized by the health care delivery industry to improve patient care?

These questions and more will have to be answered in the coming years. In order to deal with the changes that will have to take place in information systems as the health care delivery system changes, we must discuss examples of how the delivery system could change and what role the hospital will play in the new system. We must understand the status of our current information systems and how they will have to change to operate within the new delivery system. Finally, we must look at emerging technologies, their contribution to the new delivery system, and how to upgrade our existing information systems.

In the past, the traditional hospital was the focal point of most health care services. Patients went to hospitals for many services, from emergency, laboratory, and radiology to surgery, physical therapy, and mental health. Many of the services provided by the hospital are now available from independent health care facilities in the community. Ambulatory care centers, walk-up clinics, surgicenters, and independent laboratories are providing more and more services that were formerly available only from the hospital. Physicians have installed radiology equipment, laboratory equipment, and outpatient surgery facilities in their offices. In addition, many physicians participate in limited partnerships that own independent health care delivery service organizations that compete with the services offered by hospitals. Therefore, many hospitals must aggressively compete for these same customers or find alternative service offerings to guarantee fiscal stability of the facility.

Hospital executives will certainly be debating as to the best course of action for their facilities. From the financial perspective, some may want to specialize and compete, some may want to invest in partnerships that provide services in the community, some may choose to merge with a local competitor in order to share resources, some may want to participate aggressively in health maintenance organization (HMO) and preferred provider organization (PPO) relationships, and others may implement a strategy that supports all of the above.

Regardless of the strategy that is implemented to provide financial viability, the quality of patient care and customer satisfaction will be the primary focal point of each of these executives. Information systems will become an integral part of the model for patient-centered care, and traditional hospital information systems may not provide the foundation to support the changes in the health care delivery system. There is a significant difference between information systems that were developed from the premise of providing accurate and timely patient billing and accounting, or to provide the most efficient and productive laboratory, and a system that has been developed from the premise of delivering quality patient-centered care that supports the implementation of TQM/CQI plans.

It is difficult to pinpoint exactly how our health care delivery system will look in the future, but it is certain that information systems will influence the success or failure of the delivery system within each community. As the delivery system continues to change from a hospital-based system to a community-based system of independent organizations, information sharing will become a critical information systems requirement to support the basic premise of providing quality patient care. Hospitals can partner with the independent providers to create a community-based organization that results in an agreement to share appropriate patient information with all providers within the organization. The hospital that can organize the independent health care providers could emerge as the primary facility for referrals from various providers and could expand its partnerships by referring patients to other specialty service providers. The hospital can become the foundation for the community-based organization of independent providers that focuses on the continuum of care and delivers quality patient care from cradle to grave.

As hospitals organize the health care delivery system in the community and provide the vehicle for information sharing, they will be in a position to provide additional services to the providers within the organization. An appropriately designed information system may be able to provide the billing and reimbursement services for the providers, as well as providing the qualification databases for various insurance, HMO, and PPO programs. Thus, patients will receive higher quality of care as well as higher quality of service, which benefits the customer, the provider, and the hospital.

For information sharing to be successful, a consolidated database of information will have to be built. This database will contain information by patient that has been accumulated from all facilities that have provided services for the patient. The database may be clinical repositories, billing information, or qualification data, and may be accessed by individuals with the appropriate security clearances. Presently, most information that is shared between clinics, hospitals, and physicians is by actual physical transfer of paper documents by fax or mail. Although this may be a cooperative effort amongst the providers, there is significant opportunity for this system to fail. Patients have a much greater chance of lower quality care and inefficient processing of crucial information. Providers that have access to a comprehensive clinical repository of information will be able to offer the highest quality of care.

The clinical repository is only the beginning of the paperless medical record. The clinical database could integrate the entire chronological history of patient visits to various providers within the community. However, signed documents and images would still have to be transferred manually. Images from X-ray and magnetic resonance imaging (MRI) equipment and actual video presentation of patient symptoms as well as consent forms, insurance forms, and picture identification will be required to complete the paperless medical record. Upon successful implementation and integration of these various technologies, the hospital will be able to offer community providers a service to support quality patient-centered care. Hospitals that can offer the providers of health care services information that will enhance patient care and improve customer satisfaction will remain the cornerstone of community-based health care delivery systems.

Traditional Hospital Information Systems

Hospital information systems budgets have been growing as a percent of total budgets, and chief information officers and information systems directors are facing the challenge of controlling costs and improving productivity of the information systems departments. As the health care delivery system continues to change and the health care institutions react to these changes, implementation of new software applications in a timely and efficient manner becomes extremely important. Many information system managers are being asked to accomplish impossible tasks with their currently installed systems. In addition, the information systems departments that are having trouble keeping up with the changes and requests are in hospitals whose information systems budgets are higher than industry averages. Health care executives who understand the changes in our delivery system will recognize the importance of information systems for the institution's future stability, and they will be very concerned with these statistics.

Health care institutions that face this situation have similar profiles. Information systems are based on proprietary technology costing millions of dollars to procure and maintain. Application software is typically heavily modified to meet the specific needs of a hospital's requirements based on a static health care delivery system. Most of these systems were designed to provide patient accounting and billing services, and the design of the system does not offer a logical progression to patient-centered care applications. As a result, information systems managers are left with inflexible systems that require huge capital outlays to purchase and demand exorbitant ongoing maintenance costs to operate.

In addition, owing to the inflexible operating environment of the main systems, department managers have typically purchased separate systems for the specific applications to run the departments. Specialized applications for electronic billing, pharmacy, laboratory, radiology, medical records, and materiel management are in many cases installed on separate systems. The proprietary nature of each of these systems creates severe interface and communication problems for the information systems managers. The sharing and consolidation of information becomes nearly impossible. Although archaic interfaces are usually developed to provide some sort of consolidated reporting, the information is limited and the support of these numerous required interfaces is overwhelming. The health care institution must deal with inadequate consolidated reporting, an extensive backlog of requests for system changes that are extremely expensive to implement, many dissatisfied users, and departments with no information systems support.

Health care institutions that fit the profile described above could face considerable problems in the future. As the health care delivery system continues to evolve, information systems must keep pace with the changes in a timely manner. Large proprietary information systems implementations will not provide the price performance and flexibility required to support the community-based health care delivery system of the future. Hospitals that have invested millions of dollars in their current information systems must evaluate their tangible and intangible costs on a long-term basis to determine the best course of action. Tangible costs for ongoing maintenance, personnel skill sets required to support the systems with associated salaries and benefits, outside consulting contracts, depreciation and amortization, real estate costs, power consumption, redundant hardware, professional development and recruiting, and supplies must be analyzed on a long-term basis. Consideration must also be given to analysis of intangible costs such as flexibility of operating environment, implementation of prevailing industry standards, and architectural design that supports implementation of a TQM/CQI plan.

An analysis of a typical 400-bed health care facility that has installed and implemented a large proprietary system is summarized in Table [11.2]. The cost to procure proprietary hardware, application software, utilities, implementation services, and other items was approximately $6,300,000 with associated operating costs of approximately $1,750,000. The approximate operating cost and depreciation expense for this information systems environment are $2,850,000 per year. This environment may not include adequate services for the ancillary departments, and the departments are probably incurring additional data processing costs that have been incorporated in the specific departments' budgets.

The proprietary system usually has extremely limited communications capabilities for sharing of information with other systems, and the provider has either limited or no access to the information that is available on the system. Information is shared by hard copy printouts or not at all, which severely restricts the provider's opportunity to deliver high-quality patient care.

Mission 2000—Health Care Information Systems of the Future

Health care information systems of the future will have to provide information systems managers with the flexibility to respond efficiently to the rapidly changing environment. The health care delivery system of the future will be a community-based organization of independent service providers. Information sharing to promote high-quality patient-centered care will become the foundation of health care information systems of the future. Large amounts of information containing text,

Table 11.2 Cost Performance of Modified Proprietary Information System in Typical 400-bed Health Care Facility*

Capital Costs	
Hardware	$2,300,000
Utilities	100,000
Software	1,900,000
Uninterruptable power supply, etc.	400,000
Implementation	1,600,000
Total	$6,300,000
Operating Costs	
Personnel salaries	$750,000†
Benefits	140,000
Hardware maintenance	195,000
System software/utilities	140,000
Application software	300,000
Insurance, misc.	30,000
Supplies	60,000
Professional development	35,000
Recruiting	20,000
Outside services	80,000
Total	$1,750,000
Summary Depreciation Schedule	
Hardware—utilities 7 yr.	$356,000
Application software 5 yr.	380,000
Implementation—misc. 5 yr.	355,000
Depreciation expense	$1,100,000

* Information contained in the analysis is based on sample information presented by the health care consulting divisions of Ernst and Young and KPMG Peat Marwick.

† 21 Full-time equivalents including management and support staff for the information systems department.

images, and video will be required to support the health care delivery system of the future. Patients will demand higher quality service at a reasonable cost, and properly implemented information systems will provide considerable support for the realization of that goal.

The hospital can position itself as the collection agent of patient information to support the community-based health care delivery system. An organization of health care providers with the hospital as the central information point may offer the best example of a patient-centered, high-quality, low-cost health care delivery system. Health care executives and managers with a similar vision will have to understand the influence that information systems technologies can have on the success of this delivery system. Information from many sources will have to be consolidated and made available to the health care producers within the community in a real-time environment. Laboratory results from an independent laboratory can be uploaded to the hospital-based clinical repository. Information related to an outpatient surgical procedure performed on the patient at a local surgicenter can be consolidated with the recent laboratory results. MRI images with analysis reports dictated by a specialist may also be included. The physician responsible for primary care can have access to all this information from a desktop device in the office.

Hospitals that can provide this type of environment will demonstrate to the providers and the patients of the community a sincere commitment to quality patient-centered care. The providers and the patients of the community will align themselves with institutions that can deliver these high-quality services. These institutions will be positioned to receive referrals from many providers and refer their patients to specialty providers while providing comprehensive care from cradle to grave for the patient.

Implementation of advanced information systems technology will be required to support the health care delivery system of the future. Information sharing environments will require computer system implementations based on standard operating systems and communication protocols, high-speed networks utilizing fiber optic technology, relational databases, imaging, video, optical storage systems, hand-held computers, and highly available systems and disk storage systems. These advanced information systems will be designed around high-speed commodity reduced instruction set computing (RISC) and computer processing units (CPUs). Each of these significant state-of-the-art technologies and sample of the standards are outlined below.

The design of an information sharing system must be based on industry standards. Some vendors try to dictate the standards, and others conform to standards defined by independent standards organizations. It is important to evaluate each vendor's definition of standard against the criteria that the health care institution regards as relevant. An industry standards-based information system from a hardware and software perspective will provide the institution with an "open" systems environment. An open systems implementation guarantees the health care institution the greatest flexibility to implement the best products that support the goal of information sharing. Standards may be defined by IEEE, Unix International, Open Software Foundation, AT&T, OSI, and POSIX, or de facto standards like MS/DOS and UNIX emerge.

Communication of data can be conducted over industry standard hardware networks utilizing standards-based protocols like TCP/IP, Token Ring, Novell, or FDDI. Interfaces between the computer processing unit and disk storage subsystems will be done through standard interface requirements defined by the small computer interface standard (SCSI). Data can be formatted for transferral by the HL-7 definition, a health care industry standard for transferring patient information between systems.

Enabling technologies and development of the 1990s provide health care institutions with many alternatives outside the traditional information systems environment. CPUs based on RISC technology provide mainframe class computing power at a fraction of the cost. The industry has vastly improved the cost per megabyte (MB) of disk storage technology. Database technology has radically improved, and much more efficient application software development tools have become available. The operating environment on these new systems stress adherence to the standards, resulting in a more open platform, which facilitates the sharing of resources and information over a common systems network.

The operating system platform should be used on industry standards. Industry standard operating systems like UNIX for the host information sharing systems and MS/DOS and Novell for workstations and departmental computers will provide the health care institution a foundation that supports many products. Most of the application software products and industry standard communications are being developed and enhanced for these platforms. Systems based on industry standard hardware and software more open for flexibility, faster for more efficient processing of data, and less costly to purchase and maintain than comparable systems based on proprietary technology. Host systems based on the UNIX operating system will ensure compatibility with future systems and permit open connectivity with other hardware systems in the community.

The systems located throughout provider offices in the community will be linked by an open-system data communications network. Networks will become an integral component of health care systems that are designed for the sharing of patient information. Data located in systems for laboratory, pharmacy, surgicenter, radiology, physicians, and clinics will have to be formatted and transferred to the information sharing system. High-speed local area networks (LAN) and wide area networks (WAN) will be configured to transfer these large volumes of data in an efficient manner. Industry standard communications protocols will be used to facilitate the access and transfer of data and information from laboratory instruments and radiology equipment to the information system. Patient information will be made available to the appropriate provider or organization over the same network. Data communications networks must be configured with the band width to support the network traffic that will occur in this environment. Patient information inclusive of text, video, and images will require extremely high-speed network implementations. Networks capable of supporting these applications and large amounts of data will be based on fiber optic technology. Fiber optic network implementations provide support for high-speed configurations and are easily installed.

Another important component of the health care information system will be the database software that is employed to consolidate the patient information. Information from the entire community of providers will be stored on this common database; therefore the reflection of the database software must be given priority. Many relational database application software products that support large volumes of data are available on the market. Database architectures need to be evaluated for conformity to standards, speed, high availability features, user friendliness, and user interface, security, and interface capabilities for access to imaging and video. Standard query language (SQL) should be supported for simple and ad hoc access to patient information. Superior quality development tools must be available to enhance productivity of the information systems support staff. User access to all patient information must be easy, efficient, and available from this consolidated database of patient information. It is imperative that the database software platform provide the flexibility and the tools to satisfy these requirements.

The consolidated database must be capable of interfacing to or storing imaging data. Access to images over the community-based network will become an important aspect of the implementation. Imaging technology is progressing rapidly and will become an integral component of the paperless medical record. Scanning devices will be used to capture images of patient consent forms, insurance forms, and numerous other paper trails of information that need to be available on-line to enhance the efficiency of the health care providers in the community. Moreover, images from X-ray and MRI equipment will be stored and made available as a component of the medical record of the patient. It will be important to select imaging application solutions that are based on standards to work within the framework of the information sharing environment accessible at the same time as other patient information.

Video technology is rapidly being integrated into computer systems. Storage of and access to video could become an important component of the future health care information system. Access to video from computer workstations will provide another significant component of information to improve quality of care. Although the technology is available to include video access through intelligent workstations, video will probably be the last component implemented in the patient information system. This technology may have to improve to be easily integrated into the system.

Information sharing requires the storage of extremely large amounts of data in the form of text, images, and video. The hardware storage systems required to support these large amounts of data must be highly available to the user and cost-effective to implement. The information is stored on two types of media to be accessed on-line by the user. Magnetic disk subsystems will continue to be used for information that is crucial to ongoing patient care, while historical information will be stored on optical storage systems. Magnetic disk technology continues to advance, and the cost per megabyte of storage has dropped significantly. As a result, it is cost-effective to keep more patient information on-line for longer periods of time. Disk technology has also been revolutionized with the introduction of redundant arrays of inexpensive disk (RAID). RAID technology allows data to be spread on an array of disks while simultaneously a backup copy of the information is stored over the same disks (RAID 5). The backup copy of the data stores only enough information to restore the data to its original form and requires only 20 percent of the space. Therefore, one-to-one disk mirroring if unnecessary, and the cost of the RAID implementation is much less. If any one of the disks in the array fails, the user will not experience any loss of data. When the failed disk is replaced, the system will automatically restore the disk to the point of failure and continue to operate with no effect on users or the integrity of the data. These highly available disk subsystems require less space to install, less power to operate, and are less costly to maintain than the traditional implementation of magnetic disks.

The archiving of historical data, typically stored on fiche or hard copy, will be on optical disks. Optical disk technology provides for massive amounts of information on an extremely small physical medium. Although this technology is not efficient enough to be used as the storage medium for day-to-day operations, owing to slower response times, it is ideal for the archival storage and retrieval process. Patient information that is not currently required for delivery of care will be archived to the optical disk subsystems. Up to a gigabyte (GB) of information may be stored on a single optical disk the size of an audio computer disk (CD). These optical disks may be stored in a jukebox that includes many disks, providing an archival system that can contain information for many years on thousands of patients. The software that supports the jukebox and access to the archived information will be integrated to the database of patient information to allow seamless provider accessibility.

Hand-held computers, an innovative technologic advancement, will be implemented for numerous patient care services. The hand-held computers will allow nurses to have immediate access to patient care plans; home health nurses will be able to record patient information at the point of care, and phlebotomists will be able to record information for use by laboratory personnel while performing their duties. More important, hand-held computers will decrease the amount of information that has to be processed multiple times by the nursing staff. Productivity will increase, which will allow nurses to have additional time available to provide better quality patient care. Hand-held systems will be available to download information from the main system—like care plans, which can be updated by the nurse and uploaded to the host information system. Radio frequency technology will be implemented to provide on-line access to the host system by the health care provider. Hand-held computers could be the answer to the often unsuccessful implementation of bedside terminals. They are compact, fitting in the palm of a hand; therefore, they may not be inhibiting to patients and providers of care. The design of the hand-held systems and the software to support the operation will be based on minimizing the number of key strokes to record information. Innovative technology has been jointly developed by hardware and software companies to provide this functionality. Hand-held devices will become an integral part of the total health care information system designed for optimal patient-centered care.

Integration of the various technologies described above will require extremely powerful computer processors. Significant technologic advances have been made in RISC-based computing. RISC-based CPUs are now being delivered by large semiconductor facilities with unbeatable price performance. RISC CPUs can deliver the performance of traditional mainframe computer systems for a fraction of the cost. Many of the RISC-based CPUs are being designed to operate in a symmetric multiprocessing environment, and computer systems companies are integrating multiple CPUs in a single computer system. The integration of multiple CPUs in a single system requires sophisticated operating software to produce scaleable performance increases.

Implementations such as this represent the future for high-speed, low-cost data processing.

The information sharing health care system described above must be available to the providers at all times to be successful. High-quality patient-centered care cannot be delivered if the information required to support that care is not available to the providers. Financial planners and managed care administrators cannot work to hold down costs unless the information is available in a timely and efficient manner. As a result, the concept of high availability will become an important aspect of the health care information systems of the future. High availability and fault tolerant environments have been available in the mainframe world, but the cost for these systems is prohibitive to most health care institutions. However, hardware and software technology has advanced, and high-availability configurations will be costbeneficial to all health care facilities. The RISC based solutions implemented with RAID disk subsystems provide the foundation for highly available patient information systems. Coupled with redundant disk or tape controllers, uninterruptible power supplies, network redundancy, CPU-to-CPU failover, and sophisticated diagnostic software, health care facilities will be able to implement a system that will be accessible by the providers of the community 99.9 percent of the time. The cost for these implementations is not prohibitive, and upon analysis of the impact of downtime, the additional cost can easily be justified.

The skill sets of the personnel who support the future health care information systems will be profoundly different from the traditional mainframe environment described above. Application software will be provided primarily by industry specialists, which eliminates the requirement of a huge systems staff of programmers. Standards-based operating system software will be primarily supported by the vendors, and the support staff will not have to be trained for a specific proprietary product. The systems support staff will focus on the integration of information from various community-based ancillary systems, network optimization, database access, and presentation tools. The systems support staff will become an integral component of the TQM/CQI plan to deliver quality patient-centered care by facilitating access to patient information in a timely manner.

Systems based on standards cost less than proprietary systems owing to competition and integration of standards-based commodity components. Health care institutions benefit from implementing standards-based systems from the perspective of price, support, flexibility, future applications, and above all, information sharing. We have outlined the cost of a traditional mainframe system.

These systems would typically be configured with hospital-based access, limited networking capabilities, if any, limited information sharing in the form of admissions, discharge, and transfer (ADT) and results reporting, and no provider access of information on-line. To implement a common database of text-based patient information, graphics, imaging, and video would be cost-prohibitive in the mainframe environment.

The costs outlined in Table 11.3 include replacement costs for a typical 400-bed mainframe environment and approximate costs of high-speed networks, hand-held computers, and optical archiving components.

The approximate operating costs and depreciation for this information systems environment are $1,550,000 per year. Operating costs are decreased by $830,000 per year and the initial capital outlay has been decreased by 42 percent from the traditional mainframe system. Payback on the initial investment will occur in approximately four and a half years based on the savings in operating costs. Other expected results, according to KMPG Peat Marwick, are 25 percent reduction in staffing including reduced layers of management, 70 percent reduction in floor space, and network capabilities with excess capacity for future systems integration. The information will be more reliable, access to information is more efficient because users do not have to rely on information systems staff, and system downtime is limited.

Many health care institutions have installed large proprietary systems, and they may not believe that they can implement the newer technology. However, a long-term analysis of the financial considerations, improvement to quality of care, and the strategic implications for long-term viability is necessary before arriving at such a conclusion.

Health care institutions need to position their organizations for the future. As the health care delivery system evolves and new regulations are introduced, the institutions that can organize the providers of care in their respective communities will be successful. The organization of the community-based health care providers will be dedicated to constantly improving the quality of patient care. The sharing of information from each of these providers will become an integral component of this process. The institution that strategically positions its facilities as the information processor and makes that information available to providers will be the survivor of this rapidly changing system.

Table 11.3 Estimated Costs of Replacement Standards-Based Information System in 400-Bed Health Care Facility

Capital Costs	
Hardware	$850,000
Network	500,000
Software	1,200,000
UPS, optical	250,000
Implementation	500,000
Hand-held systems @ $500	100,000
Database software	250,000
Total	$3,650,000+
Operating Costs	
Personnel salaries	$500,000*
Benefits	100,000†
Hardware network maint.	75,000
System software	10,000
Application software	100,000
Insurance, misc.	20,000
Supplies	60,000
Professional development	15,000‡
Recruiting	10,000¶
Outside services	30,000‖
Total	$920,000
Estimated Summary Depreciation Schedule	
Hardware—network 7 yr.	$240,000
Application software 5 yr.	240,000
Database software 5 yr.	50,000
Implementation—misc. 5 yr.	100,000
Depreciation expense	$630,000

* Approximately 16 FTEs, including management and support staff for the information systems department. Salaries will decrease with replacement of highly specialized technical staff to productivity-oriented staff.

† Reduces as salaries decrease and fewer FTEs are required to support the system.

‡ Professional development costs decrease as the profile of information systems employees changes from programmer-analysts to information or education specialists.

¶ Recruiting costs decrease as the need to recruit highly skilled programmers and analysts declines.

‖ Outside service contracts decrease owing to the availability of quality application software products.

+ Costs estimates are based on a sample of hardware and software configurations provided by hardware and software companies in the health care industry.

Suggested Readings

Goldman, E. "Vision 2000: A View of the Emerging Delivery System." Westboro, MA: Data General Corporation, 31 March 1992.

Kissinger, K. "Downsizing." Westboro, MA: Data General Corporation, 31 March 1992.

Kramer, R., Cascio, R., and Czahor, J. "Downsizing HIS Can Save You Millions." Health Care Financial Management Association 1991 National Convention, 18 June 1991.

Packer, C. L. "Hospitals with the Best Information Systems," *Hospitals* 66 (February 1992): 56–58, 60, 62–65.

Michael Carrigan, B.S., District Manager, Health Care Sales, Data General Corporation, Irvine, California.

CASE 11
Quincy Community Health Plan

D R. LAURA SCHNEIDER, an internist at the Quincy Community Health Plan, turned on her desktop computer, clicked the cursor to a patient's name, entered a code, and instantly received a detailed account of a 69 year-old man's medical record. Without any extensive background in computers, Dr. Schneider was able to get a detailed account of the man's arthritic problems, a history of the medication prescribed to him, his detailed medical history, and a list of his previous office visits.

Dr. Schneider, had been selected as one of 15 physicians and nurses in the Quincy Community Health Plan, one of the largest health maintenance organizations in the country, to have access to the new computer system. With 20 QCHP centers in the Chicago area, Dr. Schneider's center had been a test site for the new system for the past six months. Paul Eugene, director of the project, estimated that it would take approximately five years before the organization-wide system would be operational for the more than 600,000 patients and 1,100 physicians at the 20 QCHP centers.

With market forces heating up and rising pressures to cut costs and improve quality, competition among medical providers had increased the sense of urgency for QCHP to become more efficient. Eugene recalled that senior managers had realized for some time that, despite initial costs, the new technology represented by a computerized interactive patient-record network covering the entire 20 centers, would not be a technical luxury, but an economic necessity. While only 1 or 2 percent of health care facilities around the nation have started to make this technological leap, QCHP had been warned by their management consultants that, those that fail to make the leap in the coming years will be "taken over by more aggressive competitors or disappear."

Through a central data base, all QCHP physicians would have access to patient records. They would be able to share up-to-date information on each of the 600,000 patients subscribing to the plan. All of the paper records crammed into thousands of file folders would be eliminated. Eventually the system would feed information into nation-wide data bases, and that data could be studied to determine treatment outcomes. This would provide invaluable data in helping physicians to eliminate unnecessary procedures and eradicate the need for repeating tests when results are misplaced.

Dr. Schneider remembered her first several meetings with Paul Eugene prior to the test system's installation. He noted that the system allowed the physician to walk through a diagnosis of a variety of illnesses by listing out a set of symptoms. It enabled Dr. Schneider to send prescriptions to the center's pharmacy and order diagnostic tests. It would track every prescription and test result and alert her if a patient didn't have a prescription filled or a test administered. It would remind her of allergies and other conditions about her patient. The system would also have image-processing capability for storing x-rays, CAT scans and MRI scans electronically. The fiber-optic infrastructure had the capacity for multi-media electronic physician consultations, an artificial intelligence "protocol" program that could compare past patient procedures with facts in the current case, and a capability to calculate exact costs of every variable of care of any procedure. The driving goal behind this huge undertaking was to have the right information at the right time and the right place.

Although both Dr. Schneider and Paul Eugene were convinced that the new technologies and the integration/networking capabilities of the system positioned QCHP for survival, a number of issues emerged that suggested a down side to "progress." The complexities associated with the relentless and unstoppable growth of new information technologies had raised a number of managerial concerns.

For example, Eugene remembered how difficult it was to sell the Board of Directors on such a large capital expenditure. QCHP had been burned by problems associated with the implementation of a partial—now obsolete—network several years ago. Consequently, justifying the costs was a tough job. Senior managers surveyed large local providers contemplating similar organization-wide integrated systems. Those that were surveyed were not able to determine any kind of dollar numbers regarding savings. Invariably, they claimed that this was impossible to do because so many intangibles are often associated with new technologies.

While most hospitals and health systems had computerized data systems for financial and "back office" functions—accounting, billing, supply, and communications—very few had invested in systems similar to that of QCHP. Eugene recalled that several consulting firms were approached to perform a cost-benefit analysis of the investment and each firm told senior management that QCHP didn't have much of a choice: "If QCHP is to survive, it has to make the commitment." The board was finally persuaded that the need outweighed the expense.

One issue particularly bothersome to Dr. Schneider was patient privacy. Her experience demonstrated that patients worry about confidentiality if there is a perception of wide access to the intimate details of their medical record. While some say that computerized records on the QCHP network offers far more security than paper records, the concern was commonplace. Dr. Schneider noted that this was a very real concern among patients suffering from the HIV virus.

Under the new systems neither patients nor physicians would have the option of using the traditional paper-bound form of information management. Could this, in fact, dissuade some physicians and clients from subscribing to QCHP? Would they jump to other HMOs?

In sharing these and other concerns with colleagues, Dr. Schneider noted that some clinicians regard such a task (i.e., the electronic integration of all information) as analogous not to a complicated heart transplant operation, but, rather, to a brain transplant " . . . the networking of hundreds of millions of nerves and sources of input." Would all of the seemingly infinite pieces of pertinent information regarding the business of caring for QCHP patients be available, or even recorded? As one clinician put it, " . . . a lot of information that we may need is now on paper—hopefully we'll be able access it."

While a five-year timetable may seem like a long time, Paul Eugene noted that five years for total integration of all information for an organization that has 600,000 patients and 1,100 physicians at 20 sites was a daunting task. Eugene had begun to feel a certain amount of trepidation regarding the clinicians. "I've begun to realize that this system can be installed only as fast as the clinicians will allow . . . resistance to new technology may be the Achilles heel of our future vision," he noted.

While many clinicians now working have used computers in school and their work, Eugene pointed out that in the past resistance by physicians and other clinicians had been high. This resistance might be attributed to how technology changes the ways people work and, more specifically, to how physicians practice medicine. Cutting out time-consuming searches through paper records, lowering the risk of error in diagnoses, and providing immediate up-to-date information for other clinicians will be direct outcomes of the new technology. Nevertheless, the other side of the coin might be the immediate jolt of a tidal surge of information that could well produce enough anxiety, disorientation, and chaos to slow down the positive effects of the change.

It was clear to both Dr. Schneider and Paul Eugene that the challenges associated with adjusting to the new technology was disquieting. This was especially true in Paul's case because of the recurring dreams he had been having recently. The dream was always the same. He was ill and at home. His physician was making a "house call" electronically on his home computer. Using the interactive protocol to collect information directly from Paul, the visit always ended abruptly. Having received the necessary data from Paul regarding his condition, the physician would nod somberly, and ceremoniously type "delete" on the computer at his end. Paul would then simply fade away, never to be heard from again.

Questions for Discussion

1. Apply the technologies in this case, and classify them according to the taxonomy in Table 11.1 (Information Technologies and Health Information Systems).
2. What unique managerial challenges exist for QCHP with the new information technologies described?
3. Develop a set of implementable strategies that QCHP could employ to deal with the special challenges described above.
4. How would you cultivate a "new technology culture" at QCHP that would help managers and users meet the challenges of new and emerging technologies?

GLOSSARY

Acoustic coupler   A device used in conjunction with a *modem* for changing a sequential train of pulses into sounds of a given frequency, which are received by a standard telephone receiver.

Adapter   An attachment installed in a computer to enhance its processing power or to communicate with other devices. An example of an adapter is an expanded memory card (also known as an add-on card, controller, or I/O card).

Address   A number or reference name that identifies a memory location where information is stored.

Algorithm   Sequences of logical steps that carry out specific tasks, operations, and transformation of data.

Analog   Pertaining to data in the form of continuously variable physical quantities or to devices that operate on such data, such as a mercury thermometer.

Analog computer   A computer that operates on analog data by performing physical processes on these data, in contrast to *digital computer*.

Analog-to-digital converter   An input attachment for changing continuous physical (analog) signals into discrete numbers (digital form). (A digital-to-analog converter does the opposite in electromechanical output devices.)

Application program   Standard and frequently used programs that are tailored to a user's needs (i.e., payroll, hospitals and accounts, truck lines). Programs may be supplied to the user by the manufacturer, purchased from a software house, or written by the user.

Arithmetic logic unit (ALU)   The portion of the hardware (*CPU*, see below) of a computer in which arithmetic operations are performed.

Artificial intelligence (AI)   The performance by machines of functions usually associated with the human mind—learning, adapting, reasoning, self-correction, and automatic improvement.

Assembler   A computer "translation" program that operates on symbolic input data to produce machine instructions (see *"compiler"* below).

Asynchronous   Used to refer to transmission situations where data are sent one character at a time, and the time of arrival of characters at the receiver is arbitrary.

Backup   A copy or duplicate of a program or any information stored in memory. Backup procedures prevent loss due to the destruction, damage, or modification of data.

Basic   The most popular high-level language; formed as an acronym from Beginners All-Purpose Symbolic Instruction Code.

Batch processing   Data processing in which similar input data items are grouped together and processed during a single machine run with the same program for operating convenience and efficiency.

Batch transmission   The transmission of several translations at one time, as opposed to the transmission of each translation as it occurs (conversational).

Baud   A unit of transmission speed equal to the number of signal changes in one second. The relationship of bauds to bits-per-second depends on the design of the data set. In some data sets, 1,200 bauds are equivalent to 1,200 bits per-second, a one-to-one relationship. In other data sets, the baud rate may be one-half or one-third of the bit-per-second rate.

Binary   A numbering system with two digits, 0 and 1, used by computers to store and process information.

Bit (binary digit)   The smallest element of binary machine language represented by a magnetized spot on a recording surface or a magnetized element of a storage device. Whether the bit represents a 1 or 0 (i.e., is ON or OFF) is determined by whether the magnetism was created by a positive or negative electrical charge.

Block   A physical unit of data that can be conveniently stored by a computer on an input or output device. The term is synonymous with physical record. The block is normally composed of one or more logical records or a portion of a logical record.

BPI   Abbreviation for bits per inch.

Branch   To depart from the normal sequence of executing instructions in a computer.

Buffer   Data storage area in memory that holds data intact until it can be processed or printed.

Bug   An unintentional error in programming.

Bulletin board system (BBS)   A computer set up to receive calls and act as a host system. BBSs allow computer users to communicate through message bases and to exchange files and specialized information.

Bus   A group of wires through which communication can pass between memory, CPU, and various input and output devices.

Byte   A sequence of adjacent bits operated upon as a unit.

CAD   Computer-aided design.

CD-ROM (compact disk-read only memory)   A form of optical disk that allows data to be read, but not recorded.

Carpal tunnel syndrome   A disorder found among heavy computer users consisting of damage to nerves and tendons in the hand.

Cathode ray tube (CRT)   A vacuum tube in which a beam of electrons can be focused to a small point on a luminescent screen and can be varied in position and intensity to form a pattern. The CRT can be used as an output terminal for computer systems.

Central processing unit (CPU)   The central processor of a computer system contains the internal memory unit (memory), the arithmetic logic unit (ALU), and the input/output control unit (I/O control).

Channel   A path along which signals can sent, e.g., data channel, output channel. Also, that portion of a storage medium that is accessible to a given reading station.

Character   One of a set of elementary symbols which may be arranged in groups to express information. The symbols may include the decimal digits 0 through 9, the letters A through Z, punctuation marks, operation symbols, and any other single symbol which a computer may read, store, or write.

CIO   Chief Information Officer of a hospital, company, or firm.

Chip   An integrated circuit, usually made of silicon, eight one-thousandths of an inch thick. Sometimes called a microprocessor.

Clipper chip   An encoding device that contains a "back door," allowing law enforcement officials to unscramble coded phone calls or computer data that flows through networks.

Clone   An IBM PC/XT- or AT-compatible personal computer made by a manufacturer other than IBM.

COBOL   An acronym formed from Common Business Oriented Language, a high-level language which uses statements written in English. See *Common business oriented language.*

Code   A system of symbols representing rules for handling the flow of information processing.

Coding   Writing instructions for a computer either in machine or non-machine language.

Command   That part of a program which gives the computer an instruction to do something.

Common business oriented language (COBOL)   A specific computer language by which business data processing procedures may be precisely described in a standard form. The language is intended as a means for directly presenting any business program to any suitable computer for which a COBOL compiler exists, and also as a means of communicating such procedures among individuals.

Communication multiplexer (also called communication controller)   A hardware device that allows data from two or more telephones to enter a computer's memory. It also compensates between the high internal speed of the CPU and the slower transmission speed over the communication channel.

Community health information network (CHIN)   An integrated collection of computer and telecommunication capabilities that facilitates communication of patient, clinical, and financial information among multiple

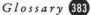

providers, payers, employers, pharmacies, and related health entities within a targeted geographic area.

Compatible Capable of connecting to or communicating with another system or component without special modification.

Compiler A computer "translation" program that operates on symbolic input so as to produce machine instructions. A compiler, more powerful than an assembler, is able to replace certain input items with series of instructions. The result is a translated and expanded version of the original program.

Computer A device capable of accepting data in the form of facts and figures, applying prescribed processes to the data, and supplying the results of these processes as meaningful information. This device usually consists of input and output devices, storage, arithmetic and logic units, and a control unit.

Computer virus A form of electronic vandalism in which a malicious program is injected into a computer system and destroys or damages information.

Console That part of a computer used for communication between the operator or maintenance engineer and the computer.

Control unit Often called the input/output control unit of I/O controller. That portion of the hardware of a digital computer which directs the sequence of operations, interprets the coded instructions, and initiates the proper commands so that the computer circuits can execute the instructions. The control unit also affects selection and retrieval of data from storage or from outside the computer.

Conversational mode A data transmission method in which every transaction originating at a remote point requires a response from the central computer's file.

CPR A computer-based patient record. Refers to an electronic medical record system that receives clinical patient treatment information in an on-line real-time mode from computers and maintains a database which acts as a central access repository for graphical and trend analysis of a patient's clinical data.

Crash When a computer goes down and everything stops until the system can reboot.

Cursor A position indicator, usually a dot of light, which shows where one is on a video screen, i.e., where insertions and deletions of data can be placed.

Cyberspace The area between the computer keyboard and the dots that appear on the monitor.

Data A collection of facts or figures.

Database All the information that exists at any time. A corporate database is all the information that exists in the company at anytime. An application database is all the information about one part of the company's activities (production, sales, financial accounting, etc.).

Data definition language (DDL) A special group of commands used in database management systems that allows the definition of the structure and contents of the database.

Data processing The collection of data, processing of the data to obtain usable information, and the communication of this usable information.

Data transfer rate The rate at which data are transferred between the peripheral unit and the central processor's memory.

Debug The process of detecting, diagnosing, and correcting errors which may occur in both software and hardware.

Digit A single symbol or character representing a quantity.

Digital computer A computer that operates on discrete data by performing arithmetic and logic processes on these data. Contrasts with *analog computer*.

Direct access Pertaining to a storage device or procedure in which access to a particular address is such that the time required to transfer a unit of information to or from the storage device is independent of the location or address which is accessed. Thus, the access time for each storage location is the same.

Direct access storage device (DASD) A device used for storage of direct access files. It can be a magnetic disk or a drum.

Directory A list of file names and the locations of files on a computer disk.

Disk drive The motor that rotates a computer's disk, plus the read/

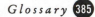

write heads and associated mechanisms, that are usually found in a mountable housing. Sometimes used to mean the entire disk subsystem.

Disk format   Refers to the method in which data is organized and stored on a floppy disk or on the hard disk of a personal computer.

Disk pack   A set of circular magnetic surfaces for storage of file information. The disk pack can be used for storage of serial or direct access files.

Diskette (floppy disk)   A flexible plastic magnetic recording medium.

Distributed processing   The use of a mix of local and nonlocal computer resources to solve a user's problem.

Documentation   An instruction manual, or its equivalent, that provides users with information on using a system. This can include system documentation (description of hardware and software) or program documentation (description of the whats and hows of a program).

DOS   An acronym formed from the words Disk Operating System. A set of programs for IBM compatibles that control the communications between computer components.

Dot matrix   A type of printer technology using a print head with pins that print out arrays of dots, forming text and graphics on the printed page.

Down, down-time   A period of time when a computer system is not functioning either through unexpected systems failure or scheduled unavailability (e.g., hardware maintenance).

Download   The process of transferring information from one computer to another.

Drive   The mechanism that allows a medium to be mounted to make its data accessible to the computer. The drive contains all electrical and mechanical components necessary to read and write data on a medium.

Drum storage   A type of addressable storage which uses magnetic recording on a rotating cylinder.

Dumb terminal   A terminal that does not possess data processing capability, but rather acts as an input or output device.

E-mail   Electronic mail (E-mail) refers to the exchange of messages via a bulletin board or on-line service. One user leaves a message on the service that is "addressed" to another user, who can later connect to the same service, read the message, and reply.

Electronic data processing (EDP)   Computer-based data system.

Emulator   The programming techniques and features that permit one computer system to execute programs written for another system.

Encryption   A security technology that protects the contents of sensitive information files or data. Typically, a data file or password is scrambled using a special "key" or set of instructions making it difficult to unscramble unless the user knows the key.

Ergonomics   The study of human factors (i.e., posture, wrist position, neck position) related to computers.

Expert system   An information system that incorporates the experience of experts in a certain area and offers it as a guide to the system's user.

External storage   Storage media separate from the machine, but capable of retaining information in a form acceptable to the computer, such as tapes, disk packs, and punched cards.

Fault-tolerance   Refers to a computer that ostensibly never fails because it has two microprocessors operating simultaneously so that if one fails, the other can process data while it's being repaired.

Fiber-optic cable   Hair-thin strands of glass used as a transmitter of electronic information.

Field   A unit of data within a record or area. A logical grouping of continuous characters.

File   A collection of records or an organized collection of data directed toward some purpose. The records in a file may or may not be sequenced according to a key contained in each record.

File server   Specialized computers that store files so they can be moved among personal computers on a network.

Flow chart   A graphic representation of a sequence of operations using symbols to represent the operation.

Formula translator (FORTRAN)   A programming system, including a language and a compiler, that allows programs to be written in a type of mathematical language. These programs are subsequently translated by a computer into machine language.

FORTRAN An acronym formed from **Fo**rmula **Tran**slator, a high level language with scientific applications.

Function keys Keys strategically placed on the keyboard and labeled F1 through F12 that perform special functions depending on the program used.

Fuzzy logic A technology that allows computers to respond to situations that fall between absolute values.

Generations of programming languages Machine languages (first generation); assembly languages (second generation); procedural languages (third generation); problem-oriented languages (fourth generation); artificial intelligence (fifth generation); and self-adapting applications or applications that learn (sixth generation).

Graphics An arrangement of lines, bars, or detailed forms generated by the computer and appearing on the CRT.

Groupware A catch-all term for programs that work within networks of personal computers and enable people to collaborate in one way or another.

Hacking Unauthorized breaking into a private computer system.

Hard copy A printed copy of machine output in a readable form, such as output from a printer.

Hard disk A rigid version of a floppy disk usually sealed in the housing of a microcomputer and not removable. Hard disks generally can hold more data than floppy disks.

Hardware The mechanical, magnetic, electronic, and electrical devices or components of a computer.

Hard-wired Physically (and usually permanently) connected to a computer.

HIN Health information network. A combination of computer software and communications facilities that permit multiple users to transmit, receive, and store all forms of health care data, including those recorded as images and voice.

HIS Health care information system.

Host computer A large central computer which provides services such as computation, data base access, special programs, or programming languages.

Information   A meaningful collection of data.

Information retrieval   The methods and procedures for recording specific information from stored data.

Input   The data to be processed.

Input device   A machine capable of accepting data and making it available for processing in a form acceptable to a computer.

Input/output control (I/O control)   The portion of the central processor of computer systems which contains electronics for supervising data flow between memory and the input/output devices connected to the central processing unit.

Instruction   A set of characters, together with one or more addresses, that defines an operation and which, as a unit, causes the computer to operate accordingly on the indicated quantities. A term associated with software operation.

Integrated system   A management information system where all information processed is regarded as a single resource that is available as needed to any information system in an organization. Typically, this means that all software applications needing data can get it from one central data base.

Intelligent terminal   A computer peripheral that provides input and output and allows some processing and storage of data.

Interactive   Describes activity in which there is immediate communication between the user and the computer system.

Interface   A communication device with both a hardware and software component used to connect systems with disparate technical characteristics.

Internal storage   Storage facilities forming an integral physical part of the computer and directly accessible to the arithmetic and control units of the computer.

Internet   A global web that connects more than thirty thousand on-line computer networks.

Interoperability   Information sharing capability among various operating entities.

IS   Information system.

IT   Information technology.

Language   A defined set of characters that is used to form symbols, words, etc., and the rules and connections for combining these into communications meaningful to a computer.

Laserdisk (or optical disk)   A recording medium that stores information as little pits burned into a special surface and read by a laser. These disks have enormous capacity with five to ten times greater capacity than magnetic disk drives.

Load   In programming, to place data into internal storage.

Loader   A program that transfers material from off-line to on-line memory.

Local area network (LAN)   An organized network of data communication pathways linking multiple computer systems, (i.e. intrahospital communications). Optical fiber, microwave, or satellite technology are high capacity carriers of data transmission for these networks.

Logging on   The procedure by which one becomes linked to a multiple-user host computer system; generally, the procedure requires a user identification name or number and a password.

Machine language   A language designed for interpretation and use without translation by a computer system.

Magnetic disk   A storage device consisting of magnetically coated disks on the surface of which information is stored in the form of magnetic spots arranged in a manner to represent binary data. The disk is usually used as a file medium.

Magnetic ink character recognition (MICR)   A check-encoding system employed by banks for the purpose of automating check handling. Using magnetic ink, checks are imprinted with characters of a type face and dimensions specified by the American Banking Association. Fourteen characters (the numbers 0–9 and four special symbols) are used to provide amount, identifying, and control information.

Magnetic tape   A continuous, flexible medium whose base material is impregnated or coated with a magnetic-sensitive material to accept data in the form of magnetically polarized spots.

Main frame   A large, fast computer that can handle multiple tasks concurrently.

Management information systems (MIS)   A specific type of data processing system that is designed to furnish management with information for assistance in decision making.

Master file   A file of semipermanent information which is usually updated periodically.

Medium   Any carrier on which data may be recorded (e.g., paper, disks, magnetic tape, punch cards, etc.).

Megabyte (mb or mbyte)   One million bytes.

Megahertz (MHz)   Millions of clock ticks per second. Clock speed affects the rate at which a microprocessor works.

Memory   Any device into which a unit of information can be copied that will hold this information in a form from which it can be obtained at a later time. Usually, memory is an internal part of the CPU.

Menu   Operator instructions that, by offering choices, guide the user through the working of a program.

Merge   To combine the items from two or more mediums onto one medium.

Microcomputer   A small but complete computer system, with a microprocessing unit (MPU) as its CPU, I/O devices, and memory.

MIPS   Millions of instructions per second.

Modem (modulator-demodulator)   A device that provides the appropriate interface between a data processing machine and a communications line. It converts data originating in digital form into analog signals that are suitable for transmission over telephone lines (and vice-versa).

Mouse   An input device for interacting with a computer. The mouse can be moved over a surface and will provide coordinate data to the computer that can be used to move a cursor on the screen.

Multitasking   An operating system's capability to run more than one application at a time.

Network   A continuing connection between two or more computers that facilitates sharing files and resources.

Off-line   Pertaining to the operation of input/output devices or auxiliary equipment not under direct control of the central processor.

On-line A system, or peripheral equipment or device in a system, in which the operation of the equipment is under control of the central processing unit. Information reflecting a current activity is introduced into the data processing system as soon as it occurs.

Open-system architecture A computer system that allows mixing and matching different vendors' hardware and software.

Operating system (OS) A set of interrelated software modules which provides the framework for the orderly assignment of a computer installation's resources to the execution of a variety of applications.

Optical character recognition (OCR) A direct data entry method that uses preprinted characters that can be read by a light source.

Optical disk See *Laserdisk*.

Optical reader A piece of hardware whose operation is based on the principle that the special shape of each character printed on the input media is capable of being identified by a reading device.

Output A copy of the text which can be read and manipulated in certain programs.

PC Personal computer.

PDA Personal Digital Assistant.

Pentium chip A 64-bit microprocessor (rather than a 32-bit processor like the 486 and 386 microprocessors). Faster than the 486 and 386 microprocessors, it has a segmented two-part memory, one for instructions and the other for data.

Peripheral Any hardware device other than the CPU. Peripherals include displays, disk drives, and printers.

Pixel The smallest information building block of an on-screen image. On a color monitor screen, each pixel is made up of one or more triads (red, green, and blue). Resolution is usually expressed in terms of the number of pixels that fit within the width and height of a complete green image.

Plotter A device for producing graphic hard copy containing lines, curves, and characters.

Port The channel or interface between the microprocessor and peripheral devices.

Printer   A device capable of producing hard copy in the form of printed material.

Printout   The printed records of a computer's operations.

Program   A sequenced set of instructions to a computer for a particular job.

Program language   A language used by programmers to write computer programs and routines.

Protocol   A set of rules for the exchange of information, such as those used for successful data transmission.

Random access memory (RAM)   The memory used to execute application programs. Also known as read-write memory or operating memory.

Read only memory (ROM)   The memory chip(s) that permanently store computer information and instructions. Also known as read-only memory.

Real-time processing   The processing of information or data at the time the data are created. The results of the processing are available quickly enough to influence the process which creates the data.

Reengineering   Information technology project reengineering looks at the end-to-end processes that are important to an organization's success and rapidly redesigns who does what. Also known as Business Process Reengineering.

Routine   A set of instructions arranged in proper sequence to direct the computer to perform a desired operation or series of operations.

Run   One performance of a program on a computer; performance of one routine, or several routines automatically linked so that they form an operating unit, during which manual manipulating by the computer operator is usually not required.

Query language   A set of commands employed by a user to extract from a database those data which meet specified criteria.

Sequential processing   A type of processing in which the records in a file are accessed serially. Also called serial processing.

Software   Various programming aids that are supplied by the manufacturer to facilitate the user's efficient operation of the equipment.

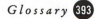

The collection of programs, routines, and documents associated with a computer.

Source language   A language that is an input to a given translation process.

Spreadsheet   On a *CRT*, a worksheet providing analysis or recapitulation of cost or other accounting data.

Software maintenance   The ongoing process of detecting and removing errors from existing programs.

Software transportability   The ability to take a program written for and working on a particular type of computer and run it without modification on a different type of computer.

Standards   Agreements on formats, procedures, and interfaces that permit the designers of hardware, software, databases, and telecommunications facilities to develop products and systems independent of one another with the assurance that they will be compatible with any other product or system that adheres to to the same standards. Standards are the single most important element in achieving integration of the information and communications resource.

Storage   A device or portion of a device that is capable of receiving data, retaining it for an indefinite period of time, and supplying it on command.

Subroutine   The set of instructions necessary to direct the computer to carry out a well-defined mathematical or logical operation; a subunit of a routine.

System   An assembly of procedures, processes, methods, routines, techniques, or equipment united by some form of regulated interaction to form an organized whole.

Systems analyst   A person responsible for the first attempts at a stepwise refinement of a problem. This consists of defining a problem in data processing terms and indicating to programmers the directions for specific data processing solutions.

Telecommunication   Using a computer to communicate with another computer via telephone lines and *modem*.

Telemedicine   A technology that enables providers to do two-way *interactive* video consultations and transmit digital images to other sites.

Terminal   A point in a system or communication network at which data can either enter or leave.

Timesharing   The use of a central processor for two or more purposes during the same overall time interval. Timesharing is done by interspersing in time the actions of the peripheral units and the central processor.

Turnkey system   A complete, running system, generally considered to meet the specified needs of a given spectrum of users.

VDT   Video display terminal.

Virtual reality   The use of electronic sensors and computer-generated images to give people the illusion of actually participating in fabricated events.

Virtual storage   A method by which the internal memory of the *CPU* can be extended almost without limit. Each program run of a computer using virtual storage is divided into segments called pages. The entire program is then stored on some direct medium, and the pages of the program are called into memory as needed for execution.

Virus   See *Computer Virus*.

Wide area network (WAN)   An organized network of data communication pathways linking multiple computer systems. Large medical centers or multi-hospital corporations may use WANs to connect clinical, administrative, and research departments in widely dispersed locations.

Window   An area of a screen that displays information. Some programs support several windows that can be viewed either simultaneously or sequentially.

Word processing   Computer-assisted production of text or documents.

Workstation   A relatively small, powerful computer system that can perform many of the same functions as a mainframe computer. Workstations can be linked to form networks that share information among many computers.

WYSIWYG   What You See Is What You Get. Refers to programs that display information on the screen the way it will appear in print.

INDEX

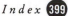

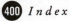

ABOUT THE AUTHORS

John Abbott Worthley is University Professor of Public Administration at Seton Hall University and an international consultant. A prolific author, he has worked in hospitals, hospices, and as a board member of a national home care foundation. His clients have included government health departments, major medical centers, health insurers, mental health facilities, nursing homes and group practices. A frequent lecturer in Europe and Asia, Dr. Worthley holds degrees from the College of Holy Cross, the University of Virginia, and the State University of New York.

Philip S. DiSalvio is the Director of the Executive Programs in Health Care Administration and Professor in the Graduate Department of Public Administration at Seton Hall University. Dr. DiSalvio has served as chief executive officer of several large health care organizations and consults extensively in the areas of management development, education and strategic planning with health care systems, medical institutions, health insurers, and non-profit organizations. He was a Robert Wood Johnson Faculty Fellow in Health Care Finance at Johns Hopkins University Medical Institutions and holds an Ed.D. from Harvard University in Administration, Planning and Social Policy.

Date Due

PRINTED IN U.S.A.   CAT. NO. 24 161   BRO DART